INTERVENTIONAL ULTRASOUND IN OBSTETRICS, GYNAECOLOGY AND THE BREAST

To those women who, after understanding the facts of their clinical condition, have allowed development of new procedures

Interventional Ultrasound in Obstetrics, Gynaecology and the Breast

Edited by

Joaquin Santolaya-Forgas

MD, PhD
Department of Obstetrics and Gynecology
University of Illinois at Chicago
Chicago, Illinois, USA

With

Didier Lémery

MD, PhD
Centre de Diagnostic Prenatal et de Médecine Foetale
Maternité de l'Hôtel Dieu
Université d'Auvergne
Clermont-Ferrand, France

**Blackwell
Science**

© 1998 by
Blackwell Science Ltd
Editorial Offices:
Osney Mead, Oxford OX2 OEL
25 John Street, London WC1N 2BL
23 Ainslie Place, Edinburgh EH3 6AJ
350 Main Street, Malden
  MA 02148 5018, USA
54 University Street, Carlton
  Victoria 3053, Australia
10, rue Casimir Delavigne
  75006 Paris, France

Other Editorial Offices:
Blackwell Wissenschafts-Verlag GmbH
Kurfürstendamm 57
10707 Berlin, Germany

Blackwell Science KK
MG Kodenmacho Building
7–10 Kodenmacho Nihombashi
Chuo-ku, Tokyo 104, Japan

The right of the Authors to be
identified as the Authors of this Work
has been asserted in accordance
with the Copyright, Designs and
Patents Act 1988.

First published 1998

Set by Setrite Typesetters, Hong Kong
Printed and bound in Great Britain
at the University Press, Cambridge

The Blackwell Science logo is a
trade mark of Blackwell Science Ltd,
registered at the United Kingdom
Trade Marks Registry

A catalogue record for this title
is available from the British Library

ISBN 0-632-03874-8

Library of Congress
Cataloging-in-publication Data

Interventional ultrasound in obstetrics,
  gynaecology, and the breast/edited by
  Joaquin Santolaya-Forgas with Didier
  Lémery
      p.   cm.
    ISBN 0-632-03874-8
    1. Ultrasonics in obstetrics.
  2. Operative ultrasonography.
  3. Generative organs, Female—
  Ultrasonic imaging. 4. Generative
  organs, Female—Surgery. I. Santolaya-
  Forgas, Joaquin. II. Lémery, Didier.
    [DNLM: 1. Ultrasonography,
  Prenatal—methods. 2. Ultrasonography,
  Interventional—methods. 3. Fetal
  Diseases—ultrasonography. 4. Genital
  Diseases, Female—ultrasonography.
  5. Breast Diseases—ultrasonography.
  WQ 209 I6172 1998]
  RG527.5.U48I58   1998
  618'.047543—dc21
  DNLM/DLC
  for Library of Congress   98-12984
                                        CIP

DISTRIBUTORS
Marston Book Services Ltd
PO Box 269
Abingdon, Oxon OX14 4YN
(Orders: Tel: 01235 465500
          Fax: 01235 465555)

USA
Blackwell Science, Inc.
Commerce Place
350 Main Street
Malden, MA 02148 5018
(Orders: Tel: 800 759 6102
              781 388 8250
          Fax: 781 388 8255)

Canada
Login Brothers Book Company
324 Saulteaux Crescent
Winnipeg, Manitoba R3J 3T2
(Orders: Tel: 204 224 4068)

Australia
Blackwell Science Pty Ltd
54 University Street
Carlton, Victoria 3053
(Orders: Tel: 3 9347 0300
          Fax: 3 9347 5001)

For further information on
Blackwell Science, visit our website:
www.blackwell-science.com

Contents

List of contributors

ALFRED Z. ABUHAMAD *Director of Maternal Fetal Medicine, Eastern Virginia Medical School, 825 Fairfax St, Norfolk, Va 23507, USA.*

CLIVE ALDRICH *Department of Obstetrics and Gynaecology, University College London, Medical School, 86–96 Chenies Mews, London WC1E 6HX, UK.*

JANE ARRINGTON *Chief sonographer, Tidewater Perinatal Center, 1080 First Colonial Rd, Virginia Beach, Va 23454, USA.*

JACQUES BECO *Département de Gynecologie-Obstétrique, Université de Liège, Boulevard du 12ème de Ligne, 4000 Liège, Belgium.*

ALEXANDRA BENACHI *Centre for Fetal Care, Royal Postgraduate Medical School, Institute of Obstetrics and Gynaecology, Queen Charlotte's and Chelsea Hospital, Goldhawk Road, London W6 0XG, UK.*

ISAAC BEN-NUN *Department of Obstetrics and Gynecology and IVF Unit, Meir General Hospital, Kfar-Saba, Israel; and Tel Aviv University Medical School, Israel.*

ANDRE BIENIARZ *University of Illinois School of Medicine, Maternal Fetal Medicine Division, Department of Obstetrics and Gynecology (M/C 808), 840 S. Wood Street, Chicago IL 60612, USA.*

REVAY BOTCHORISHVILI *Department of Obstetrics, Gynecology and Reproductive Medicine, Polyclinique de l'Hôtel Dieu, 13 Bd Charles de Gaulle, 63033 Clermont-Ferrand, France.*

JEAN-ALAIN BOURNAZEAU *Department of Obstetrics, Gynecology and Fetal Medicine, Université de Clermont-Ferrand, l'Hôtel Dieu, 63033 Clermont-Ferrand, France.*

MAURICE A. BRUHAT *Department of Obstetrics, Gynecology and Reproductive Medicine, Polyclinique de l'Hôtel Dieu, 13 Bd Charles de Gaulle, 63033 Clermont-Ferrand, France.*

BARBARA K. BURTON *Division of Genetics and Metabolism, University of Illinois at Chicago, Director of the Center for Medical and Reproductive Genetics, Michael Reese Hospital and Medical Center, Chicago, Illinois 60616-3390, USA.*

STUART CAMPBELL *Department of Obstetrics and Gynaecology, St George's Hospital, London, UK.*

MICHEL CANIS *Département of Obstetrics, Gynecology and Reproductive Medicine, Polyclinique de l'Hôtel Dieu, 13 Bd Charles de Gaulle, 63033 Clermont-Ferrand, France.*

JOSÉ COHEN *Perinatology Research Branch, NICHD, Georgetown University Medical Center, Department of Obstetrics and Gynecology, 3800 Reservoir Road NW, 3PHC, Washington, DC 20007, USA.*

ANNE-FRANÇOIS DE POERCK *Centre Hospitalier Molière-Longchamp, Département de Sénologie, 142 rue Marconi, 1190 Brussels, Belgium.*

MARC DOMMERGUES *Maternité Port Royal-Baudelocque, 123 Boulevard Port, Royal 75014, Paris, France.*

YVES DUMEZ *Maternité Port Royal-Baudelocque, 123 Boulevard Port, Royal 75014, Paris, France.*

MARK I.EVANS *Department of Obstetrics and Gynecology, Molecular Medicine and Genetics, Wayne State University, Detroit, Michigan, USA.*

VIVIANE FEILLEL *Service de Sénologie, Centre Jean Perrin, Rue Montalembert BP 392, 63011 Clermont-Ferrand, France.*

MOSHE D.FEJGIN *Department of Obstetrics and Gynecology and IVF Unit, Meir General Hospital, Kfar-Saba, Israel; and Tel Aviv University Medical School, Israel.*

NICHOLAS M.FISK *Centre for Fetal Care, Royal Postgraduate Medical School, Institute of Obstetrics and Gynaecology, Queen Charlotte's and Chelsea Hospital, Goldhawk Road, London W6 0XG, UK*

REGINE GAETJE *Department of Obstetrics and Gynaecology, Johann Wolfgang Goethe-University Clinic, Theodor-Stern-Kai 7, 60596 Frankfurt am Main, Germany.*

MAURIZIO GALASSO *Perinatology Research Branch, NICHD, Georgetown University Medical Center, Department of Obstetrics and Gynecology, 3800 Reservoir Road NW, 3PHC, Washington, DC 20007, USA.*

DANIEL GAUTHIER *Division of Maternal-Fetal Medicine (MC 808), Department of Obstetrics and Gynecology, University of Illinois at Chicago, College of Medicine, 820 South Wood Street, Chicago, Illinois 60612, USA.*

FABIO GHEZZI *Perinatology Research Branch, NICHD, Georgetown University Medical Center, Department of Obstetrics and Gynecology, 3800 Reservoir Road NW, 3PHC, Washington, DC 20007, USA.*

RICARDO GOMEZ *Perinatology Research Branch, NICHD, Georgetown University Medical Center,*

Department of Obstetrics and Gynecology, 3800 Reservoir Road NW, 3PHC, Washington, DC 20007, USA.

LUÍS F.GONÇALVES *Perinatology Research Branch, NICHD, Georgetown University Medical Center, Department of Obstetrics and Gynecology, 3800 Reservoir Road NW, 3PHC, Washington, DC 20007, USA.*

ALAIN ISNARD *Centre République, 99 Avenue de la République, 63100 Clermont-Ferrand, France.*

BERNARD JACQUETIN *Centre de Diagnostic Prenatal et de Médecine Foetale, Maternité de l'Hôtel Dieu, Université d'Auvergne, Avenue Vercingétorix BP 69, 63003 Clermont-Ferrand, France.*

RICHARD JAFFE *Department of Obstetrics and Gynecology, Columbia Presbyterian Medical Center, 622 West 168th Street, New York, NY 10032, USA.*

ERIC JAUNIAUX *Department of Obstetrics and Gynaecology, University College Hospital, London, UK.*

DAVOR JURKOVIC *Department of Obstetrics and Gynaecology, King's College Hospital, London, UK.*

S.MICHAEL KINSELLA *Sir Humphry Davy Department of Anaesthesia, St Michael's Hospital, Southwell Street, Bristol BS2 8EG, UK.*

CLAUDINE LAFAYE *Service de Sénologie, Centre Jean Perrin, Rue Montalembert BP 392, 63011 Clermont-Ferrand, France.*

DIDIER LÉMERY *Centre de Diagnostic Prenatal et de Médecine Foetale, Maternité de l'Hôtel Dieu, Université d'Auvergne, Avenue Vercingétorix BP 69, 63003 Clermont-Ferrand, France.*

SYLVIE LÉMERY *Service de Sénologie, Centre Jean Perrin, Rue Montalembert BP 392, 63011 Clermont-Ferrand, France.*

JODI P.LERNER *Department of Obstetrics and Gynecology, Columbia Presbyterian Medical Center, 622 West 168th Street, New York, NY 10032, USA.*

GERARD MAGE *Department of Obstetrics, Gynecology and Reproductive Medicine, Polyclinique de l'Hôtel Dieu, 13 Bd Charles de Gaulle, 63033 Clermont-Ferrand, France.*

FRANÇOIS N.MASSON *Department of Obstetrics, Gynecology and Reproductive Medicine, Polyclinique de l'Hôtel Dieu, 13 Bd Charles de Gaulle, 63033 Clermont-Ferrand, France.*

ANA MONTEAGUDO *Director of Obstetrics at Bellevue Hospital, New York University Medical Center, 550 1st Avenue, Room 9N28, New York, NY 10016, USA.*

HERNÁN MUNOZ *Perinatology Research Branch, NICHD, Georgetown University Medical Center, Department of Obstetrics and Gynecology, 3800 Reservoir Road NW, 3PHC, Washington, DC 20007, USA.*

CAMRAN NEZHAT *Center for Special Pelvic Surgery, The Medical Quarters, 5555 Peachtree-Dunwoody Road, Suite 276, Atlanta, Georgia 30342, USA.*

CEANA NEZHAT *Center for Special Pelvic Surgery, The Medical Quarters, 5555 Peachtree-Dunwoody Road, Suite 276, Atlanta, Georgia 30342, USA.*

FARR NEZHAT *Center for Special Pelvic Surgery, The Medical Quarters, 5555 Peachtree-Dunwoody Road, Suite 276, Atlanta, Georgia 30342, USA.*

KYPROS H.NICOLAIDES *Harris Birthright Research Centre for Fetal Medicine, King's College Hospital Medical School, London, UK.*

PHILIPPE PEETRONS *Centre Hospitalier Molière-Longchamp, Head of Medical Imaging Department, 142 rue Marconi, 1190 Brussels, Belgium.*

MARIE HÉLÈNE POISSONNIER *Hôpital Saint-Vincent-de-Paul, 82, Avenue Denferts Rochereau, 75674 Paris, France.*

LOTHAR W.POPP MD *Clinic Dr, Guth, Juergensallee 44, 22609 Hamburg, Germany.*

JEAN-LUC POULY *Department of Obstetrics, Gynecology and Reproductive Medicine, Polycliniques de l'Hôtel Dieu, 13 Bd Charles de Gaulle, 63033 Clermont-Ferrand, France.*

DENIS QUERLEU *Clinique Universitaire de Gynecologie Obstétrique et Pathologie de la Reproduction, Pavillon Paul Gelle, 91 Avenue Julien Lagache, 59100 Roubaix, France.*

RODIN RAMBOATIANA *Département d'Anesthesie Réanimatian, Centre Hospitalier, 33 Blaye, France.*

CHARLES RODECK *Department of Obstetrics and Gynaecology, University College London, Medical School, 86–96 Chenies Mews, London WC1E 6HX, UK.*

ROBERTO ROMERO *Perinatology Research Branch, NICHD, Georgetown University Medical Center, Department of Obstetrics and Gynecology, 3800 Reservoir Road NW, 3PHC, Washington, DC 20007, USA.*

JOAQUIN SANTOLAYA-FORGAS *Division of Maternal-Fetal Medicine (MC 808), Department of Obstetrics and Gynaecology, University of Illinois at Chicago, College of Medicine, 820 South Wood Street, Chicago, IL 60612, USA.*

PIERRE SCHOEFFLER *Département d'Anesthesie-Réanimation, Centre Hospitalier Universitaire, BP 69, 63003 Clermont-Ferrand, France.*

DAVID SHERER *Perinatology Research Branch, NICHD, Georgetown University Medical Center, Department of Obstetrics and Gynecology, 3800 Reservoir Road NW, 3PHC, Washington, DC 20007, USA.*

FRANÇOIS SUZANNE *Maternité de l'Hôtel-Dieu, Avenue Vercingétorix, BP69, 63003 Clermont-Ferrand, France.*

DAVID TALBERT *Centre for Fetal Care, Royal Postgraduate Medical School, Institute of Obstetrics and*

Gynaecology, Queen Charlotte's and Chelsea Hospital, Goldhawk Road, London W6 OXG, UK.

ILAN E.TIMOR-TRITSCH MD *Director of Obstetrical and Gynecological Ultrasound, New York University Medical Center, 550 1st Avenue, New York, NY 10016, USA.*

ARMELLE TRAVADE *Centre République, 99 Avenue de al République, 63100 Clermont-Ferrand, France.*

PHILIPPE VANLIEFERINGHEN *Centre de Diagnostic Prenatal et de Médecine Foetale, Maternité de l'Hôtel Dieu, Université d'Auvergne, Avenue Vercingétorix BP 69, 63003 Clermont-Ferrand, France.*

ANNIE VERHAEREN *Centre Hospitalier Molière-Longchamp, Département de Radiologie, 142 rue Marconi, 1190 Brussels, Belgium.*

YVES VILLE *Fetal Medicine Unit, St George's Hospital Medical School, Blackshaw Road, London SW17 0QT, UK.*

RONALD J.WAPNER *Tide Water Perinatal Center, 1080 First Colonial Rd, Suite 305, Virginia Beach, Va 23454, USA.*

STEVEN L.WARSOF *Eastern Virginia Medical School, Department of Obstetrics and Gynecology, Division of Maternal Fetal Medicine, 825 Fairfax Avenue, Norfolk, Virginia 23507–1912, USA.*

ARMAND WATTIEZ MD, *Department of Obstetrics, Gynecology and Reproductive Medicine, Polyclinique de l'Hôtel Dieu, 13 Bd Charles de Gaulle, 63033 Clermont-Ferrand, France.*

LAIRD WILSON *University of Illinois School of Medicine, Maternal Fetal Medicine Division, Department of Obstetrics and Gynecology (M/C 808), 840 S. Wood Street, Chicago IL 60612, USA.*

Preface

Analysis of chromosomes and specific alterations on DNA sequences, detection of infections or alterations in biochemical and histological parameters from organs, tissues or cells obtained by ultrasound-guided sampling procedures has important applications in many areas of medicine. In the medical care of women, there has been a wide development of ultrasound-guided techniques with roles in the diagnosis and sometimes treatment of conditions directly related to her reproductive and urinary systems. Thus far, applications of these techniques have already broken ground, by broadening the horizon for ultrasound morphologists and many other professionals. Ultrasound-guided techniques have allowed precise intracavitary studies as well as sampling from alternative sites of the uterus, ovaries, breast or products of conception. As described in this volume, interventional ultrasound has also allowed for minimally invasive surgical treatment of a variety of diseases related to the woman's reproductive system or the fetus.

In this book, the major indications and variations of the ultrasound-guided techniques as they refer to the field of obstetrics and gynecology are described. Each chapter has been written by an expert in the field of ultrasound and related techniques. The authors have had considerable experience in establishing and performing the procedures. Their experience in the ultrasound room is particularly valuable for those who intend to perform these techniques. This book is organized to give detailed methods for the preparation and use of these techniques. The emphasis of this book, however, is not on theory, but on practical techniques, and it is anticipated that by following the methods described here, you too will be able to practice interventional ultrasound successfully!

I am indebted to the contributing authors who have shared their expertise and time to make this book possible. I am also grateful to Ms Anupama Kushwaha for her excellent copyediting work and to Dr Joaquin Diaz Recasens, Dr Umberto Nicolini and Dr Antonio Scommegna for their invaluable input throughout my medical career.

Joaquin Santolaya-Forgas

Thirty years: the real beginning of an independent and mature professional life for any doctor after medical school, residency and fellowship. How many young obstetricians remember that the very first acts in interventional fetal medicine are as old as they are. How many can remember that Sir William Liley performed the first fetal transfusion 30 years ago using X-rays while they have known only ultrasound.

Lead by fetal medicine, interventional ultrasound has been widespread in all the fields of women's medicine during the past twenty years. Nowadays minimal invasive procedures can be performed because of the help of real-time high-definition ultrasound. Ultrasound is now merging with endoscopy to create new concepts in fetal medecine or surgery. Would William Liley have imagined such evolution thirty years ago?

Interventional ultrasound can initiate and build up a new friendship. When Joaquin Santolaya and I met in Chicago in 1992 it became obvious that the hours and days (and sometimes nights) of discussions we had about our common passion would link us for a long time. Even if the initiation of this book is mine, I would like to thank him for the major part of editing work he did for this book.

Interventional ultrasound procedures cannot be improvised thus we had a common problem: how to teach it well…. We had had a dream: what a chance it would have been for us if we could have learnt each procedure with one of the best specialists. It would have been necessary to travel all over the world for half a life or to have had all these experts around us ....

This is the reason why we decided to convince some our friends and colleagues, known worldwide for their techniques, to help us in realizing our project. We wanted a handbook of techniques covering in one book all the fields of a woman's reproductive life. All the contributors have made every effort to share with the reader all details, descriptions, traps and tricks about the techniques they know best. We hope this book will be a tool to which any OB-GYN or radiologist can refer to before performing or learning a new ultrasound-guided invasive procedure.

The pregnancy of this book has lasted long, delivery was difficult, we hope the baby will be successfull. Finally, for Sylvie, Nicolas, Marie and Emmanuelle: whatever would be the events of life, thank you for being mine.

Didier Lémery

Section 1
Obstetrics

Chapter 1/Patient counselling, ethical and legal issues

BARBARA K.BURTON

This chapter reviews the basic principles of genetic counselling as well as special questions relevant to the counselling of patients considering invasive obstetrical and gynaecological procedures. Some of the many ethical and legal issues raised by the technologies discussed in later chapters are also addressed.

Genetic counselling

Many of the procedures discussed in the later chapters of this book are performed for purposes of prenatal diagnosis in patients identified as being at increased risk for birth defects or genetic disorders. It goes without saying that an integral component of the care of such patients is genetic counselling. Concepts regarding what constitutes appropriate genetic counselling vary widely. Some erroneously believe that genetic counselling is equivalent to genetic advice-giving. This could not be further from the truth. There is virtually never a circumstance that justifies a purely directive approach to counselling patients in the process of reproductive decision-making. There is an overwhelming consensus among geneticists and genetic counsellors that the appropriate approach to genetic counselling is the non-directive one [1]. The American Society of Human Genetics has issued the following statement defining the appropriate goals and content of genetic counselling.

> Genetic counselling is a communication process which deals with the human problems associated with the occurrence, or the risk of occurrence, of a genetic disorder in a family. This process involves an attempt by one or more appropriately trained persons to help the individual or family to (1) comprehend the medical facts, including the diagnosis, probable course of the disorder, and the available management; (2) appreciate the way heredity contributes to the disorder, and the risk of recurrence in specified relatives; (3) understand the alternatives for dealing with the risk of recurrence; (4) choose the course of action which seems to them appropriate in view of their risk, their family goals, and their ethical and religious standards, and to act in accordance with that decision; and (5) to make the best possible adjustment to the disorder in an affected family member and/or to the risk of recurrence of that disorder.

Several important observations can be made from this statement. The first is that there is considerably more to genetic counselling than simply quoting to a patient her recurrence risk. At the outset, the patient must fully understand the medical condition, birth defect or disorder that is being addressed. This means she must not only understand the diagnosis but also its significance, including natural history, variability (what's the worst it could be?, what's the best it could be?) and available treatment. Imparting such understanding to a patient may not be a difficult task when dealing with couples who have already had an affected child or close relative and have lived with the condition; however, it can be quite daunting in dealing with patients from the general population who have been identified through such mechanisms as routine carrier testing or prenatal screening as being at increased risk for a specific condition that they have often never heard of. This will become an increasing challenge as carrier testing becomes more widespread for conditions such as cystic fibrosis and as maternal serum screening markers and ultrasonography become increasingly more sophisticated and more widely utilized. In attempting to help a patient understand the implications of a particular diagnosis, it is important to take advantage of a variety of resources. Printed materials designed for patients and families and articles from the medical literature can frequently be helpful. Disease-specific foundations, such as the Spina Bifida Association, Cystic Fibrosis Foundation and many others, can often provide information and put patients in touch with families actually affected with individual disorders. In the case of very rare conditions in the USA, the National Organization for Rare Disorders (NORD) can often serve the same function. Of course, direct patient-to-patient contacts can often be arranged within an individual genetic centre as well. Patients carrying a fetus with a congenital anomaly or birth defect syndrome often benefit from consultation with the specialists, such as neonatologists, paediatric surgeons, neurosurgeons, etc., who would be involved in the infant's care after birth. This can allow them to obtain a realistic picture of what such care will involve, which helps in decisions regarding whether or not to terminate a pregnancy. In continuing pregnancies, such consultation is extremely helpful in allowing parents to feel more prepared and in control of their own circumstances.

In emphasizing the importance of discussing the diagnosis and its implications with a patient, it is implied that the physician or counsellor has knowledge of the correct diagnosis and that the diagnosis is accurate. It has frequently been said that the most common mistake made in genetic counselling is that very accurate and appropriate counselling is provided for the wrong diagnosis. This can have disastrous consequences. Therefore, prior to initiating any counselling, the physician must take every step possible to ensure that an accurate diagnosis has been established. Diagnoses reported by patients in themselves or other family members should not be accepted at face value. Confirmation of diagnosis first involves exploring the patient's medical history and family history in further detail. If the findings described in a patient or family member seem inconsistent with the diagnosis reported, this should alert the physician to investigate the diagnosis further. Medical records should be obtained for documentation of diagnosis whenever possible, even when the situation seems quite straightforward. At times further diagnostic evaluation of the patient or family member should be suggested. The physician must be certain to consider all findings in an individual patient prior to providing counselling. Consider, for example, the patient who reports that she had pulmonic stenosis that was surgically corrected during childhood, a finding verified by review of medical records. In the absence of any other family history of congenital heart disease, the patient with isolated pulmonic stenosis has approximately a 3% risk of having a child affected with a similar cardiac defect. Suppose, however, that the same patient had a webbed neck and short stature, findings suggestive of the diagnosis of Noonan syndrome, a dominantly inherited disorder, but was unaware of the diagnosis because her only significant problem had been her heart disease. If the physician failed to note these additional findings or was unaware of their significance, very inappropriate and inaccurate counselling could be provided. Rather than a 3% risk, this same patient would have a 50% risk of recurrence and this risk would not only encompass congenital heart disease but potentially other problems such as short stature and mental retardation as well.

The third component of genetic counselling involves a discussion of the patient's options for dealing with a risk of occurrence or recurrence of a disorder. The specific options available will vary depending on the individual circumstances. For patients at increased risk of a genetic disorder by virtue of their family history or carrier testing or at increased risk of congenital malformations because of maternal conditions (such as diabetes) or medications (such as anticonvulsants), the importance of preconceptional counselling cannot be overestimated. Only then will the patient have the full range of options open to her, including not having any children if she feels the risks are too great. Depending on the individual circumstances and the mode of transmission of the disorder in question, other options that might be discussed include simply taking the risk and accepting the outcome, adoption, prenatal diagnosis with selective termination of pregnancy, artificial insemination by donor, *in vitro* fertilization with ovum donation or perhaps even *in vitro* fertilization with preimplantation diagnosis. Regardless of the counsellor's own personal view of any of these options, if they are available he or she is ethically bound to discuss them with the patient. It will then be the patient's *own* view of the risks, family goals and ethical and religious beliefs that will ultimately dictate which course of action is taken. Finally, the counsellor should help the patient to make the best possible adjustment to the risks they are facing or the decision they have made. This may involve providing ongoing counselling and support, referral to support groups or mental health professionals or simple reaffirmation of the fact that whatever course of action a patient feels is best for herself and her family undoubtedly *is* best. If physicians or counsellors cannot provide this kind of support, regardless of their own personal beliefs, they should not be involved in this undertaking. Patients confronting the extraordinarily difficult and often agonizing experience of having a child with a birth defect or genetic disorder should not have to endure the additional stress of feeling the judgement or disapproval, however subtly conveyed, of the healthcare professional whose task is to provide care for them.

However, although the goal should be to adhere to a non-directive approach in providing genetic counselling, most experienced counsellors are aware that a purely non-directive posture may be difficult to achieve. A patient's decision can be significantly influenced in very subtle ways. Patients receiving what on the surface appears to be the same information may perceive the circumstances differently and arrive at a very different decision based on the way in which the information is presented. To minimize the risk of introducing bias, physicians and counsellors should be careful not to use value-laden terms in providing counselling. Risks should rarely be characterized as 'high' or 'low' since what is high to one patient may be low to another. It is far preferable to present numerical risks and then to assist the patient in putting these into perspective by presenting some comparison risks. For example, a patient's risk of having a fetus with a particular anomaly may be 5% or 1 in 20. It can be pointed out that this also means that the chance that the fetus does not have the anomaly is 95%. Furthermore, this 5% risk of a specific anomaly can be compared with the general population risk of 2–3% of having a baby with at least one major malformation. The same approach can be used in discussing procedure-related risks, e.g. the risk of procedure-induced fetal loss can be compared with the risk that such a loss would occur in the absence of any intervention.

Most of the discussion of counselling principles thus far has made reference to the patient as opposed to the couple. In cases in which there is an involved husband or partner, it is always preferable to provide counselling to the couple together. This relieves the woman of the burden of relaying very complex information to her partner, allows the couple to provide emotional support to one another and provides each member of the couple with the opportunity to hear the information presented in an unedited fashion.

While some genetic counselling is an integral part of the patient education that occurs during the course of regular medical care, complex counselling issues are best addressed by medical geneticists and trained genetic counsellors. Therefore, obstetricians, radiologists and others involved in prenatal diagnosis and in fetal therapy should work closely with a medical genetic centre. While this is of prime importance for ensuring accurate and appropriate genetic counselling, it goes without saying that it is also critically important for providing the laboratory support essential to genetic diagnosis.

Counselling patients prior to interventional ultrasound

Very careful consideration must be given to the circumstances under which it is appropriate for a physician to offer a particular invasive procedure, with any degree of risk to mother or fetus, to an individual patient. The very act of offering a procedure to a patient implies that acceptance of that offer would be an appropriate alternative. This issue is particularly important in offering procedures associated with a relatively high or unknown risk. Since our capabilities to intervene in obstetrics and gynaecology are rapidly expanding, such circumstances will arise with increasing frequency as new techniques of visualization, diagnosis and treatment are introduced. Until a substantial base of data is accumulated regarding the long-term risks of such intervention, these new procedures should be restricted to patients who have the greatest likelihood of benefiting from them. For example, first-trimester embryoscopy with unknown risks might reasonably be offered to a patient with a 25% risk of specific fetal malformations that could not be diagnosed in any other way, but it would be clearly inappropriate to even offer the procedure to a woman at 1% risk of spina bifida due to family history or valproic acid exposure. In the latter case, not only is the chance that a detectable malformation is present quite low but there are other methods available for prenatal diagnosis which have risks that have been more clearly defined.

In counselling patients regarding the risks of invasive procedures, it is essential that a discussion of all known risks be accompanied by discussion of what is unknown. If a physician says to a patient 'there are no known risks', this very definitely does not mean the same thing as 'the risks are unknown'. The patient should be aware of the extent of the data on which risk assessment is based and the limitations of the data. New techniques are often introduced into medical practice on the basis of early reassuring risk studies that often lack the power to detect uncommon complications, even ones that are very serious. This is largely unavoidable and there is nothing inherently unethical about the introduction of procedures with potentially unknown risks, given appropriate patient selection. However, patients may erroneously assume that the fact that a procedure is in use clinically means that its risks and long-term complications are clearly understood. This is very rarely the case.

Although the emphasis thus far in the discussion of counselling patients prior to invasive procedures has focused on risks, both known and unknown, there are many other important components to such counselling. These include a realistic appraisal of possible and likely benefits, accuracy of diagnostic tests to be utilized, and a discussion of alternatives. Such counselling should not take place on the ultrasound table. The patient must be given the time and opportunity to carefully consider all of the issues related to any such decision before she can truly provide informed consent.

Prior to initiating a procedure during which there may be unanticipated or adverse findings, the physician should consider how this will be addressed with the patient. Although some discussion of the findings may be necessary during the course of the procedure, a detailed discussion is best conducted with the patient at eye level in a face-to-face encounter. In addition to considering the possibility of adverse findings, the physician should also be prepared for the occurrence of complications during invasive procedures and should give thought to how such occurrences will be communicated to the patient.

Counselling in fetal medicine

Invasive procedures performed during pregnancy differ from procedures performed in any other medical setting since there are two patients potentially at risk, the mother and the fetus. Although the physician's primary obligation is to the mother, he or she must, in pregnancies destined to continue, also do everything possible to safeguard the health of the fetus. There are some circumstances in which there are several alternative procedures available that could potentially accomplish the same reproductive goal. For example, following counselling regarding her risk of fetal chromosome anomalies, a 37-year-old patient may have made the decision to pursue prenatal diagnosis with selective termination in the case of a positive diagnosis. Although such a patient should be informed of all diagnostic procedures currently performed in such circumstances, with their individual risks and benefits, it is not a violation of the tenets of non-directive counselling for the physician to recommend one procedure over another if he or she feels it is the safest method of achieving the patient's own reproductive goals. Those who raise such an argument fail to distinguish the appropriateness of non-directive counselling in presenting reproductive options from its inappropriateness in medical decision-making. Few would argue that it is appropriate for a physician to approach a patient with hypertension, lay out the various options including non-treatment and treatment with a variety of agents and then, in a non-directive fashion, ask the patient to choose. Although such an approach would preserve patient autonomy, it would clearly not be in the patient's best interest for the physician not to make a specific recommendation in such a case. Some might fallaciously argue that the 37-year-old woman at 18 weeks' gestation who wants prenatal diagnosis for chromosome anomalies should be non-directively offered amniocentesis and percutaneous umbilical blood sampling (PUBS) and then allowed to choose. This would be clearly inappropriate, however, since the 1 week shorter time to diagnosis associated with PUBS is not a great enough advantage to justify the added risk associated with the procedure. With regard to the choice between chorionic villous sampling (CVS) and traditional amniocentesis, the issue is somewhat more complex since, although the risks associated with CVS are clearly greater than those associated with amniocentesis, the diagnosis is achieved an average of 4–6 weeks earlier in pregnancy and termination in the first trimester is generally easier than in the second. It may be difficult for the physician to weigh these relative risks and benefits for a patient at high risk of having an abnormality detected and it would therefore be more appropriate for the patient to do so. Many factors, such as the patient's past pregnancy experience and the perceived importance of procedure-induced fetal loss or fetal defects, among others, will influence the patient's decision. However, for low-risk patients, such as those in the 35–39-year-old age group, the situation is quite different since 98–99% of these patients will have normal test results and would never face the possibility of termination even if second-trimester amniocentesis were selected. Except in unusual circumstances, the risk of CVS for such patients clearly outweighs the benefits.

Counselling patients who have been offered new techniques for fetal therapy, such as open or endoscopic surgery or gene therapy, is perhaps the most challenging task of all. Many procedures that might theoretically have the potential to make things better for the fetus or newborn also have the clear potential to make things worse. Since most of the fetal conditions potentially approached with such interventions are individually quite uncommon, there will rarely be a large body of data on which to base patient counselling regarding potential risks and benefits. Patients should clearly understand that they are participating in research when choosing to undergo such procedures. When there is a reasonable possibility that a fetal condition could be successfully treated postnatally, there is little justification for intervention *in utero*. Physicians must temper their instinct to explore new horizons that might possibly result in benefit with a realistic appraisal of what probably will occur. Not everything that can be done should be done.

Ethical issues

Ethical dilemmas abound in this area of medicine and will only grow as the technical capabilities of interventional ultrasound increase. It would be impossible to touch on all of the potential ethical issues related to such topics as prenatal diagnosis, preimplantation diagnosis, fetal therapy and malignant pelvic or breast tumours, so only a few examples are addressed. One of the most significant of these has already been touched on in the earlier discussion of counselling issues, i.e. when it is ethical for a physician to offer a new invasive

technique, with a relatively high or unknown risk, to a patient. The potential for harm is so great in such circumstances that utmost care should be utilized in arriving at an answer to this question. The burden of responsibility cannot and should not be shifted to the patient by saying that the patient will be told that the risks are unknown. The very act of offering a procedure to a patient makes a statement that accepting it is a reasonable choice. If it were not reasonable or recommended, then a competent physician surely would not offer it, even under the clearly defined label of research. Proper preliminary investigation in pregnancies destined for termination or in animal models and appropriate patient selection followed by fully informed consent would appear to be the most critical elements in satisfying the physician's ethical obligation in this regard. Such criteria cannot always be satisfied, however. For example, PUBS, shunt surgery and needle aspiration of breast and pelvic cysts were first performed without the benefit of human data regarding the possible long-term risks of the procedures. There would obviously be no way of gathering such data since experience with animals does not always reflect what will occur in human beings. The initial patients involved in these undertakings must therefore have chosen to participate with the understanding that there was no available information with regard to whether or not these procedures would result in long-term consequences in the patients or in the children born subsequently. Recognizing that some adverse effects may require many years to identify, the burden on the physician to counsel patients appropriately is very great indeed. In this arena, as in every other, physicians must be careful to make a distinction for the patient between what they think the risks may be and what they know.

Prenatal diagnosis

An ethical dilemma that may arise with increasing frequency in the future relates to the issue of controversial indications for prenatal diagnosis. This has come up most commonly in the past in the case of couples requesting prenatal diagnosis for sex selection unrelated to the existence of X-linked disease. Although the use of medical techniques for such non-medical purposes draws an immediate negative response from most medical professionals in the western world, who find the practice morally repugnant, the same is not necessarily true in other cultures. Furthermore, even though surveys in the USA suggest that most practitioners of prenatal diagnosis find sex selection 'unacceptable' [2], this does not necessarily mean that they would not allow it as an option for their patients. The approach to such requests in clinical practice appears to vary widely. Wertz and Fletcher [3] conducted an international survey of geneticists and genetic counsellors and found that 42% of the respondents overall would either perform prenatal diagnosis for sex selection or would refer the couple to another centre offering this service. There was considerable variation in response from nation to nation. Although there was a clear consensus against this practice among most European nations, it is of interest that 62% of respondents from the USA indicated that they would either perform prenatal diagnosis for sex selection or refer. A similarly high percentage of geneticists from Hungary and India indicated that they would comply with such a request.

It is relatively easy to mount an ethical argument against the use of an invasive medical procedure with a small but finite risk for sex selection by emphasizing that gender is not a genetic disorder and that such procedures should be utilized only for the diagnosis of pathological conditions. A similar argument could be extended in opposition to the use of prenatal diagnosis to select for other normal human traits, such as eye colour or hair colour, if this ever becomes possible. The distinction between such normal variability and conditions such as Down's syndrome and spina bifida seems readily apparent but the lines begin to blur as milder conditions gradually lend themselves to diagnosis. There can even be debate as to what constitutes a disorder as opposed to a polymorphic trait. For example, most physicians consider albinism to be a disorder because of the existence of a medical complication, namely visual impairment, in a large percentage of affected individuals. Many patients with albinism have argued quite vocally, however, that this should be considered a recessively inherited trait (like blue eyes) and not a disorder. If albinism could be diagnosed prenatally, should it be? What about late-onset disorders, such as Alzheimer's disease, or conditions that confer increased risk of disease (like familial hypercholesterolaemia) but do not invariably result in harm? It seems clear that this issue will become increasingly

complex as time goes on but, at present, it is appropriate to assume that the patients and families confronted with living with such disorders are in the best position to determine whether or not a condition is 'severe' enough to justify prenatal diagnosis.

The issue of whether or not to provide prenatal diagnosis for sex selection could become a moot point if non-invasive methods of diagnosing fetal chromosome anomalies, such as those involving separation of fetal cells from the maternal circulation, eventually become available. It is likely that such techniques would also yield information regarding fetal sex. Since any patient could be carrying a fetus with a chromosomal abnormality, it would be difficult to deny a test with no risk to any patient, including those with no specific indications, providing the patient was willing to pay the cost of the testing. Her use of the information subsequently would be impossible to control, as it is now following CVS or amniocentesis. The only real way to restrict the practice of sex selection would be to bar the disclosure of fetal sex in cases with normal test results. Most geneticists would find this objectionable since it would be a violation of the patient's right of access to her own medical records.

The same type of ethical dilemma may arise in patients undergoing *in vitro* fertilization for infertility as the techniques of preimplantation diagnosis are further developed. In many cases more embryos are available for transfer to the uterus than will be utilized in a given cycle. If the sex of the embryos could be reliably determined, would selection on this basis for transfer to the uterus be viewed in the same negative light as sex selection by prenatal diagnosis? It is likely that it would not be. The two are clearly not comparable in the sense that abortion would not be involved in preimplantation sex selection. Although not widely utilized, there does not appear to be the same negative view of preconceptional sex selection through such techniques as sperm separation as has been observed in response to requests for prenatal diagnosis with selective termination of the unwanted sex.

Abortion

Another obvious ethical dilemma that arises in any discussion of prenatal diagnosis relates to abortion choices. Although the ethics of abortion can be debated on a global scale, and the ethics of selective abortion may be particularly problematic because of the eugenic implications, the debate should not be carried into the care of the individual patient. The decision of whether or not to undergo an abortion in the face of a fetal anomaly or genetic disorder frequently presents an agonizing dilemma to the patient. Although sensitive to the patient's plight, it should not present a dilemma to the physician. The physician's own personal views on the abortion issue are irrelevant to the individual patient's decision of what is best for her and for her family in a particular case. In a society in which abortion is a legal option, the physician is obligated to present it to the patient as an alternative in an objective and non-directive fashion and to support her in whatever decision she makes. The physician is not obligated to participate in the performance of abortions but is surely obligated to refer the patient to a practitioner or facility where an abortion may be obtained. If physicians are not able to perform this function in a supportive and compassionate fashion, they should not be practising in a setting in which they will be called upon to do so.

While those patients who choose to terminate an abnormal pregnancy should be provided with maximal support, since their grief and sense of loss is often overwhelming, it is equally important that patients confronted with the diagnosis of a fetal abnormality do not feel compelled by the physician to undergo an abortion. Continuation of pregnancy in the face of a fetal abnormality, even a lethal one, must be presented as a valid alternative. There has been some suggestion in the past that women in the USA may perceive social pressure to terminate pregnancy following diagnosis of a serious fetal abnormality [4]. While presenting termination as an option, it is never appropriate for the physician to 'recommend' abortion in such circumstances unless there is a clear risk to the life or health of the mother. Furthermore, the patient should be helped to understand that it is her feelings that matter most in the abortion decision, not those of society, other family members or even her own husband. The feelings of the physician surely matter not at all. The patient will live with her decision forever. The physician will move on momentarily to another patient in another crisis facing yet another dilemma.

Multiple gestations

Complex and unique ethical dilemmas may arise in caring for patients with multiple gestations in which one fetus is abnormal and the other or others are not. Selective termination of the abnormal fetus can be offered as an option in such cases, but is associated with greater risk to the mother than in the case of termination of a singleton and is also associated with some risk to the normal twin. Therefore, careful consideration must be given to the potential consequences of such an attempt. In the case of a disorder that is invariably lethal at birth, such as anencephaly or bilateral renal agenesis, it would be inappropriate in most circumstances to place the normal twin at any increased risk, provided the parents want the pregnancy to continue. In the case of non-lethal but serious abnormalities, such as Down's syndrome or spina bifida, the patient must weigh the increased risk associated with a selective termination attempt of losing the normal twin against her wish not to give birth to the affected twin. When the first reports of selective termination appeared in the medical literature, they were challenged on ethical grounds from a number of directions. Somerville [5] argued that the principles governing a woman's right to abortion, defined as evacuation of the uterus incidentally resulting in fetal demise, did not apply to 'killing a fetus *in utero* without its evacuation'. It would appear that most physicians providing prenatal diagnosis do not share this view, since the end result of both undertakings is the same. None the less, there is less acceptance of selective termination for many indications than there is for termination of a singleton gestation [2,3].

Ethical issues of a somewhat different nature arise in consideration of selective termination of normal fetuses in a multifetal gestation. This typically follows treatment for infertility and the purpose of termination is quite different under these circumstances, since the goal is typically to improve the chances of survival for the remaining living fetuses. Evans *et al.* [2] surveyed physicians, ethicists and clergy on this issue and found that there was support for selective termination in pregnancies involving four or more fetuses in which the chances of successful outcome would be very small without intervention. There was a general lack of support for purely elective selective termination in pregnancies involving twins or triplets if the only reason for the procedure was that the parents did not want to have more than one child.

Legal issues

It is virtually impossible to provide a comprehensive discussion of the legal issues related to interventional procedures in obstetrics and gynaecology since the laws related to this issue vary from nation to nation. Therefore, only an overview of some of the most significant legal issues is presented here.

Medical malpractice

A legal issue of pressing concern to physicians involved in invasive obstetrical procedures and interventions, particularly in the USA, is that of medical malpractice. The field of obstetrics and gynaecology has been the subject of intense legal scrutiny and an ever-increasing number of lawsuits. Generally speaking, to prevail in a malpractice lawsuit a plaintiff must demonstrate that the physician breached the standard of care and that this action (or inaction) caused injury. Since the standard of care is so rapidly changing in the field of obstetrics and gynaecology, the physician must be continuously alert to new developments.

PRENATAL DIAGNOSIS

Most malpractice lawsuits involving prenatal diagnosis can be divided into several basic categories. The first of these includes those alleging failure to obtain, or appropriately respond to, relevant clinical information. This would include failure to obtain an adequate family history or other relevant information leading to failure to identify factors that place the patient at increased risk of a specific birth defect or genetic disorder; failure to arrive at an accurate diagnosis in a patient who presents with findings that could reasonably lead to a diagnosis; failure to provide accurate genetic counselling; and failure to offer prenatal diagnosis to patients at increased risk of having a child with a detectable disorder. A closely related but somewhat different allegation would involve the failure to secure fully informed consent prior to a diagnostic procedure.

During recent decades, there have been a number of claims of 'wrongful birth' allegedly resulting from the failure of the physician to warn a woman of a known reproductive risk, thereby depriving her of the option of not having children or of having prenatal diagnosis. Claims alleging that the physician has a duty to inform women 35 years or older of the age-associated risk of Down's syndrome (*Becker* v. *Schwartz*, 1978) and to inform Ashkenazi Jewish couples of their risk for Tay–Sachs disease (*Howard* v. *Lechner*, 1977) have been upheld by the courts. Wrongful birth actions in such circumstances are brought by parents against physicians and seek to recover extraordinary medical and educational expenses and special costs of caring for the handicapped child. In contrast, a number of 'wrongful life' actions have been filed with the affected child as a plaintiff alleging that he or she would not have been born were it not for the negligence of the physician and that this would have been preferable. In most cases, courts in the USA have not recognized such a claim, thereby averting the need to measure the value of life impaired by a genetic handicap against non-existence. There have been exceptions, however, and several states in recent years have recognized this course of action. For example, the Supreme Court of California recognized a wrongful life action on behalf of a child born with hereditary deafness after a physician failed to diagnose the same condition in an older sibling. Similarly, a Washington court held that a child born with fetal hydantoin syndrome after a physician reassured a woman with a seizure disorder that her fetus was not at risk had the right to sue for wrongful life. There is no claim under English law for wrongful life and this has been tested and confirmed in a court case [6].

NEGLIGENCE IN THE PERFORMANCE OF INTERVENTIONAL ULTRASOUND TECHNIQUES

A second general category of malpractice actions are those alleging negligence in the performance of invasive procedures that result in a complication causing damage to the patient. The patient clearly has a legal right to expect that procedures will be performed using proper equipment by a skilled operator or at least under the supervision of a skilled operator. While it may be difficult in many cases to distinguish a complication that is an inherent risk of a procedure from one resulting from negligence, it is imperative that patients be informed in advance of all known complications that may occur.

MISDIAGNOSIS

The final common category into which malpractice lawsuits related to interventional ultrasound fall is that involving allegations of error resulting in misdiagnosis or no diagnosis. This encompasses errors occurring within the laboratory as well as inappropriate handling of samples before they reach the laboratory. It could also include failure to identify a significant abnormality by ultrasound examination or diagnosis of an abnormality not actually present. Clearly not all laboratory errors or misdiagnoses are a result of negligence, just as not all procedure-related complications are a result of negligence. For example, there are inherent inaccuracies in many of the tests used for prenatal diagnosis. Patients should be clearly informed of the accuracy of individual tests and possible reasons for inaccuracies prior to undergoing any diagnostic procedure.

Fetal research

Although a number of states have passed laws restricting fetal research and there is a ban on federal funding for fetal research in the USA, there are currently no legal restrictions on prenatal diagnostic procedures performed during pregnancy. As diagnosis moves to the preimplantation embryo, the situation becomes considerably more complex. The legal complexities related to the status of the embryo affect not only preimplantation genetic diagnosis but also *in vitro* fertilization in general. Ethical and legal issues related to preimplantation diagnosis have recently been reviewed by Robertson [7]. Many of these derive from a societal lack of consensus regarding the moral status of the embryo. Despite the ethical considerations, Robertson concluded that there are currently few legal barriers to preimplantation genetic diagnosis or even to genetic research with embryos, whether followed by transfer or discard. There are laws in several states that restrict the disposal of embryos, but even in these states embryo biopsy with transfer or long-term storage is not prohibited.

Abortion

Abortion is currently legal in the USA in all states and the woman's right to choose abortion, as originally established by *Roe* v. *Wade*, has been repeatedly upheld in a number of court challenges. At the same time, other court decisions have opened the door to placing restrictions on this right, which is clearly not viewed by the majority of jurists as an unconditional legal right. As a result, there is increasing state-to-state variation in laws governing abortion, which deal with such issues as waiting periods, parental notification and gestational age limits. Virtually all states impose a limit on the gestational age at which abortions can be performed, even in the face of fetal abnormalities, and this varies from state to state. Additional legal challenges to the right to choose continue to be mounted and it cannot be assumed that all options currently available to patients in the USA will always be there.

There is wide variation in the legal status of abortion throughout Europe, ranging from the most restrictive laws of Ireland, which totally prohibit pregnancy termination even in the face of fetal handicap, to the more liberal policies in the UK and the even more liberal policies in eastern Europe. The UK Abortion Act 1967 provided for legal termination of pregnancies involving fetal handicap up to the legal age of viability, which was historically defined as 28 weeks but more recently reduced in practice to 24–25 weeks. More recently, the Human Fertilization and Embryology Act 1990 removed any restriction based on gestational age for terminations based on fetal handicap.

References

1 Ad Hoc Committee on Genetic Counseling of the American Society of Human Genetics. Genetic counselling. *Am J Hum Genet* 1975;27:240–242.
2 Evans MI, Drugan A, Bottoms SF *et al*. Attitudes on the ethics of abortion, sex selection and selective termination among health care professionals, ethicists and clergy likely to encounter such situations. *Am J Obstet Gynecol* 1991;164:1091–1099.
3 Wertz DC, Fletcher JC (eds). *Ethics and Human Genetics: A Cross-cultural Perspective*. Springer, Heidelberg, 1989.
4 Rothman BK. *The Tentative Pregnancy*. Viking, New York, 1986.
5 Somerville MA. Selective birth in twin pregnancy. *N Engl J Med* 1981;305:1218.
6 Brahams D. No claim in English law for wrongful birth. *Lancet* 1982;i:691–692.
7 Robertson JA. Ethical and legal issues in preimplantation genetic screening. *Fertil Steril* 1992;57:1–11.

Chapter 2/Overview of interventional ultrasound: tricks and traps of ultrasound guidance

STEVEN L. WARSOF, JANE ARRINGTON and
ALFRED Z. ABUHAMAD

Ultrasound has revolutionized the practice of obstetrics. Prior to ultrasound the clinician had no way to examine the fetus and had to use signs, symptoms, clinical judgement and experience. Today, however, the precision needed in modern obstetrics cannot rely on these factors alone. The use of ultrasound for pregnancy dating, evaluation of at-risk pregnancies, following fetal growth, and diagnosing fetal anomalies and abnormalities of the placenta and amniotic fluid volume have been well documented. This chapter first reviews the basis of ultrasound physics and technology, and then uses this knowledge to understand the basic techniques of ultrasound guidance for invasive procedures. Finally we discuss problems commonly encountered in applying these techniques.

Physics of ultrasound

Sound travels in oscillating waves with alternating cycles of compression and rarefaction of particles. The distance sound travels in one of these cycles is referred to as the wavelength. The frequency of a sound wave is the number of oscillating cycles per second (c.p.s.). Ultrasound is defined as a frequency greater than 20 000 c.p.s. or 20 000 Hz (20 KHz). The frequency of ultrasound used in clinical practice is between 2 and 10 MHz (1 000 000 c.p.s. = 1 MHz).

Ultrasonic imaging is produced by converting sound waves into electric energy. This is accomplished by a transducer, which is a device with the ability to transform energy from one form to another. An ultrasound transducer uses the properties of a piezoelectric crystal to transform electrical energy into a sound wave. Similarly, it has the ability of changing a sound wave back into electrical energy. This is known as the piezoelectric phenomenon, which was first described by the Curies in 1888. When the piezoelectric crystal receives an electrical stimulation, it produces an alteration in the crystal lattice structure that causes the crystal to vibrate and produce sound waves. Similarly, when the crystal is struck by a sound wave, the vibration in the lattice produces electrical energy that can be amplified, recorded and displayed on a cathode ray tube or video monitor.

Most ultrasound transducers consist of many piezoelectric crystals arrayed in precise geometric patterns and electronically sequenced. At a precise moment, each crystal receives its electrical signal and emits an ultrasound wave. In continuous-wave techniques, crystals are continuously transmitting or receiving sound waves. This technology is useful for continuous-wave Doppler applications. However, imaging is accomplished with pulsed-wave technology where multiple crystals fire short bursts of sound waves in a specific order. In order to prevent electrical interference between the crystals, each crystal spends the vast majority of the time receiving rather than transmitting signals. Commonly, a transducer has a transmit-to-receive ratio of 1 : 1000, meaning it transmits sound only 0.1% of the time and receives returning signals for the remainder of the time. Sequential stimulation also allows continued updating of the ultrasound picture, thus allowing update of the information on the video monitor leading to real-time imaging.

The image itself is created when the transmitted sound wave travels through a medium and strikes an object with a different density, such as soft tissue, amniotic fluid, cartilage or placenta. When this occurs, some of the incident wave energy is reflected back while the remainder of the energy wave is transmitted through the object, but in an attenuated fashion. Fluid–tissue and fat–muscle interfaces reflect as much as 1% of the sound energy. A gas–tissue interface, however, is 99.99% reflective and thus stops any sound wave from passing through. This makes the use of sonic coupling gel or oil necessary. The time interval between transmission of the signal and reception of the reflected wave and the intensity of the reflected wave are the parameters that produce the image. The brightness of the signal is correlated with tissue density and can be converted into various shades of grey or colour by a scan converter. The merging of hundreds of returning signals make up the eventual real-time grey-scale image.

Advances in technology have allowed fine differentiation of the intensity of the returning sound wave. Whereas in its earliest form only large differences in tissue density were detected, such as between fluid and bone, now small differences in tissue density can be differentiated, such as between fetal liver and lung. This ability to differentiate tissue density is referred to as contrast resolution. Modern equipment also has the ability to eliminate spurious or artefactual noise. This low-noise capability allows for sharp contrast between liquid and solid interfaces and improves diagnostic capabilities.

The clarity of the ultrasound image is frequently based on lateral and axial resolution. The lateral resolution of the ultrasound image is determined by the ultrasound wave's beam width. The beam width increases with distance from the transducer. Therefore, in general, the greater the distance from the transducer, the poorer the lateral resolution. This problem can be overcome with electronic beam focusing, which decreases this tendency for the ultrasound wave beam to widen. The axial resolution is determined by the beam frequency. The lower the beam frequency, the greater the depth of penetration. In general, the higher the beam frequency, the better the spatial or axial resolution. It is the spatial resolution that allows visualization of small anatomic detail.

Artefacts

This book emphasizes the use of real-time ultrasound in invasive techniques. Regardless of whether one is performing a simple amniocentesis, chorionic villous sampling (CVS), or a cordocentesis, the principles of ultrasound-guided invasive procedures are all similar. It is first necessary, therefore, to analyse many commonly seen artefacts in real-time imaging and then to identify how these artefacts may compromise one's ability to perform an ultrasound-guided procedure.

The most commonly seen artefact, which is often taken for granted, is the 'reverberation artefact'. This is caused by returning sound waves from superficial structures that are reflected back into the body at the tissue–scanner interface. This bouncing back and forth between internal interfaces at the scanning interface can occur multiple times. As the sound waves bounce back and forth multiple times, it is displayed as a grey shading in the anterior field (Fig. 2.1). This is frequently named 'near-field artefact' and may also be confused with the appearance of an anterior placenta in the inexperienced operator's hands. If placental localization is faulty, then even the most basic invasive procedure cannot be safely performed. Frequently, an amniocentesis is referred with the note 'unable to perform procedure due to anterior placenta' when in fact this is merely near-field artefact. This artefact is usually overcome by decreasing the near-field gain.

A second type of reverberation artefact is frequently referred to as the ring-down or 'comet-tail' artefact. This is an important artefact in invasive procedures as it is frequently associated with metallic structures, such as needles. It was first identified with metallic surgical clips and copper intrauterine devices (IUD's) but is now most commonly seen with a needle or probe tip. Recognizing

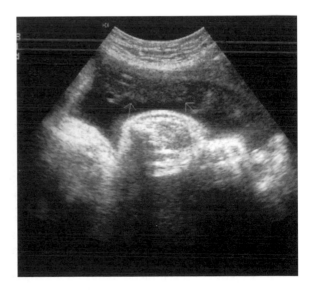

Fig. 2.1 Near field reverberation artefact is shown by arrows. The grey shading is due to bouncing back and forth of sound waves at the tissue–scanner interface.

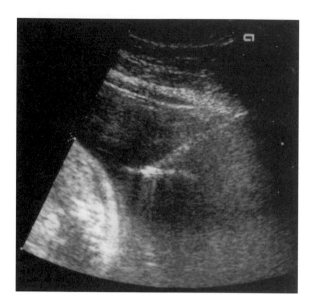

Fig. 2.2 'Ring artefact' at the tip of the needle during an ultrasound guided amniocentesis procedure.

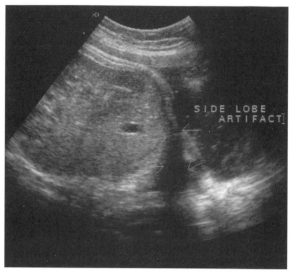

Fig. 2.3 The 'Chinese hat' or shadowing artefact is due to refraction of the sound waves at the edge of structures.

this ring-down artefact can be useful in identifying the precise location of the needle tip. It is caused by sound waves bouncing back and forth at various metal–tissue interfaces (Fig. 2.2).

The 'mirror-image' artefact is important in invasive procedures as it displays a virtual image in the wrong location. This mirror-image artefact is rarely seen with newer ultrasound equipment, and is mentioned for historical purposes.

Shadowing artefacts are commonly seen. Although they may cause problems in identifying fetal structures, they are not very problematic during invasive procedures. They may be caused by reflection, absorption or refraction of the sound waves. The first two are caused by sound waves being blocked completely by extremely sonoreflective structures, such as bone or calcification. Air also causes shadowing, but a hazier or less distinct pattern. Refractive shadowing is an artefact seen at the edge of structures. This is very similar to side-lobe or 'Chinese hat' artefact (Fig. 2.3).

Beam-thickness artefact may be problematic for invasive procedures. This is caused by attempting to make a three-dimensional object lie flat on the two-dimensional ultrasound screen. Objects near, but outside of, the imaged plane can interfere with low echo level. This problem may be lessened by the operator scanning

perpendicularly across the area in question, so that the three-dimensional structure becomes clearer.

Invasive procedures

Despite the above artefacts, ultrasound-guided invasive procedures initially appear simple. A two-dimensional image is identified, the target seen and all one simply needs to do is guide the needle percutaneously to the target. However, one hears with numbing regularity that the procedure was unsuccessful because of inability to visualize the needle.

In order to maximize success, the operator must have enough experience to use the correct transducer, the correct instruments and, the proper gain settings, and there must be appropriate coordination between the operator and the imager.

Although amniocentesis is the most commonly used ultrasound-guided procedure in obstetrics, numerous other procedures have been developed based upon the ability of ultrasound to guide an instrument within the body. These different procedures are detailed throughout the remainder of the book but briefly include the following.

1 Diagnostic amniocentesis, or sampling of amniotic fluid, was the first ultrasound-guided procedure to be

introduced into obstetrics. This was originally developed to aid in the management of Rhesus isoimmunization. With the subsequent advances in cytogenetics and the recognition of the association of elevated α-fetoprotein levels with some congenital abnormalities, mainly open neural tube and ventral wall defects, amniocentesis was quickly adapted to the role of second-trimester prenatal diagnosis of chromosomal abnormalities and many congenital anomalies. It is also useful in the third trimester for the diagnosis of fetal lung maturity and to rule out *in utero* fetal infection. Therapeutic amniocentesis under ultrasound guidance allows for relief of severe polyhydramnios and in the treatment of the 'stuck twin' syndrome.

2 Fetoscopy, direct fetal visualization, was also guided by ultrasound until the target could be visualized.

3 CVS, whether performed transcervically or transabdominally, uses ultrasound to guide either a plastic cannula or a needle into the placental bed for sampling.

4 Percutaneous umbilical blood sampling (PUBS), also referred to as cordocentesis, relies on ultrasound guidance of the needle to the umbilical cord, thus allowing for puncture of an umbilical vessel for direct haematological or biochemical analysis of the fetus.

5 Fetal blood transfusions are performed under ultrasound guidance, initially through the peritoneum and subsequently intravascularly through the umbilical cord, intrahepatic portion of the umbilical vein or directly intracardiac. *In utero* transfusions have been described in a simple or exchange fashion.

6 Additional fetal diagnostic procedures have been described that utilize ultrasound-guided procedures, including fetal skin or liver biopsies.

7 Ultrasound-guided procedures have been described for fetal treatment, including the placement of a double pigtail catheter into the fetal bladder in the setting of genitourinary outlet obstruction. Fetal surgery has also been attempted to treat progressive hydrocephalus and pleural and peritoneal fluid accumulations.

8 Ultrasound-guided procedures have also been employed in gynaecological and general surgery both diagnostically, such as percutaneous organ biopsies, as well as therapeutically for drainage of cysts and other fluid collections.

9 Ultrasound guidance has also been employed for egg collection in various assisted reproductive techniques, such as classical *in vitro* fertilization or associated procedures such as gamete intrafallopian transfer or zygote intrafallopian transfer.

10 In the future these procedures will be important for fetal gene treatment or stem cell transplants.

Although each of these procedures have their technical differences, which are discussed in their respective chapters, they are all similar in their use of ultrasound guidance. The experience and skills gained with any one of these techniques should be applicable to all of the others.

Technical aspects

The evolution of amniocentesis techniques over the last quarter of a century provides insight into all invasive procedures. When amniocentesis was originally introduced it was performed in a blind technique. The operator was guided by either palpation of the fetus *in utero* or the hands-on 'touch technique', where the operator tried to feel the needle crossing the different tissue layers. Unfortunately, both these techniques were fraught with hazard and dry or bloody taps were common and caused by the inadvertent placement of the needle into the placenta, uterine wall or fetus. It is probably fortunate that there was little documentation as to why there were so many 'dry taps'. There have also been a number of fetal injuries reported from these early procedures.

In order to avoid fetal injury, fetal head elevation and suprapubic amniocentesis was then introduced as an added safety method. With the introduction of ultrasound, patients began to present for their procedure with an 'X' on the abdomen where an ultrasound-determined fluid pocket was discovered. When first introduced, ultrasound guidance was frequently performed anywhere from several minutes to several days prior to the procedure. Unfortunately, the fetus was constantly moving and these initial attempts at ultrasound guidance were in reality identical to the blind technique.

With improvement in skills, equipment and experience, the ultrasound machine and the operator came closer together in time and location. Finally, skill, equipment, operator and machine were able to merge in one room: one team was able to identify the fluid pocket and perform the procedure immediately afterwards. Even so, the tendency was to put the transducer down just prior to the procedure. For the most part, where this technique persisted the most frequent problem was having enough trained personnel at hand.

The final development was that of continuous ultrasound guidance, where the transducer remains on the skin in order to provide a continuous ultrasound image and consequently a continuous guidance for needle injection. This technique allows for instantaneous correction of needle direction and depth of insertion to take into account the always changing intrauterine environment. To anyone who has participated in this technical evolution it is now practically unthinkable to perform any invasive procedure without continuous ultrasound guidance. Furthermore, it is now apparent how crude and fraught with potential danger the earlier techniques were.

Two variations of the continuous ultrasound-guided procedure exist. In the single-operator technique, a single skilled individual performs the procedure with his/her dominant hand while guided by the transducer held in the other hand. Usually an assistant is available to withdraw the stylet and aspirate the fetal sample. This 'single-operator' technique allows for the closest cooperation between scanning and 'needling' as it is done by the same individual. Unfortunately, this leaves the task of actual aspiration to a frequently uninitiated assistant. This can lead to inadvertent movement or dislodging of the needle at the time of aspiration, thus increasing the hazard of the procedure. Although this is not a major problem during amniocentesis, it can cause dislodging of the needle or cord laceration during the PUBS procedure.

The two-operator technique is preferred at our centre, where an ultrasonographer performs the ultrasound guidance while the operator places the needle. In this way, the operator manipulates the needle with necessary finesse to reach the desired target. However, this technique is dependent on a close relationship between the scanner and the operator. This is especially true for the more technically precise procedures such as PUBS. The operator and scanner must be able to communicate well and almost to anticipate each other's fine movements.

As stated earlier, transducers come in various sizes and shapes. Original real-time equipment employed linear scanners. Later, sector-scanning transducers were introduced. Both of these were able to visualize the needle tip but were suboptimal in their ability to visualize the needle in its entirety. This was related to the configuration

of the transducer head. The linear transducers were too large and the sector transducers too small, leading to inappropriate near-field sizes. Transducers were then developed with 'needle ports'. Unfortunately, this provided little help. Similarly on-screen biopsy needle guide lines were used with limited success. Curvilinear transducers are the latest transducer configuration and appear to be best suited for invasive procedures.

Some operators advocate using a fixed needle guide on the transducer head in order to assure the needle path. This technique, however, locks the needle and transducer together, so once the procedure has started the transducer cannot be moved. At our institution a free-hand technique is preferred that allows for fine tuning of the needle position. As the needle and transducer are not locked together, the scanner has the ability to adjust its position and to intermittently check fetal heart rates and other aspects of the uterine environment without interfering with the needling itself.

There are three free-hand techniques based upon the orientation of the needle and the transducer. The first is a perpendicular offset approach, where the transducer is placed off the sterile field at 90° to the path of the needle (Fig. 2.4). This is only practical with a protuberant or pregnant abdomen. We have not found this procedure to be very successful, as the distance between the transducer and its target is frequently outside the focal length of the transducer. The second technique is frequently referred to as 'parallel' or 'side-on' approach (Fig. 2.5), where the needle is introduced at the midpoint of the side of the transducer. Although this technique usually assures the operator what is below the transducer, it is unlikely to see more than a single point on the needle shaft. The point seen is not necessarily the tip of the needle, but is only the position where the needle shaft crosses the plane of the ultrasound beam. We have had the most success with an 'end-on' approach to ultrasonic guidance (Fig. 2.6). With this technique, the target is identified and the needle is introduced at the short end of the transducer. The angle of entry can vary and the transducer can be rocked along the abdominal wall. It is important, however, for the operator to be familiar with the focal plane of the transducer. Each transducer may have a different focal plane. It is unusual for the focal plane to be in the precise middle of the transducer; therefore, the operator should overcome the logical tendency to

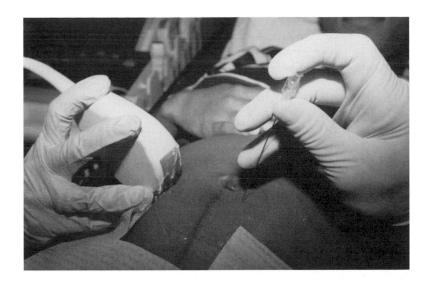

Fig. 2.4 Perpendicular offset approach for ultrasound guidance of the needle.

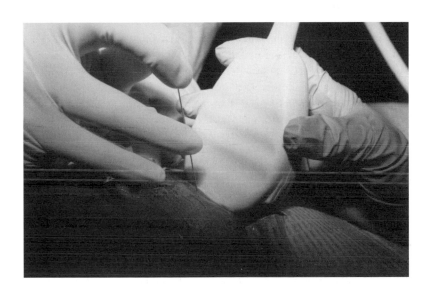

Fig. 2.5 Side-on approach for ultrasound guidance of the needle.

introduce the needle in the middle of the transducer. Instead, the operator should be familiar with each transducer and able to identify its 'sweet spot' (determined using phantoms or during easy procedures); this will reliably provide assurance that the needle in its entirety will be visualized. It is also important that the needle be directed on line with the transducer for maximum needle visibility. For this reason, we usually recommend that if a needle smaller than 22 gauge is used then it should be of increased rigidity; otherwise, the chance

of the needle bending when crossing through tissue or of not going in the desired direction because of tissue density can be problematic.

The use of phantoms to gain experience is quite helpful, both for the 'single-operator' and the two-operator technique. This allows the operator to gain considerable expertise without jeopardizing a pregnancy. Although sophisticated phantoms are commercially available, we advocate simply putting targets in a jug of ultrasound gel. The jug can then be scanned and needle-guided

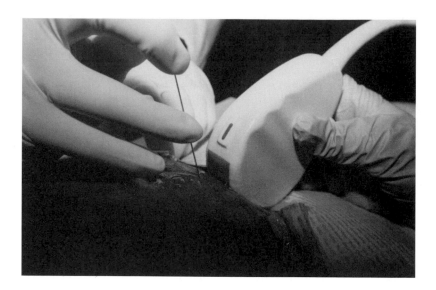

Fig. 2.6 End-on approach for ultrasound guidance of the needle.

procedures performed on the phantom. Targets can be in near field, mid field or far field. Operator and scanner quickly learn how to accommodate each other.

Before leaving the technical issue of invasive procedures we should address the issue of optimizing machine settings in order to enhance visualization. Some ultrasound machines are set at the factory and the operator has limited ability to enhance visualization. More sophisticated equipment gives the operator many choices to try to enhance visualization. We employ a series of changes in our equipment to enhance needle visualization. If machines have colour capacity then colour enhancement can sometimes be used to visualize the needle better. Computerized post-processing can be used with alterations in the settings to increase contrast and enhance the needle tip relative to surrounding tissue and fluid. Image preprocessing has not been very helpful. Total Gam Curve (TGC) settings will need to be adjusted to meet individual patient needs regarding the depth of the target, the patient's body habitus and sonogenicity. Frequently, the exact 'knobology' depends greatly on the operating team's personal preferences. Over the past several years, we have performed ultrasound-guided procedures with different machines of various sophistication and have had excellent success with all of them using curvilinear transducers.

Some manufacturers have promoted the use of sono-enhanced needles. Usually this implies a needle with fine ridging near the needle tip or multiple holes along its shaft. Although we have used these sono enhancements in the past, we have found them to be unnecessary for the most part.

Maintaining sterility in ultrasound-guided procedures is of paramount importance. Procedures have been performed with various degrees of sterile technique, ranging from using only sterile gloves to full operating-room procedures, including scrub suits, sterile gowns, hats and masks. In our experience, anticipated brief procedures are performed in a regular scanning room in our office. A sterile field is created with Betadine preoperatively. Sterile gloves are used but no particular clothing. The transducer is placed in a sterile glove, allowing for imaging over the sterile field. Sterile coupling gel is applied to the transducer head. With transabdominal CVS or PUBS on previable fetuses, we add the additional precaution of placing the transducer in a sterile shroud and the scanner also employs sterile gloves. With fetal blood transfusions, PUBS after fetal viability, or other involved procedures, we perform the procedure in the labour and delivery room (L&D) in order to respond rapidly if an emergency arises. Scrub suits, masks and hats are added in this setting.

Local anaesthetics are not used for simple amniocentesis procedures. It is frequently felt that the local anaesthetic may be more painful than the procedure itself. With more involved procedures and with

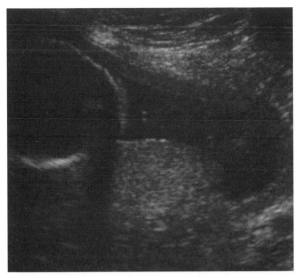

(a)

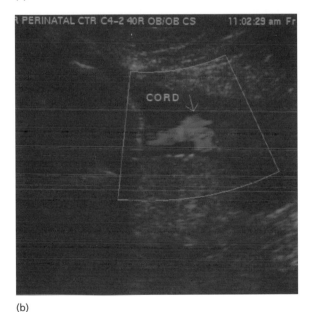

(b)

Fig. 2.7 a,b: Colour Doppler imaging may be helpful to differentiate empty/filled pockets of amniotic fluid.

transabdominal CVS, local anaesthetics are used. This serves two very useful purposes: the first is obviously as a local anaesthetic; secondly, it gives the operator an opportunity to guide the local anaesthetic needle toward the intended path. The small anaesthetic needle serves as a good initial marker for the final procedure.

Systemic prophylactic antibiotics have been advocated, although we would only use them for particularly difficult or high-risk situations.

A realistic target size for ultrasound-guided procedures should be set. Some would advocate deferring amniocentesis when the pocket of fluid is less than 1×1 cm. Our experience, however, is that if the target can be visualized, then a needle can be directed into that place. A final word of caution: colour Doppler imaging may be helpful to differentiate empty pockets of amniotic fluid from tempting targets that appear to be pockets of fluid which actually may be filled with loops of cord (Fig. 2.7). Detailed informed consent should be obtained prior to any procedures and risks and benefits need to be explained, with a clear-cut understanding by patients and medical team exactly what steps will be taken in an emergency.

Conclusions

The development of diagnostic ultrasound has opened the field of invasive ultrasound-guided procedures with a myriad of applications. The free-hand, two-operator, end-on technique is preferred in our centre. Local anaesthetic is used in complex procedures and CVS, but not in routine procedures. Prophylactic antibiotics are used only in high-risk situations. Developing skills and technique with a phantom will be helpful to gain confidence. The most important aspect of all invasive procedures is experience and teamwork between operator and scanner. This is critical.

Acknowledgements

We would like to thank the many highly skilled sonographers that we have worked with over the years, and who have made these procedures technically feasible.

Chapter 3 / Ultrasound-guided techniques in fetal medicine

KYPROS H. NICOLAIDES and YVES VILLE

All ultrasound-guided diagnostic and therapeutic invasive procedures in fetal medicine are best done transabdominally by using essentially the same technique. Such an approach ensures that the risks associated with the introduction of a new surgical technique will be minimized: if thoraco-amniotic shunting is performed in a similar fashion to amniocentesis, then whenever either technique is carried out, the operator becomes better at both.

Another prerequisite for invasive procedures is that the operator should have extensive experience in ultrasound scanning; although it is possible for the operator to be guided by another sonographer, coordination is inevitably better with one cerebellum rather than two.

Invasive procedures can be performed with curvilinear, sector or linear-array transducers, and either the free-hand technique or needle guides can be used. We prefer a curvilinear transducer because it combines the advantages of both linear-array and sector systems (the needle is visualized throughout its length and the image of the tip is sharp). Furthermore, the free-hand technique is preferred because it allows freedom for manipulation if the position of the target is suddenly altered by a uterine contraction or fetal movements.

An ultrasound scan is first performed to define the position of the fetus, placenta and adnexal vessels or masses. In general, we prefer a lateral entry into the uterus irrespective of whether the placenta is anterior or posterior. In this position visualization and manipulation of the guided instrument is easier. At the lower pole of the uterus, access is limited by the maternal iliac bones, whereas at the upper pole, access is limited by her umbilicus. Therefore potential sites of skin puncture are from 1 o'clock to 5 o'clock on the left and 7 o'clock to 11 o'clock on the right (Fig. 3.1); these sites are examined systematically to find the most suitable location.

The transducer is held in the left hand of a right-handed operator; the desired target is identified and the transducer is aligned in such a way that the target is in the centre of the screen while the proposed site of entry in the maternal abdomen is visualized at the edge of the screen. Starting from the 'five past seven' position, the transducer, which is always kept at right angles to the operating table, is gradually rotated for systematic examination of all potential sites of entry and identification of the most suitable one. Subsequently, the right index finger is placed on the maternal abdomen, about 2–3 cm away from the edge of the transducer, and pressed firmly toward the uterus. Provided the finger and transducer are within the same plane, the indentation caused is clearly visible, allowing the operator to simulate needle insertion.

The chosen site of entry on the maternal abdomen is cleaned with antiseptic solution and, when required, local anaesthetic is infiltrated under ultrasound guidance down to the myometrium. This initial step also provides an overview of the needle pathway and allows correction of the angle of entry with the puncture needle.

The needle or instrument is then introduced into the uterus, ensuring that the whole length is visualized continuously. This is best achieved when the needle is directed at 45° from the horizontal plane of the transducer (Fig. 3.2). Once the needle has entered the skin, the transducer, maintained in the same vertical plane, should be angled to clearly visualize the initial shaft of the needle and to correct its angle before entering the myometrium.

In amniocentesis, even when the placenta is posterior, a lateral entry into the uterus is preferable to an anterior one because in this position the pool of amniotic fluid is always deeper. This is also true for chorionic villous sampling: even with a posterior placenta, almost always there is a lateral extension of

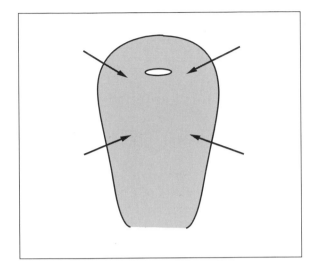

Fig. 3.1 Preferred entries to the uterus.

the placenta so that it is unnecessary and risky to enter the amniotic cavity before reaching the target. For cordocentesis, when the placenta is anterior or lateral, the needle is introduced transplacentally into

Fig. 3.2 Technique for ultrasound-guided procedures.

an umbilical vessel, which is visualized longitudinally (Fig. 3.3). Care is taken to avoid going through the chorionic plate and the amniotic cavity before puncturing the cord because inadvertent puncture of a chorionic plate vessel, which lacks Wharton jelly support, could cause catastrophic haemorrhage. When the placenta is posterior, the needle is introduced transamniotically and the cord is punctured at right angles to the longitudinal axis of the cord, close to its placental insertion; occasionally, when fetal parts obscure the cord insertion, appropriate external pressure may be needed to change the position of the fetus. For fetal skin biopsy (dermatocentesis), the needle is introduced at right angles to the longitudinal axis of the fetus and since, contrary to the commonly held view, there is scarring of the fetus it is best that the biopsies are taken from the fetal buttocks or scalp. In fetal liver biopsy (hepatocentesis), the needle, at right angles to the longitudinal axis of the fetal abdomen, is directed to the right hypochondrium. For fetal bladder aspiration (urodochocentesis), or vesico-amniotic shunting, the needle/canula is introduced into the bladder at right angles to the fetal trunk and care is taken to avoid puncturing the umbilicus: in this respect, an anterolateral approach is recommended. Similarly, for intraperitoneal fetal blood transfusions, the needle is introduced

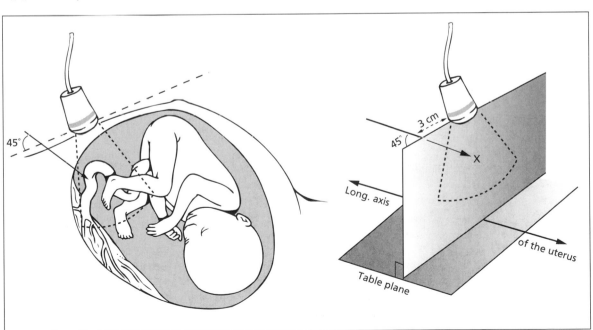

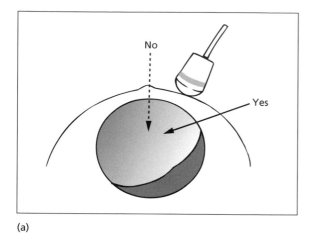

(a)

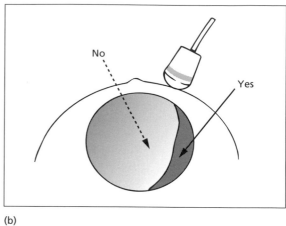

(b)

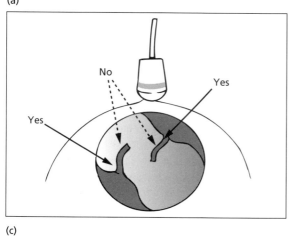

(c)

Fig. 3.3 (a–c) Cordocentesis.

anterolaterally into the lower fetal abdomen. For thoraco-amniotic shunting, the thorax is best approached posterolaterally (if the shunts are introduced anteriorly, the fetus often pulls them out). If drainage of the contralateral lung is also needed, the appropriate fetal position is achieved by rotating the fetal body using the tip of the canula.

Chapter 4 / Anaesthesia for interventional ultrasound in obstetrics

PIERRE SCHOEFFLER and RODIN RAMBOATIANA

Greater resolution and increased specificity explain the developments in prenatal ultrasonography. Ultrasound not only makes an early diagnosis of many lesions possible but also enables an increased number of lesions to be treated percutaneously during pregnancy. Most of these treatments, though 'non-invasive', require anaesthesia for the mother and fetus because of the elevation of plasma concentrations of endogenous catecholamines caused by maternal anxiety, surgical stimulation and postoperative pain. Increased secretion of catecholamines can compromise the fetus by lowering placental blood flow and by predisposing to preterm labour.

In order to limit these events, anaesthesia is required with special attention to the physiological changes of pregnancy.

Physiological changes of pregnancy

Many of the maternal physiological changes that occur during pregnancy can influence the conduct of anaesthesia. They involve the cardiovascular, pulmonary and gastrointestinal systems, as well as airway anatomy and coagulation factors.

Cardiovascular system

The maternal cardiac output at term increases by 30–40%, the plasma volume by 50% and the red cell mass by 30%. The systemic vascular resistances are reduced [1,2].

Aortocaval compression becomes clinically significant in the supine position after 10 weeks' gestation, reducing venous return, cardiac output and uteroplacental perfusion. Inferior vena cava compression by the enlarged gravid uterus is associated with venous stasis in the lower extremities and with an increased risk of thrombophlebitis. Alterations in the level of several coagulation factors (increase in factors VIII, XII and fibrinogen, decrease in factors XI and XIII) may potentiate the risk of venous thrombosis [3].

Respiratory function

Minute alveolar ventilation increases during pregnancy, leading to respiratory alkalosis [4]. This is compensated by renal excretion of bicarbonate in order to maintain normal acid–base balance. Consequently, pregnancy creates a decreased ability to buffer an acidotic state.

While maternal oxygen consumption increases, functional residual capacity decreases, explaining why hypoxia occurs rapidly in cases of apnoea.

Gastrointestinal tract

As the uterus expands, the stomach is shifted to a more cephalad and horizontal position. Hence, the angle of the gastro-oesophageal junction alters, reducing the competency of the oesophageal sphincter. At the same time, gastric acid production increases. Both factors predispose to passive regurgitation and aspiration of gastric contents during general anaesthesia.

Pharmacology of anaesthetic drugs

The increase in cardiac output, glomerular filtration and volume of distribution on the one hand and the decrease in plasma protein level on the other lead to dramatic alterations of the pharmacokinetics of anaesthetic drugs during pregnancy [5]. Due to modifications of their hormonal state (especially an increased level of progesterone), pregnant women are also more sensitive to the effects of general and local anaesthetic drugs [6,7].

After crossing the placental barrier, these drugs may

influence the fetus directly. Placental transfer and fetal drug concentration depend on lipid solubility, ionization, fetal pH, portal clearance, plasma protein binding and metabolism. Furthermore, administration of drugs to pregnant women may induce teratogenic effects and no agent has been shown to be safer than another. However spinal anaesthesia, when appropriate, minimizes fetal drug exposure.

Through their effects on the haemodynamics and respiratory physiology of the mother, anaesthetic agents can have an indirect action on the fetus. Fetal well-being may also be affected by alterations in uterine tone and/or placental blood flow. Many drugs can increase uterine tone, e.g. ketamine in doses larger than 1.1 mg/kg. Toxic concentrations of local anaesthetics (resulting from accidental intravascular injection) cause direct uterine artery vasoconstriction [8].

Anaesthetic techniques

Monitoring and positioning

Appropriate intraoperative monitoring consists of pulse oxymetry, non-invasive blood pressure estimation and electrocardiographic display. Fetal heart rate and uterine activity must also be monitored throughout the whole procedure. In our centre complete monitoring is used in every patient even if local anaesthetic infiltration of the abdominal wall is the only anaesthetic technique used.

During positioning of the patient, left uterine tilt is essential in order to limit aortocaval compression and to ensure optimal uterine blood flow.

Preoperative period

An informative visit will take place a few days before the procedure in order to explain in detail every aspect and the risk of the anaesthesia.

Systematic preoperative screenings are not mandatory, although assessment of haemostasis (prothrombin time and partial thrombin time, fibrinogen level and platelet count) is justified because of the frequent abnormalities of coagulation factors in pregnancy. A preoperative electrocardiogram is useful if β-mimetic tocolytic drugs are to be administered in the postoperative period for prophylactic control of uterine contractions.

PREMEDICATION

Premedication with a benzodiazepine on its own or associated with a narcotic will help relieve maternal anxiety. Prophylactic indomethacin, 100 mg *per rectum*, may help prevent preterm labour [9].

In order to prevent gastric acid aspiration, an antacid is given *per os*, in combination with metoclopramide and cimetidine.

Local and regional anaesthesia

For these percutaneous procedures, local anaesthesia by skin infiltration is the simplest choice [10]. This technique is very easy to use and avoids the risk of maternal aspiration associated with general anaesthesia. However all local anaesthetics cross the placenta and diffuse into the fetal circulation [11]. High plasma concentrations of local anaesthetics after accidental intravenous injection may depress the fetal cardiovascular system.

The use of large-size needles or/and multiple placement attempts despite sonographic guidance may result in stimulation of the maternal autonomic nervous system. This catecholamine secretion directly increases uterine arterial resistance and therefore lowers placental blood flow and causes uncoordinated uterine contractions, which may lead to preterm labour. Although epidural or intrathecal regional anaesthesia provides the mother with better comfort, these techniques may lower maternal blood pressure, decrease uterine blood flow and induce a risk of fetal asphyxia [12]. If hypotension occurs, it must be corrected with vascular fluid loading and with an indirect-acting agent such as ephedrine, which raises maternal blood pressure but has no effect on uterine vascular resistances [8].

Neither local nor regional anaesthesia administered to the mother provides anaesthesia of the fetus. Late in gestation, the fetus responds to stimuli such as noise, pressure or touch [10]. An unanaesthesized fetus responds to any surgical manipulation by a dramatic stimulation of the autonomic nervous system. Direct infiltration of small amounts of lidocaine into the fetal surgical site will not always cause an entirely efficient fetal anaesthesia and does not ensure an immobile fetus. Fetal anaesthesia can be obtained by sedation of the mother with benzodiazepines and opiates; however, these drugs may depress maternal ventilation leading to fetal hypoxaemia, acidosis and cardiac depression [13]. Hypercarbia of the mother will also raise her catecholamine concentration, resulting in a reduction of uterine blood flow.

General anaesthesia

General anaesthesia allows more accurate control of maternal ventilation and blood pressure. Maternal anaesthesia will also provide appropriate fetal anaesthesia.

INDUCTION

The usual 'full stomach' precautions must be observed during the induction of general anaesthesia, including a rapid sequence induction, with cricoid compression before systematic endotracheal intubation.

Maternally administered intravenous anaesthetics have indirect effects on the fetus. Due to maternal hypotension and release of catecholamines during airway instrumentation, there is a fall in intervillous blood flow following rapid sequence induction of anaesthesia with thiopental [14].

MAINTENANCE

Nitrous oxide in oxygen and halogenated agents provide adequate maternal relaxation and fetal anaesthesia. The halogenated anaesthetic agents can theoretically affect the fetus by changing maternal haemodynamics. However, the drop in blood pressure induced by low or moderate concentrations of these agents is offset by an increase in urine blood flow secondary to uterine relaxation together with a decrease in uterine vascular resistances [15].

Intraoperative narcotics and benzodiazepine also may be used. These drugs are commonly used to reduce maternal adrenergic responses to surgical stimulation that are deleterious for placental blood flow. Narcotics given to the mother will also produce fetal analgesia and lack of movement. Benzodiazepines provide the fetus with amnesia, which may decrease fetal response to subsequent stressful stimuli [10,16]. Fetal immobility can also be obtained from muscle relaxants administered to the mother or directly to the fetus, e.g. pancuronium, 0.5 mg, injected into fetal gluteal muscle will provide 2

or 3 hours' immobility [17]. Reversal of neuromuscular blockade with anticholinesterases such as neostigmine can increase uterine tone.

Uterine relaxation is important for both operative comfort and placental blood flow and can be obtained from halogenated agents like halothane, enflurane, isoflurane or desflurane. These anaesthetic agents, at low to moderate doses, also lower uterine vascular resistances, helping to maintain uteroplacental blood flow. No one halogenated agent has a particular advantage over the others.

In order to maintain normocarbia, a capnograph is absolutely required to adjust maternal ventilation parameters during the anaesthetic procedure. Hyperventilation, and resulting hypocarbia, produce a vasoconstriction that impairs uterine blood flow. The second consequence of hyperventilation is a respiratory alkalosis, resulting in a leftward shift of the haemoglobin dissociation curve and a decrease in oxygen availability for the fetus [18]. On the other hand, hypercarbia due to hypoventilation will also raise maternal catecholamine concentrations, resulting in reduced uterine blood flow.

Postoperative period

The β-tocolytics are to be used with strict monitoring of the maternal electrocardiogram. Fetal heart rate and uterine activity must also be checked during the whole postoperative period. When necessary, adequate pain relief decreases maternal plasma catecholamines and helps prevent the onset of premature labour.

References

1 Berkowitz RL, Berkowitz GS. Invasive hemodynamic studies during normal pregnancy. *Obstet Gynecol* 1990;**75**: 1041–1042.
2 Capeless EL, Clapp JF. Cardiovascular changes in early phase of pregnancy. *Am J Obstet Gynecol* 1989;**161**:1449–1453.
3 Fletcher AP, Alkjaersig NK, Burstein R. The influence of pregnancy upon blood coagulation and plasma fibrinolytic function. *Am J Obstet Gynecol* 1979;**134**:743–751.
4 Bonica JJ. Maternal respiratory changes during pregnancy and parturition. In: Marx G. (ed.) *Parturition and Perinatology*. Philadelphia: Davis, 1973:9.
5 Notarianni LJ. Plasma protein binding of drugs in pregnancy and in neonates. *Clin Pharmacokinet* 1990;**18**:20–36.
6 Butterworth JF, Walter FO, Lysak SZ. Pregnancy increases

median nerve susceptibility to lidocaine. *Anesthesiology* 1990;72:962–965.

7 Palahniuk RJ, Shnider SM, Eger EI. Pregnancy decreases the requirement for inhaled anesthetic agents. *Anesthesiology* 1974;41:82–83.

8 Greiss FC, Still J, Anderson SG. Effects of local anesthetic on the uterine vasculature and myometrium. *Am J Obstet Gynecol* 1983;124:889–894.

9 Longaker MT, Golbus MS, Filly RA, Rosen MA, Chang SW, Harrison MR. Maternal outcome after open fetal surgery. *JAMA* 1991;265:137–141.

10 Rosen MH. Anesthesia for fetal surgery. In: Shnider SM, Levinson G (eds) *Anesthesia for Obstetrics*, 2nd edn. Baltimore: Williams & Wilkins, 1987:206.

11 Santos AC, Pedersen H, Morishima HO, Finster M, Arthur GR, Covino BG. Pharmacokinetics of lidocaine in nonpregnant and pregnant ewes. *Anesth Analg* 1988;67: 1154–1158.

12 Wright RG, Shnider SM. Hypotension and regional anesthesia. In: Shnider SM, Levinson G (eds) *Anesthesia for Obstetrics*, 2nd edn. Baltimore: Williams & Wilkins, 1987:293.

13 Levinson G, Shnider SM. Anesthesia for surgery during pregnancy. In: Shnider SM, Levinson G (eds) *Anesthesia for Obstetrics*, 2nd edn. Baltimore: Williams & Wilkins, 1987:188.

14 Jouppila P, Kuikka J, Jouppila R, Hollmen A. Effect of induction of general anesthesia for cesarean section on intervillous blood flow. *Acta Obstet Gynecol Scand* 1979;58:249–254.

15 Gregory GA, Wade JG, Beihl DR, Ong BY, Sitar DS. Fetal anesthetic requirement (MAC) for halothane. *Anesth Analg* 1983;62:9–14.

16 Ralston DH, Shnider SM. The fetal and neonatal effects of regional anesthesia in obstetrics. *Anesthesiology* 1978;48:34–39.

17 Hickle RS. Administration of general anesthesia. In: Firestone LL, Lebowitz PW, Cook CE (eds) *Clinical Anesthesia Procedures of the Massachusetts General Hospital*, 3rd edn. Boston: Little, Brown & Co, 1988:136.

18 Delaney AG. Anesthesia in the pregnant woman. *Clin Obstet Gynecol* 1983;26:795–814.

Chapter 5 / Fetal anaesthesia and analgesia

S. MICHAEL KINSELLA and JOAQUIN SANTOLAYA-FORGAS

Introduction

Pain is an unpleasant subjective sensation usually associated with actual or potential tissue damage. Besides this subjective component, nociception is also associated with behavioural and neurohormonal autonomic responses. If a subject is not able to communicate verbally, only these latter responses, which can be observed or measured, can be used to gauge the extent of nociception. When the fetus is considered, we may never 'prove' that he or she can feel pain [1]. Even so, the humanitarian approach assumes that if there is a potential for pain, as shown by objective responses to stimuli that induce pain in adults and children, then anaesthesia or analgesia should be provided for the fetus also.

Our changing attitude to the neonate is a good example. Only a decade ago, it was considered by many clinicians that the neonate could not feel pain in qualitatively the same way as the child or adult [2]. Anand and Aynsley-Green showed that surgical stress responses lasted longer in preterm than full-term neonates and were greater in magnitude compared with adults [3,4]. However major changes in clinical practice were set in motion after they published a randomized control trial of anaesthesia for ligation of patent ductus arteriosus in premature neonates, using either nitrous oxide, which is weakly analgesic, or nitrous oxide plus fentanyl, a powerful opioid analgesic [5]. Wilkinson [6], in the correspondence following this paper, stated that to withhold the fentanyl analgesia in the control group was unethical, but the authors pointed out that the use of nitrous oxide alone was a standard anaesthetic technique in many centres [7]. There followed editorials in anaesthetic, paediatric as well as general journals [8] arguing that the same considerations used for the provision of analgesia for adults and children should

also be applied to neonates. This important work has led to much more liberal use of systemic and regional analgesia for surgery in infants and neonates [9].

However, the neurological development of the preterm infant parallels that of the fetus. The fetus is able to interact with his or her environment in a complex fashion [10], including responses to unpleasant stimuli. Logic dictates that if anaesthesia and analgesia are provided for premature neonates in intensive care from the start of viability, as young as 24 weeks, then the same considerations should definitely apply to fetuses of similar or later gestation. At what gestation this should start is unclear: the philosophical debate continues [11,12].

Adverse effects of nociception in the fetus

Fetal anaesthesia as a part of invasive therapy and surgery may be desirable for two reasons: the avoidance of physiological responses to unmodified nociception, and because of possible long-term psychological responses (pain memory).

The stress response is a hormonal consequence of tissue damage. Although it has not been proved to have any adverse consequence in the adult, in the neonate it has been linked to poor outcomes [13]. Anand et al. [5] found that two of eight preterm neonates who did not receive fentanyl analgesia for their surgery, but none of eight who did, developed intraventricular haemorrhages. They postulated that fluxes of blood glucose and plasma osmolality in the first group could explain subsequent intraventricular haemorrhage, although they stated that causation could not be proved. Several complications were more common or found only in the no-opioid group, including increased ventilation requirements, episodes of bradycardia, hypotension and metabolic acidosis. This suggests that the stress response induced cardiovascular instability in these infants. The majority of the infants in the nitrous oxide–fentanyl group, but none of the nitrous oxide-only infants, developed impairment in body temperature control. A later trial that compared low- and high-dose opioid anaesthesia for cardiac surgery demonstrated a significantly higher mortality, together with more marked stress responses, in the low-dose group [13].

A wide variety of cardiorespiratory fluctuations may also occur during painful stimulation in neonates [2]. Anand *et al.* [5] found well-developed stress responses in neonates at an average gestational age of 28 weeks. The stress response to fetal blood sampling has recently been examined by Giannakoulopoulos *et al.* [14] in fetuses having blood sampling. The site of cord puncture was either at the intrahepatic umbilical vein or at the placental cord insertion, the former approach necessitating passage of the needle through the abdominal wall and the liver capsule. The choice of site for vessel puncture depended on technical factors only, and the fetuses were comparable in other respects. When the intrahepatic route was used for blood transfusions, a median increase of 183% was found in plasma cortisol and 590% in β-endorphin between samples taken at the beginning and the end of the procedure. With transfusion via the placental cord insertion, no change in cortisol and β-endorphin concentrations was found before and after the procedure. Vigorous body and breathing movements were noted by these workers with needling using the intrahepatic route but not using the placental cord insertion. The authors noted the hormonal response in fetuses as early as 23 weeks of gestation.

In a subsequent study, the same workers measured middle cerebral artery Doppler Pulsatility index in two groups of fetuses, one having needle puncture of the trunk and one of the umbilical cord [15]. The former group had a reduction in Pulsatility index, whereas there was no change in the latter. This effect in reponse to needle trauma may have an analogy with the redistribution of blood to essential organs including the brain, and away from the carcass, during acute stress in animals [15].

Taddio *et al.* [16] found higher pain scores during routine vaccination in 4–6-month-old boys who had been circumcised at birth compared with uncircumcised boys, indicating long-lasting effects of prior painful experience. Besides behavioural differences, long-term psychological sequelae have been postulated after circumcision without anaesthesia [2]. Premature neonates have a greater flexion response and increased sensitization after noxious stimulation compared with full-term neonates. At present, there is no evidence for a 'carry-over' effect of intrauterine surgical experiences having long-term effects after delivery.

In the past one of the reasons for a reluctance to provide powerful analgesia for neonatal surgery has been the possibility of inducing side-effects. In some respects these considerations may be less important for fetal surgery: concerns over impairment of temperature control [5] or respiratory depression induced by powerful opioids do not apply to the fetus.

Monitoring of responses

Cycles of fetal activity and quiet develop in the third trimester, although they become clearly defined only after 36 weeks' gestation [17]. The fetus may be aroused into the active state by stimulation, either innocuous (e.g. vibroacoustic) or noxious. Vigorous motor activity follows needling of the body wall [14,18]. In paediatric practice, a pain scale for infants based on observation of responses to a stimulus has been developed [19]. This depends on motor responses of the body, crying and facial expressions. Some of these changes may be detectable *in utero*, either directly or using ultrasound. Spontaneous and induced truncal, limb, breathing or eye movements will be abolished with fetal anaesthesia. Although provoked movements during fetal procedures might not always be due to nociception, absence of movement in response to noxious stimuli implies adequate anaesthesia, unless neuromuscular blockers have been used.

Autonomic responses except for heart rate are not amenable to external measurement in the human fetus. If the fetus is adequately anaesthetized, it will not respond with an increase in heart rate. Analysis of heart rate variability has been proposed as an indicator of anaesthetic depth in adults [20]. There are limitations to the application of this monitoring, as different anaesthetic agents induce specific changes. Whether such an approach is applicable to the fetus is debatable, given the further variable of gestation-dependent changes in heart rate control.

Monitoring of fetal physiological state is an issue

that has been addressed for fetal surgery. Invasive transabdominal monitoring has been developed in an animal model of endoscopic surgery. This allows the measurement of heart rate, oxygen saturation with pulse oximetry, temperature and amniotic pressure [21]. For a resumé of fetal monitoring during open fetal surgery, the reader is referred to papers from the San Francisco group led by Harrison [22,23].

In future, modifications of the hormonal stress response to fetal procedures induced by anaesthesia might be studied as an adjunct to blood sampling for other purposes. The influence of different anaesthetic techniques on the stress response would also be very amenable to study in animal models with the use of umbilical catheters, especially the time course of responses in the postoperative period.

Requirements for anaesthesia

The requirement for anaesthesia or analgesia will depend on the type of procedure and its site, invasiveness and duration of surgery. The umbilical cord at its placental insertion is not innervated and there is no evidence for nociceptive stimulation when it is needled. Blood sampling or transfusion via the intrahepatic vein involves piercing the body wall with the needle, and locating the correct site takes longer with this approach than at the cord insertion [14]. Similar considerations will apply to placing catheters and shunts in the urinary tract, chest or head. There are likely to be more developments in endoscopic surgery [21,24]; at the end of the spectrum is major open surgery carried out via hysterotomy [22].

Published work has so far concentrated on two areas. Neuromuscular blockers (muscle relaxants) have been used to help the operator perform invasive procedures, and empirical regimens of maternal sedation were described at the same time. Open fetal surgery necessitates maternal general anaesthesia and there are data on the anaesthetic inhalational agents used to maintain this condition. With the advent of more extensive intrauterine therapy using ultrasound or fetoscopy, a middle ground between these extremes will develop. On the one hand, maternal drug administration may be inadequate, and on the other may not be indicated. This is the territory of fetal anaesthesia and analgesia.

The available routes of systemic drug administration to the fetus are either by direct parenteral administration or indirectly by administration to the mother and consequent placental transfer. The approach to fetal anaesthesia is often conditioned by maternal requirements, but the class of drug may also necessitate one or other route. Neuromuscular blockers are strongly ionized compounds that do not cross the placenta freely, and hence the ability to use them in the mother at Caesarean delivery without clinically significant paralysis in the neonate. Direct administration to the fetus is necessary. In contrast, inhalational agents are absorbed and largely eliminated at the alveolar–capillary interface in the lungs and maternal therapy is the only option. Most other anaesthetic and analgesic agents, being diffusible across lipid membranes, cross the placenta and can be administered either way.

Concerning maternal administration, the goal should be to administer appropriate anaesthesia to the mother for her own needs. In some cases this may be adequate for fetal requirements also. However when transfer to the fetus is not adequate, direct administration should be considered. Only when this option is not feasible should deliberate maternal overdosage be contemplated.

Systemic therapy by direct fetal administration: routes

Just as intravenous therapy in adults has developed with the introduction of indwelling cannulae and catheters, so intravenous therapy in the fetus may follow the same route [25] (see Chapter 12). This would allow intermittent injections or even continuous infusions of short-acting anaesthetic agents if so desired. The feasibility of intraosseous infusions has also been explored [23]. Other potential routes of administration include intramuscular and intraperitoneal. The original descriptions of neuromuscular blockade to ensure fetal immobility were via the intramuscular route [26–29] using d-tubocurarine or pancuronium. These agents come in solution and there is a limit to the volume of agent that it is desirable to inject. However, this objection might be overcome by using an agent such as vecuronium, which is available in crystalline form and therefore can be made up in concentrated solutions. Drugs might also be given intraperitoneally; this site might act as a 'depot', with relatively slow absorption and therefore more prolonged duration.

Wherever possible, consideration should be given to administration of anaesthetic agents using the access that has been placed for the therapeutic procedure, so as to avoid the risk of extra needling.

Local anaesthesia

Local anaesthesia for the fetus is readily achievable during open surgery by infiltration along the incision [30]. With closed surgery, the limited access reduces the options for local anaesthesia, but two approaches are possible. One is infiltration of local anaesthetic at the puncture site during tube or catheter insertion. Alternatively, local anaesthetic block of nerve trunks, such as the intercostal nerves during chest drain insertion, might be feasible with a fetoscopic approach. However, the precision needed may not be possible using ultrasound guidance.

High spinal anaesthesia has been used in fetal lambs, with very effective blockade of the marked stress response to major fetal thoracic surgery that included cardiac bypass [31].

Anaesthetic and analgesic agents

Inhalational agents

Fetal anaesthesia for surgery in humans has usually been provided with halothane [32]. The potency of halothane in ovine fetuses at 130–135 days' gestation (full term is 145–150 days) has been studied directly. Gregory *et al.* [33] found that fetal motor responses to a painful stimulus were abolished at an average blood halothane concentration of 48 mg/litre and maternal responses at 133 mg/litre; this equated to a calculated MAC* of 0.33% and 0.69% respectively (Fig. 5.1). This suggests that fetal anaesthesia may be adequate at approximately 0.5 times maternal MAC. They found in two animals that MAC increased over the first 8 hours after birth to reach a plateau of 1.1%, associated with declining levels of progesterone. The decrease in MAC during pregnancy (Table 5.1) [35] is thought to be due to increased levels of progesterone [36] and this probably accounts for the low MAC during intrauterine life.

Biehl *et al.* [37,38] found that while ewes breathed a

* Minimum alveolar concentration (MAC) is the concentration of an inhalational agent in the alveolus that abolishes the motor response to a painful stimulus in 50% of cases [34].

constant inspired concentration of either 1.5% halothane (Fig. 5.2) or 2% isoflurane (Fig. 5.3), there was a lag in the rise of fetal arterial concentrations behind those in the mother. Fetal and maternal levels stabilized at 50–60 min, the fetal always remaining lower than maternal. Using the values for halothane MAC provided by Gregory *et al.* [33], fetal and maternal MAC-equivalent would be achieved at approximately 13 and 28 min respectively of halothane anaesthesia.

Gregory *et al.* [33] found no significant decrease in fetal systolic arterial pressure at either fetal or maternal MAC. This finding is in contrast to the majority of other studies. Biehl *et al.* [39] found a significant 27% fall in fetal mean arterial pressure at 8 min after the start of administration of 1.5% inspired halothane while the fetal arterial halothane concentration was 0.74 times fetal MAC, but cardiac output and regional blood flow were maintained. Palahniuk and Shnider [40] similarly found a decrease in fetal mean arterial pressure at MAC or 1.5 times MAC halothane and isoflurane administered to the mother, but with no change in hind limb arterial blood gases. Two times MAC halothane or isoflurane (1.46% halothane and 2.02% isoflurane) [40] were found to produce fetal hypoxia and acidosis mediated through maternal hypotension and reduced cardiac output. They did not find any difference between halothane and isoflurane but cautioned against deep maternal inhalational anaesthesia. Biehl *et al.* [38] found a significant decrease in fetal axillary artery pH after 48 min of 2% isoflurane anaesthesia and a 27% reduction in cardiac output from baseline at 60 min. This was in contrast to their earlier study where they found that halothane was not associated with fetal acidosis [37] and they concluded that halothane was the preferred agent to isoflurane.

The effects of inhalational anaesthesia on the acidotic sheep fetus have also been studied. After asphyxia had been induced with partial umbilical cord occlusion, 1.5% halothane was found to reduce cerebral oxygen delivery and aggravate acidosis [41]. A further study showed that although 1.5% halothane reversed asphyxia-induced fetal hypertension, brain blood flow was maintained (fetal blood halothane 46 mg/litre, 0.32 vol%) [42]. When uterine artery occlusion was used to induce asphyxia prior to 1% halothane [43] or 1% isoflurane anaesthesia [44], cerebral oxygen delivery was maintained but acidosis was aggravated.

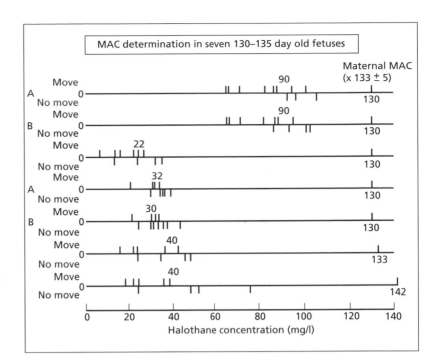

Fig. 5.1 Individual minimum alveolar concentration (MAC)-equivalent determinations in seven fetal sheep and their mothers: blood halothane concentrations at which movement in response to pain was abolished on 50% of occasions. (From Gregory *et al.* [33] with permission.)

Table 5.1 Minimum alveolar concentration in ewes. (Data from Palahniuk *et al.* [35], with permission.)

	Non-pregnant	Pregnant	Change from non-pregnant to pregnant
Halothane	0.97	0.73	−25%
Isoflurane	1.58	1.01	−40%

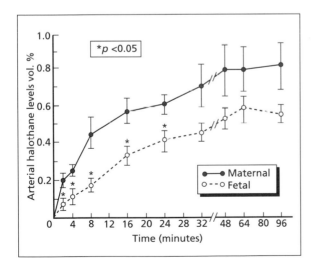

Fig. 5.2 Maternal and fetal arterial halothane concentrations during constant administration of 1.5% inspired halothane. (From Biehl *et al.* [37] with permission.)

To summarize, in the chronically instrumented sheep with a normal fetus, high concentrations of inhalational agents given to the mother induce maternal hypotension and fetal hypotension and acidosis. Halothane may cause less of a problem than isoflurane. Further acidosis is produced in the situation where the fetus is already asphyxiated.

These experiments, however, may not reflect adequately the effects of inhalational agents in the context of fetal surgical interventions; for instance, major procedures are unlikely to be performed in a fetus with pre-existing acidosis. Sabik *et al.* [31] came to a radically different conclusion on the use of halothane during fetal intervention from those who recommend it. They compared ovine fetal effects of maternal 1% halothane anaesthesia during fetal instrumentation with the effects of ketamine anaesthesia, as well as with control results taken from chronically instrumented unanaesthetized animals. Compared with the chronically instrumented

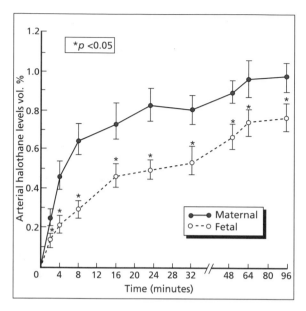

Fig. 5.3 Maternal and fetal arterial halothane concentrations during constant administration of 2% inspired isoflurane. (From Biehl *et al.* [38] with permission.)

sheep, both forms of anaesthesia were associated with reduced fetal cardiac output and placental blood flow but the extent of this was much greater in the halothane group than the ketamine group. Furthermore, placental blood flow as a percentage of cardiac output was reduced by halothane, shunting blood away from the placenta and leading to significant hypercarbia. The extent of fetal acidosis and mortality was related to the duration of anaesthesia.

With these findings in mind, there is an urgent need to perform further comparative studies of anaesthetic techniques at the time of fetal surgery or complex procedures.

Intravenous anaesthetic, sedative and opioid agents

Intravenous anaesthetics and sedative agents such as the benzodiazepines, being highly lipid soluble, will cross the placenta freely if given to the mother. However, after a single maternal dose, concentrations in blood perfusing the fetal brain will always be significantly lower than maternal arterial levels. This is due to dilution of umbilical venous blood firstly in the inferior vena cava and then in the right atrium. Thus, unless significant

maternal sedation or anaesthesia is accepted fetal anaesthesia will not be achieved [18,45,46]. Furthermore, with any parenteral single-dose technique with quick absorption, such as via intravenous or intramuscular routes, after a fairly rapid peak the maternal and fetal plasma levels will begin a steady decline.

As far as duration of action is concerned, there is an advantage to loading the maternal circulation rather than administration to the fetus. Lipid-soluble agents can cross the placenta freely in either direction including from fetus to mother. Maternal uterine blood flow is twice that of umbilical blood flow, ensuring rapid removal; if an appropriate dose is given directly to the fetus, the amount of drug will not lead to a significant increase in maternal blood levels and the concentration gradient will always effectively be zero on the maternal side. Transplacental clearance to the mother will be extremely rapid after fetal administration, and single intravenous injections given to the fetus will have an evanescent effect. For a more prolonged action, such drugs would have to be given as an intravenous continuous infusion or multiple doses, or via some other parenteral fetal route.

Opioids have a much greater spread of lipid solubilities. There is a 3000-fold difference between morphine and buprenorphine. Low lipid solubility may be the limiting factor in the transfer of morphine across the placenta. Umans and Szeto [47] infused morphine or methadone to pregnant ewes in doses that were equipotent for their sleep-suppressant effect when given directly to the fetuses. Morphine had only one-third the fetal effect of methadone when given maternally, which the authors suggested was due to slow maternal–fetal transfer. This was confirmed in a further study [48]. The effect of morphine in the fetuses was also prolonged compared with methadone, presumably because of similarly slow fetomaternal transplacental clearance [47]. Direct comparisons of opioids, in the high doses needed to reduce stress responses, must be performed before we can draw any further conclusions as to comparative usefulness.

Other agents

Neuromuscular blockers (muscle relaxants)

The indication for muscle relaxants is usually to produce fetal immobility during transfusion and other procedures.

Fetal movements may cause dislodgement of the needle, with consequences such as cord tamponade or umbilical artery spasm. These risks may be less when the intrahepatic umbilical vein is used. However, as previously mentioned counteracting this is the marked increase in fetal body movements with the latter approach as a result of increased nociception [14].

The use of muscle relaxants in the fetus was initiated by de Crespigny and co-workers [26,27] (Table 5.2). They administered 3 mg/kg D-tubocurarine into the thigh muscle under ultrasound guidance to aid needling of the intrahepatic umbilical vein or inferior vena cava, usually for the purpose of blood transfusion. Escape of part of the injected fluid into the amniotic fluid was observed in one case and only partial paralysis resulted. At delivery, there was no evidence of local damage in the leg. Seeds *et al.* [28] used intramuscular pancuronium 0.5 mg/kg, which they considered to be an equivalent dose to 3 mg/kg D-tubocurarine. The intravenous route was used soon after [49]. Not surprisingly, paralysis with this method of administration is quicker, more reliable and shorter. Moise *et al.* [51] found that paralysis tended to be shorter with increasing gestation, even though doses were adjusted for estimated fetal weight. They suggested that this reflected more efficient metabolism of pancuronium as fetal development progresses. Although this relationship was not confirmed on statistical analysis, a strong relationship

was found between increased duration and decreased fetal haematocrit, which allows tailoring of the dose of relaxant to the particular circumstances:

Duration in hours = 5.24 + 10.3 × adjusted dose (mg/kg) − 0.16 × haematocrit

The future may also see the use of shorter-acting agents such as atracurium [18].

Chestnut *et al.* [53] compared the cardiovascular effects of D-tubocurarine 3 mg/kg and pancuronium 0.5 mg/kg in fetal sheep; D-tubocurarine decreased fetal heart rate and mean arterial pressure, whereas pancuronium increased both these variables. They concluded that pancuronium is a more appropriate agent than D-tubocurarine for fetal paralysis. Fan *et al.* [52] preferred pipecurium to pancuronium because of fetal tachycardia caused by the latter drug. Fetal heart rate variability and accelerations decrease after intravenous pancuronium [46,52] and sinusoidal patterns may be seen [46].

It is essential to remember that muscle relaxants do not produce any central depressant effects and there is no evidence that they obtund the stress response. References to the fetus 'awakening' after the drug wears off [46] imply a misconception that the fetus was sedated or asleep while the drug was working, but of course the fetus is merely unable to move in response to stimulation. Muscle relaxants may assist

Table 5.2 Onset and duration of neuromuscular blockers in the fetus.

Reference	No. of cases (no. of procedures)	Route	Drug	Dose (mg/kg) based on estimated fetal weight	Onset (min)		Duration (hours)	
					Mean	Range	Mean	Range
de Crespigny *et al.* [26]	5 (12)	i.m.	D-Tubocurarine	3	—	<30	—	3–5
Seeds *et al.* [28]	4 (6)	i.m.	Pancuronium	0.5 mg—all cases	—	<1	—	<2
Moise *et al.* [29]	44	i.m.	D-Tubocurarine	3	3.2	1–15	9.0	4.7–16
	4	i.m.	D-Tubocurarine	1.5	5.1	4–6.5	3.8	2–4.8
	12	i.m.	Pancuronium	0.3	3.8	1.5–16	6.8	2–11.5
Copel *et al.* [49]	4 (5)	i.v.	Pancuronium	0.1	—	—	0.7	0.5–1.25
Byers *et al.* [50]	—	i.v.	Pancuronium	0.1	—	—	—	1–3
Pielet *et al.* [46]	18	i.v.	Pancuronium	0.05–0.1	—	Rapid	—	0.42–3.5
Moise *et al.* [51]	12 (34)	i.v.	Pancuronium	0.2–0.3	—	—	—	1.2–7
Fan *et al.* [52]	8	i.m.	Pancuronium	0.2	4.6		1.9	
	8	i.m.	Pipecuronium	0.2	4.5		2.0	

i.m., intramuscular; i.v., intravenous.

the obstetrician to perform surgery safely, but they are not a substitute for fetal anaesthesia or analgesia!

Blood gases and circulating volume

Carbon dioxide

Increases in maternal blood P_{CO_2} will increase fetal carbon dioxide because it is eliminated down a concentration gradient, and therefore fetal acidosis will occur. When deep general anaesthesia is used for fetal surgery, controlled ventilation should be provided to avoid this.

The traditional method of deep maternal sedation with large doses of depressant drugs used for less extensive fetal procedures [18,45,46] also risks maternal hypercarbia, as well as hypoxia and aspiration of regurgitated stomach contents. Although the maternal 'intrusion' might seem less than with a general anaesthetic, paradoxically any hypoventilation is not amenable to correction. Berkowitz *et al.* [18] described women going to sleep and developing considerable abdominal wall movement, necessitating waking them. This movement may well have been associated with respiratory obstruction. Therefore, a more appropriate approach might be to use patient-controlled sedation [54], which precludes oversedation. The woman self-administers small boluses of a drug; propofol is very suitable as, used in this way, the half-life is short. If the patient is too drowsy to press the button, no further drug is administered and the depth of sedation decreases.

Oxygen supply

Oxygen supply to the fetus depends on two components: maternal arterial P_{O_2} and uteroplacental blood flow.

Fetal umbilical P_{O_2} and haemoglobin saturation have been shown, at Caesarean section under epidural anaesthesia, to correlate with the maternal inspired oxygen concentration [55]. During maternal general anaesthesia, fetal oxygenation is also maximum when the maternal inspired gas contains 100% oxygen [56].

Long-term maternal oxygen administration has been used in hypoxic growth-retarded fetuses with suggestion of clinical benefit [57,58]. Cordocentesis has shown that fetal oxygen levels are increased into the normal range [57,58]. Oxygen has potent circulatory effects,

however, and attention must be paid not only to the alterations during maternal administration but also upon withdrawal. The response to hypoxia is a diversion of blood flow to essential organs at the expense of the carcass, and vice versa for an increase in oxygen levels: a reduction in vascular resistance to the carcass [59]. If supplementary oxygen is withdrawn suddenly, there is the potential for a worsening of supply to vital organs. Bekedam *et al.* [59] found that fetal heart rate decelerations sometimes occurred in growth-retarded fetuses when 40 min of maternal oxygen administration was stopped.

Uteroplacental blood flow is dependent on perfusion pressure and resistance. Maternal systemic hypotension is deleterious to the fetus during open surgery [31], but is easy to detect and treat. Aortic compression, however, is not detectable with standard maternal monitoring. Neither is it as amenable as inferior vena cava compression to prevention with the use of lateral pelvic tilt [60]. As severe aortic compression with an uncontracted uterus affects approximately 1 in 10 women while supine in an unpredictable fashion (the incidence rises to 30% with uterine contractions) [60,61], consideration should be given to direct monitoring during long procedures either with continuous [60] or intermittent blood pressure in the leg [61] or toe pulse waveforms [61].

Uterine vascular resistance is particularly influenced by uterine baseline tone and contractions, and tocolysis is considered in the next section. For the venous-equilibration type of placenta, such as the sheep, fetal umbilical vein P_{O_2} is linked by a diffusion gradient to the same variable in the maternal uterine vein. According to the Fick principle, uterine vein oxygen content (and therefore partial pressure) will depend on arterial oxygen content and uterine blood flow if oxygen extraction is constant:

Venous content = (arterial content − consumption)/flow

It was found by Sabik *et al.* [31] that ovine fetal outcome was improved by ensuring that the P_{O_2} of uterine venous blood was maintained above 45 mmHg. Whether a similar relationship holds true for human surgery is not clear. The venous-equilibration model may not be accurate here, as increases in fetal oxygenation with maternal oxygen administration are greater than the predicted increase in uterine venous P_{O_2} based on arterial oxygen content changes [55].

Tocolysis

One of the most significant problems related to fetal surgery is not the surgery itself but the inability to prevent preterm delivery of the fetus following the surgery. Uterine or fetal surgery is invariably followed by significant uterine contractions, particularly nocturnal, lasting for 3–5 days post-surgery. One of the major effects of uterine and/or fetal surgery in primates is a marked increase in maternal oestrogen levels [62,63]. This is due to the stress of the surgery on the fetus which results in enhanced release of dehydroepiandrosterone (DHEA) from the fetal adrenal glands. The DHEA is in turn converted to oestrogen by the placenta. An enhanced oestrogen environment contributes to the appearance of uterotonic factors such as maternal oxytocin, by increasing oxytocin synthesis and lowering the threshold for release.

Tocolysis during fetal surgery is a pharmacological effect of all of the currently used inhalational agents. This is of benefit during uterine manipulation, surgery and especially uterine closure. However, this effect is not sustained after administration finishes, and other agents such as magnesium sulphate or β-agonists have been used to continue tocolysis. These agents can be associated with severe maternal toxicity [64–66].

Other agents have a better therapeutic profile but do not yet have the same clinical track record. The formation of prostaglandins after damage to the amnion is a potent cause of the increased uterine activity after fetal surgery, and this may be blocked with inhibitors of prostaglandin synthesis. Initially, indomethacin was only used preoperatively during human surgery [32], but now has been used postoperatively in monkeys [30] and humans [67].

Parenteral nitroglycerin, which has a smooth muscle relaxant effect via nitric oxide formation, has been suggested as a possible uterine relaxant after fetal surgery [22]. Nitroglycerin has many of the attributes of an ideal tocolytic agent, as it is relatively non-toxic, able to be administered by infusion and 'loaded' to therapeutic blood levels rapidly and non-cumulative with rapid offset of therapeutic effects. Its role is yet to be determined [68].

Newer approaches to suppression of post-surgical uterine contractions are very promising. Aromatase inhibitors can be given to block oestrogen formation and thus the induction of uterotonic factors by oestrogen [63,69]. The problem with the use of aromatase inhibitors is the potentially deleterious effect on the fetal brain development and sexual differentiation. However, this is unlikely to be a problem if the aromatase inhibitor is administered short term (2–3 days). Nocturnal uterine contractions in primates are driven by maternal oxytocin. Therefore the use of an oxytocin antagonist, which blocks the action of oxytocin at the receptor, can be used for controlling post-surgical nocturnal uterine contractions. Oxytocin antagonists are a new generation of tocolytics that are particularly attractive since their side-effects are minimal compared to the commonly used tocolytics. Examples of such antagonists are Atosiban [70] and TT-235 aka ANTAG III [71]. In addition, morphine is a potent inhibitor of oxytocin release in primates [72] thus the use of morphine as a post-surgical analgesic has the additional benefit of suppressing oxytocin release.

Intravenous fluids

Currently, advice on maternal fluid administration after hysterotomy and fetal surgery in humans is conditioned by the fear of maternal pulmonary oedema after high doses of tocolytic agents [73]. If improvements in this aspect of therapy are possible, then fluids might be given as clinically indicated. When pregnant sheep are given oral and intravenous fluids preoperatively and peroperatively, both mother and fetus benefit in terms of blood pressure and placental perfusion [31]. Umbilical artery Doppler Systolic/Diastolic ratio decreased after a maternal intravenous fluid load [74], possibly through a decrease in fetal blood viscosity secondary to haemodilution. Transfer of water and electrolytes across the placenta will occur freely. The corollary of this is that in the situation of fetal anaemia, care must be taken not to overdo fluid administration to the mother because of the chance of fetal haemodilution.

Conclusions

Fetal anaesthesia is easy to achieve in terms of the sensitivity of the fetus to drugs. However, the difficulty of access to the fetus has meant that administration has usually been achieved indirectly via the mother. This may have led to regimens that were suboptimal for both individuals. With potential developments in the systems available to deliver therapy directly to the fetus, tailoring of the anaesthetic to the fetus rather than depending on transfer from the mother is an exciting prospect. The necessity will increase with the advent of more extensive intrauterine procedures, not requiring maternal general anaesthesia but with greater nociception than the simple procedures that characterized the early development of fetal medicine.

Many anaesthetic and analgesic drugs are likely to have only a brief duration of action in the fetus if given as a single intravenous dose. The exception may be morphine because of its limited lipid solubility. High concentrations and prolonged exposure to inhalational agents may cause fetal problems during open surgery. An acceptance of these doses has been necessary because of the reliance on the tocolytic action of halothane. Development of reliable tocolytic agents with a greater safety margin is necessary. Maternal sedation should ideally reflect the mother's own needs, and reduced interference in maternal cardiovascular and respiratory control will benefit the fetus.

There is a growing acceptance that prelabour factors are more commonly implicated in cerebral palsy than birth asphyxia [75]. The fetus may be susceptible to physiological derangements as a result of surgical stress, which could damage his or her immature organs; if anaesthesia can reduce the stress response it may have an importance besides any humanitarian considerations.

References

1 Richards T. Can a fetus feel pain? *Br Med J* 1985;**291**:1220–1221.

2 Anand KJS, Hickey PR. Pain and its effects in the human neonate and fetus. *N Engl J Med* 1987;**317**:1321–1329.

3 Anand KJS, Brown MJ, Bloom SR, Aynsley-Green A. Studies on the hormonal regulation of fuel metabolism in the human newborn infant undergoing anaesthesia and surgery. *Horm Res* 1985;**22**:115–128.

4 Anand KJS, Brown MJ, Causon RC, Cristofides ND, Bloom SR, Aynsley-Green A. Can the human neonate mount an endocrine and metabolic response to surgery? *J Pediatr Surg* 1985;**20**:41–48.

5 Anand KJS, Sippell WG, Aynsley-Green A. Randomised trial of fentanyl anaesthesia in pre-term babies undergoing surgery: effects on the stress response. *Lancet* 1987;**i**:243–248.

6 Wilkinson DJ. Anaesthesia and surgery in children. *Lancet* 1987;**i**:750.

7 Anand KJS, Sippell WG, Aynsley-Green A. Anaesthesia and surgery in children. *Lancet* 1987;**i**:750–775.

8 Rogers MC. Do the right thing. Pain relief in infants and children. *N Engl J Med* 1992;**326**:55–56.

9 de Lima J, Lloyd-Thomas AR, Howard RF, Sumner E, Quinn TM. Infant and neonatal pain: anaesthetists' perceptions and prescribing patterns. *Br Med J* 1996;**313**:787.

10 Liley AW. The foetus as a personality. *Aust N Z J Pyschol* 1972;**6**:99–105.

11 Glover V, Fisk N. Do fetuses feel pain? We don't know; better to err on the safe side from mid-gestation. *Br Med J* 1996;**313**:796.

12 Lloyd-Thomas AR, Fitzgerald M. Do fetuses feel pain? Reflex responses do not necessarily signify pain. *Br Med J* 1996;**313**:797–798.

13 Anand KJS, Hickey PR. Halothane–morphine compared with high-dose sufentanil for anesthesia and postoperative analgesia in neonatal cardiac surgery. *N Engl J Med* 1992;**326**:1–9.

14 Giannakoulopoulos X, Sepulveda W, Kourtis P, Glover V, Fisk NM. Fetal plasma cortisol and β-endorphin response to intrauterine needling. *Lancet* 1994;**344**:77–81.

15 Teixeira J, Fogliani R, Giannakoulopoulos X, Glover V, Fisk NM. Fetal haemodynamic stress response to invasive procedures. *Lancet* 1996;**347**:624.

16 Taddio A, Goldbach M, Ipp M, Stevens B, Koren G. Effect of neonatal circumcision on pain responses during vaccination in boys. *Lancet* 1994;**344**:291–292.

17 Arduini D, Rizzo G, Giorlandino C, Valensise H, Dell'Acqua S, Romanini C. The development of fetal behavioural states: a longitudinal study. *Prenat Diagn* 1986;**6**:117–124.

18 Berkowitz RL, Chitkara U, Wilkins I, Lynch L, Mehalek KE. Technical aspects of intravascular intrauterine transfusions: lessons learned from thirty-three procedures. *Am J Obstet Gynecol* 1987;**157**:4–9.

19 Taddio A, Nulman I, Goldbach M, Ipp M, Koren G. The use of lidocaine–prilocaine cream for vaccination pain in infants. *J Pediatr* 1994;**124**:643–648.

20 Komatsu T, Kimura T, Sanchala V, Shibutani K, Lees DE. Evaluation of spectrum analysis of heart rate variations during anesthesia. *Anesthesiology* 1986;**65**:A139.

21 Luks FI, Deprest JA, Vandenberghe K, Brosens IA, Lerut T. A model for fetal surgery through intrauterine endoscopy. *J Pediatr Surg* 1994;**29**:1007–1009.

22 Harrison MR, Adzick NS. Fetal surgical techniques. *Semin Pediatr Surg* 1993;**2**:136–142.

23 Jennings RW, Adzick NS, Longaker MT, Lorenz HP, Estes JM, Harrison MR. New techniques in fetal surgery. *J Pediatr Surg* 1992;**27**:1329–1333.

24 Estes JM, MacGillivray TE, Hedrick MH, Adzick NS,

Harrison MR. Fetoscopic surgery for the treatment of congenital anomalies. *J Pediatr Surg* 1992;27:950–954.

25 Lemery D, Urbain MF, Micorek JC, Jacquetin B. Fetal umbilical cord catheterization under ultrasound guidance. *Fetal Ther* 1988;3:37–43.

26 de Crespigny LCh, Robinson HP, Ross AW, Quinn M. Curarisation of fetus for intrauterine procedures. *Lancet* 1985;i:1164.

27 de Crespigny LCh, Robinson HP, Quinn M, Doyle L, Ross A, Cauchi M. Ultrasound-guided fetal blood transfusion for severe Rhesus isoimunization. *Obstet Gynecol* 1985;66: 529–532.

28 Seeds JW, Corke BC, Spielman FJ. Prevention of fetal movement during invasive procedures with pancuronium bromide. *Am J Obstet Gynecol* 1986;155:818–819.

29 Moise KJ, Carpenter RJ, Deter RL, Kirshon B, Diaz SF. The use of fetal neuromuscular blockade during intrauterine procedures. *Am J Obstet Gynecol* 1987;157:874–879.

30 Brodner RA, Markowitz RS, Lantner HJ. Feasibility of intracranial surgery in the primate fetus. Model and surgical principles. *J Neurosurg* 1987;66:276–282.

31 Sabik JF, Assad RS, Hanley FL. Halothane as an anesthetic for fetal surgery. *J Pediatr Surg* 1993;28:542–547.

32 Longaker MT, Golbus MS, Filly RA, Rosen MA, Chang SW, Harrison MR. Maternal outcome after open fetal surgery. A review of the first 17 human cases. *JAMA* 1991;265:737–741.

33 Gregory GA, Wade JG, Biehl DR, Ong BY, Sitar DS. Fetal anesthetic requirement (MAC) for halothane. *Anesth Analg* 1983;62:9–14.

34 Eger EI II, Saidman LJ, Brandstater B. Minimum alveolar anaesthetic concentration: a standard of potency. *Anesthesiology* 1965;26:756–763.

35 Palahniuk RJ, Shnider SM, Eger EI. Pregnancy decreases the requirements for inhaled anesthetic agents. *Anesthesiology* 1974;41:82–83.

36 Datta S, Migliozzi RP, Flanagan HL, Krieger NR. Chronically administered progesterone decreases halothane requirements in rabbits. *Anesth Analg* 1989;68:46–50.

37 Biehl DR, Cote J, Wade JG, Gregory GA, Sitar D. Uptake of halothane by the foetal lamb *in utero*. *Can Anaesth Soc J* 1983;30:24–27.

38 Biehl DR, Yarnell R, Wade JG, Sitar D. The uptake of isoflurane by the foetal lamb *in utero*: effect on regional blood flow. *Can Anaesth Soc J* 1983;30:581–586.

39 Biehl DR, Tweed WA, Cote J, Wade JG, Sitar D. Effect of halothane on cardiac output and regional flow in the fetal lamb *in utero*. *Anesth Analg* 1983;62:489–492.

40 Palahniuk RJ, Shnider SM. Maternal and fetal cardio-vascular and acid–base changes during halothane and isoflurane anesthesia in the pregnant ewe. *Anesthesiology* 1974;41:462–472.

41 Palahniuk RJ, Doig GA, Johnson GN, Pash MP.

Maternal halothane anesthesia reduces cerebral blood flow in the acidotic sheep fetus. *Anesth Analg* 1980;59:35–39.

42 Yarnell R, Biehl DR, Tweed WA, Gregory GA, Sitar D. The effect of halothane anaesthesia on the asphyxiated foetal lamb *in utero*. *Can Anaesth Soc J* 1983;30:474–479.

43 Cheek DBC, Hughes SC, Dailey PA *et al*. Effect of halothane on regional cerebral blood flow and cerebral metabolic oxygen consumption in the fetal lamb *in utero*. *Anesthesiology* 1987;67:361–366.

44 Wycke Baker B, Hughes SC, Shnider SM, Field DR, Rosen MA. Maternal anesthesia and the stressed fetus: effects of isoflurane on the asphyxiated fetal lamb. *Anesthesiology* 1990;72:65–70.

45 Spielman FJ, Seeds JW, Corke BC. Anaesthesia for fetal surgery. *Anaesthesia* 1984;39:756–759.

46 Pielet BW, Socol ML, MacGregor SN, Dooley SL, Minogue J. Fetal heart rate changes after fetal intra-vascular treatment with pancuronium bromide. *Am J Obstet Gynecol* 1988;159:640–643.

47 Umans JG, Szeto I II I. Effects of opiates on fetal behavioural activity *in utero*. *Life Sci* 1983;33:S639–S642.

48 Szeto HH, Umans JG, McFarland J. A comparison of morphine and methadone disposition in the maternal–fetal unit. *Am J Obstet Gynecol* 1982;143:700–707.

49 Copel JA, Grannum PA, Harrison D, Hobbins JC. The use of intravenous pancuronium bromide to produce fetal paralysis during intravascular transfusion. *Am J Obstet Gynecol* 1988;158:170–171.

50 Byers JW, Aubry RH, Feinstein SJ *et al*. Intravascular neuromuscular blockade for fetal transfusion. *Am J Obstet Gynecol* 1988;158:677.

51 Moise KJ, Deter RL, Kirshon B, Adam K, Patton DE, Carpenter RJ. Intravenous pancuronium bromide for fetal neuromuscular blockade during intrauterine transfusion for red-cell alloimmunization. *Obstet Gynecol* 1989;74: 905–908.

52 Fan SZ, Susetio L, Tsai MC. Neuromuscular blockade of the fetus with pancuronium or pipecuronium for intra-uterine procedures. *Anaesthesia* 1994;49:284–286.

53 Chestnut DH, Weiner CP, Thompson CS, McLaughlin GL. Intravenous administration of D-tubocurarine and pancuronium in fetal lambs. *Am J Obstet Gynecol* 1989;160: 510–513.

54 Cook LB, Lockwood GG, Moore CM, Whitwam JG. True patient-controlled sedation. *Anaesthesia* 1993;48:1039–1044.

55 Ramanathan S, Gandhi S, Arismendy J, Chalon J, Turndorf H. Oxygen transfer from mother to fetus during cesarean section under epidural anesthesia. *Anesth Analg* 1982;61: 576–581.

56 Bogod DG, Rosen M, Rees GAD. Maximum F_{IO_2} during Caesarean section. *Br J Anaesth* 1988;61:255–262.

57 Nicolaides KH, Campbell S, Bradley RJ, Bilardo CM, Soothill PW, Gibb D. Maternal oxygen therapy for intrauterine growth retardation. *Lancet* 1987;i:942–945.

58 Battaglia C, Artini PG, D'Ambrogio G, Galli PA, Segre A, Genazzani AR. Maternal hyperoxygenation in the treatment of intrauterine growth retardation. *Am J Obstet Gynecol* 1992;**167**:430–435.

59 Bekedam DJ, Mulder EJH, Snijders RJM, Visser GHA. The effects of maternal hyperoxia on fetal breathing movements, body movements and heart rate variation in growth retarded fetuses. *Early Hum Dev* 1991;**27**:223–232.

60 Kinsella SM, Whitwam JG, Spencer JAD. Aortic compression by the uterus: identification with the Finapres digital arterial pressure instrument. *Br J Obstet Gynaecol* 1990;**97**:700–705.

61 Abitbol MM, Monheit AG, Poje J, Baker MA. Nonstress test and maternal position. *Obstet Gynecol* 1986;**68**:310–316.

62 Wilson L Jr., Parsons MT, Flouret G. Forward shift in the initiation of the nocturnal estradiol surge in the pregnant baboon. Is this the genesis of labor? *Am J Obstet Gynecol* 1991;**165**:1487–1498.

63 Nathanielsz PW, Binienda Z, Wimsatt J, Fifueroa JP, Massmann A. Patterns of myometrial activity and their regulation in the pregnant monkey. In: McNellis D, Challis JRG, MacDonald PC, Nathanielsz PW, Roberts JM, eds. *The onset of labor: cellular and integrative mechanisms.* Ithaca, New York: Perinatology Press, 1988:359–372.

64 Elliott JP, O'Keeffe DF, Greenberg P, Freeman RK. Pulmonary edema associated with magnesium sulfate and betamethasone administration. *Am J Obstet Gynecol* 1979;**134**:717–718.

65 Elliott JP. Magnesium sulfate as tocolytic agent. *Am J Obstet Gynecol* 1983;**147**:277–284.

66 Watson NA, Morgan B. Pulmonary oedema and salbutamol in preterm labour. Case report and literature review. *Br J Obstet Gynaecol* 1989;**96**:1445–1448.

67 Harrison MR, Adzick NS. The fetus as a patient. Surgical considerations. *Ann Surg* 1991;**213**:279–291.

68 Cauldwell CB, Rosen MA, Harrison MR. The use of nitroglycerin for uterine relaxation during fetal surgery. *Anesthesiology* 1995;**83**:A929.

69 Wilson L Jr., Pak SC, Santolaya J, Parsons M. Induction of estradiol synthesis and nocturnal uterine contractions by dehydroepiandrosterone and their inhibition by an aromatase inhibitor. *41st Annual Meeting of the Society for Gynecologic Investigation*, Chicago, IL, March 22–25, 1994:Abst# 14.

70 Goodwin TM, Paul RH, Silver H *et al.* The effect of the oxytocin antagonist atosiban on preterm labor uterine activity in the human. *Am J Obstet Gynecol* 1994;**170**:474–478.

71 Wilson L Jr., Flouret G, Parsons M, Fejgin M, Pak SC. Oxytocin antagonists. In: D. Wienstein, S. Gabbe, eds. *First World Congress on Labor and Delivery.* Bologna, Italy: Monduzzi Editore, 1995:155–162.

72 Kowalski W, Parsons MT, Pak SC, Wilson L Jr. Morphine inhibits nocturnal oxytocin secretions and uterine contractions in the pregnant baboon. *Biol Reprod* 1998;**58**:971–976.

73 Harrison MR. Fetal surgery. *Am J Obstet Gynecol* 1996;**174**:1255–1264.

74 Giles WB, Lah FX, Trudinger BJ. The effect of epidural anaesthesia for Caesarean section on maternal uterine and fetal umbilical artery blood flow velocity waveforms. *Br J Obstet Gynaecol* 1987;**94**:55–59.

75 Nelson KB, Ellenberg JH. Antecedents of cerebral palsy. Multivariate analysis of risk. *N Engl J Med* 1986;**315**:81–86.

Chapter 6/Coelocentesis: a new invasive technique for very early prenatal diagnosis

DAVOR JURKOVIC, ERIC JAUNIAUX and STUART CAMPBELL

Introduction

In 1991, two independent teams, based respectively at King's College Hospital and St Bartholomew's Hospital Medical College, reported the first data on the biochemistry of the coelomic fluid [1,2]. Both teams showed that coelomic fluid could be successfully aspirated by transvaginal puncture between 6 and 12 weeks of gestation and that the coelomic fluid had different biochemical characteristics from those of early amniotic fluid and maternal serum. The aim of the first reports by the St Bartholomew's team was to establish normal ranges of α-fetoprotein (AFP) concentrations in early fetal fluid and to emphasize the importance of identifying the site of amniocentesis in the first trimester [3]. Since 1991 we have been investigating the physiological role of coelomic fluid in maternofetal exchange at the time of gestation when fetal blood cannot be obtained. We have also been exploring the potential role of coelomic fluid for the prenatal diagnosis of chromosomal and genetic disorders. Advantages of very early prenatal diagnosis are obvious and there is a great need for a method that can be used in the first trimester. Unfortunately, due to increased fetal risks, both early amniocentesis and chorionic villous sampling are not being used before 10 weeks' gestation. Coelocentesis is theoretically less traumatic to the fetus and early placenta and may therefore be a safer method in very early pregnancy. In this chapter, we discuss the use of coelocentesis for both physiological studies and early prenatal diagnosis.

Embryology

Transvaginal transducers provide optimal visualization of the early anatomic structures that were classically described by embryologists (Fig. 6.1). The extraem-

bryonic coelom develops during the fourth week after the last menstrual period [4,5]. It surrounds the blastocyst, which is composed of two cavities separated by the bilaminar embryonic disc, i.e. the amniotic cavity and the primary yolk sac. At the end of the fourth week of gestation, the developing exocoelomic cavity splits the extraembryonic mesoderm into two layers: the somatic mesoderm, lining the trophoblast; and the splanchnic mesoderm, covering the secondary yolk sac and the embryo. At approximately 31 days' menstrual age, the gestational sac measures 2–3 mm in diameter and can be detected by transvaginal ultrasound imaging [6]. At the end of the fifth week of gestation, the secondary yolk sac is well developed and has a wide communication with the ventral part of the flat trilaminar embryo. From 6 weeks onwards the gestational sac contains the amniotic and exocoelomic (chorionic) cavity, which can be visualized on the scan. The exocoelomic cavity is much larger than the amniotic cavity at this stage. Its mean volume doubles between 6 and 8 weeks to reach a maximum of 5–6 ml at 9 weeks and then starts to decrease gradually. The amniotic cavity is very small until 7 weeks' gestation. It starts to expand rapidly after that and from 9 weeks onwards the amniotic cavity takes up most of the gestational sac volume. Fast expansion continues until the end of the first trimester, when amniotic and chorionic membranes eventually become fused thus completely obliterating the exocoelomic cavity.

Technique of coelocentesis

Coelomic aspiration is performed under ultrasonographic guidance using a high-frequency transvaginal probe. The vagina has to be carefully cleansed with an antiseptic solution such as chlorhexidine gluconate 0.05% and cetrimide 0.5% to minimize the risk of bacterial contamination. The probe is covered with a sterile rubber

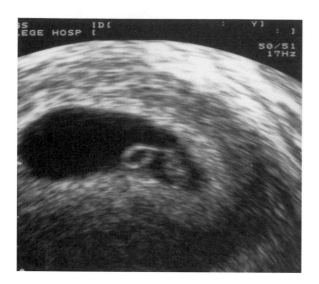

Fig. 6.1 Transvaginal ultrasonic view of the gestational sac at 10 weeks' gestation.

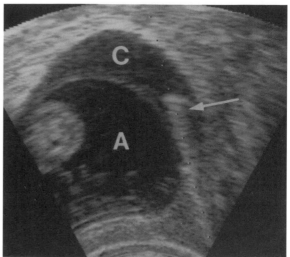

(a)

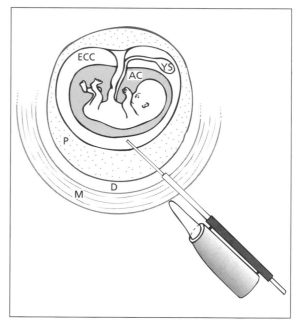

(b)

Fig. 6.2 (a) Coelocentesis at 10 weeks' gestation. (b) Schematic representation.

sheath and a transvaginal scan performed to locate the fetus, amniotic membrane, extraembryonic coelomic cavity and yolk sac. There is no need for anaesthesia. A needle guide is then attached to the shaft of the probe and a 20-gauge needle introduced into the coelomic cavity under ultrasound control, taking care to avoid puncture of the amniotic membrane or yolk sac (Fig. 6.2). The needle should be introduced into the uterus centrally through the anterior wall far from the main uterine vessels, which run alongside its lateral borders. In this way the risk of inadvertent bowel puncture is also reduced. The only pelvic organ close to the needle route is the urinary bladder and care should be taken to avoid puncturing it. Although an accidental bladder puncture is unlikely to be associated with significant complications, it is better avoided.

Success of coelocentesis depends on the position of the needle tip in relation to the amniotic membrane and the yolk sac. The needle should always be nearly parallel to the amniotic membrane, otherwise the membrane tends to attach to the needle tip and obstruct coelomic fluid aspiration. The yolk sac is attached to the umbilical cord by the vitelline duct. Both structures are relatively mobile and also tend to adhere to the needle tip during aspiration. To avoid this the needle should be placed as far as possible from either structure and the position of

the needle tip should be monitored continuously during aspiration.

The exocoelomic cavity can be visualized from 5 to 12 weeks' gestation and coelomic fluid is aspirated

Table 6.1 Success rate of coelocentesis at different gestational ages.

Gestation (weeks)	No. of patients	Success (%)
6	6	6 (100%)
7	13	12 (92%)
8	13	12 (92%)
9	18	17 (94%)
10	17	17 (100%)
11	12	5 (42%)
12	21	2 (10%)
Total	100	71 (71%)

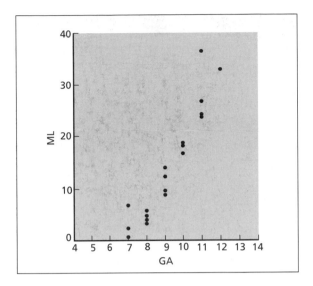

Fig. 6.4 Volume of amniotic fluid between 7 and 12 weeks of gestation measured after transvaginal aspiration of the entire exocoelomic cavity.

with a high success rate, close to 100% in pregnancies between 6 and 10 weeks (Table 6.1). The amniotic cavity can be clearly identified from the beginning of the seventh week of gestation and amniotic fluid can be obtained in all cases from 8 weeks. The volume of fluid obtained from the exocoelomic cavity varies from 2 to 8 ml at 6 and 10 weeks, respectively, whereas amniotic fluid volume samples increase exponentially from 3 to 30 ml between 7 and 12 weeks (Figs. 6.3 & 6.4). However, for diagnostic purposes only 0.5–2.5 ml

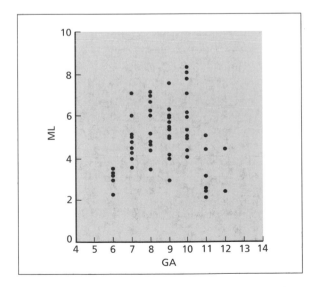

Fig. 6.3 Volume of coelomic fluid between 6 and 12 weeks of gestation measured after transvaginal aspiration of the entire exocoelomic cavity.

of coelomic fluid is usually aspirated. The pressure during aspiration should be low. High pressure or aspiration of large fluid volumes is more likely to drag the yolk sac or amniotic membrane towards the needle, which will result in a failed procedure. In all cases, exocoelomic fluid is yellow coloured and more viscous than amniotic fluid, which is always clear. This may help recognition of inadvertent puncture of the amniotic cavity during coelocentesis, although we have not experienced this complication as yet.

Physiological role of coelomic fluid

Biological substances present in the maternal circulation in early pregnancy must cross the villous barrier to reach the embryonic compartments. When the definitive placenta forms at the end of the first trimester, materno-fetal transfers may also occur at the level of the free amniotic membranes. Maternal or placental proteins filtered in the extraembryonic coelomic cavity are probably absorbed by the secondary yolk sac, which is in direct continuity with the primitive digestive system throughout embryonic development.

A highly significant difference in total protein levels is found between the exocoelomic and the amniotic

Table 6.2 Comparison of coelomic versus amniotic fluid protein composition.

Protein	Coelomic fluid	Amniotic fluid
Total protein (g/l)	3.5 ± 0.7	0.2 ± 0.2
α-Fetoprotein (kIU/l)	21 816 ± 12 667	27 096 ± 11 822
Albumin (g/l)	1.7 ± 0.5	ND
Prealbumin (g/l)	0.04 ± 0.02	ND
IgG (mg/dl)	32 ± 21	ND
Human chorionic gonadotrophin (mIU/ml)	165 607 ± 78 543	1752 ± 1451

ND, not determined.

fluids, suggesting that the thin membrane separating these two compartments, which later becomes the amniotic epithelium, is not permeable to molecules with a high molecular weight (Table 6.2). The total protein concentration in matched samples decreases gradually from maternal serum to coelomic and then amniotic fluid [1,4,5]. Between 6 and 12 weeks of gestation, the mean level of total protein in coelomic fluid is 18 times lower than in maternal serum and 54 times higher than in the amniotic cavity [6]. Total protein concentrations in the coelomic fluid are not influenced by changes in maternal serum protein levels during the first trimester. The total protein concentration in the exocoelomic cavity increases with advancing gestation while it decreases in the maternal serum. Furthermore, no correlations are found between AFP, albumin and prealbumin levels in coelomic fluid and those in maternal serum, indicating that the placental transfer rate of these specific proteins is probably independent of their respective concentrations on each side of the placental barrier. During the first trimester, albumin concentration in maternal serum demonstrates a relative decrease due to increased maternal blood volume and haemodilution, while globulin and fibrinogen concentrations demonstrate both absolute and relative increases. During the same period, the levels of total protein and prealbumin increase in coelomic fluid while the levels of albumin do not vary significantly [6].

AFP is produced by the secondary yolk sac up to 10 weeks of gestation and by the embryonic liver from 6 weeks until delivery. Although its molecular mass is high (70 kDa), it is found in similar concentrations on both sides of the amniotic membrane (Table 6.2). Analysis of concanavalin A affinity molecular variants of AFP have demonstrated that both exocoelomic fluid and amniotic fluid AFP molecules are mainly of yolk sac origin while maternal serum AFP molecules are mainly of fetal liver origin [3]. These results suggest that human secondary yolk sac has also an excretory function and secretes AFP towards embryonic and extraembryonic compartments. In humans, molecules of AFP are also synthesized by the vitelline duct (which has the same cellular constitution as the yolk sac) and are excreted in the amniotic fluid at the level where the duct fuses with the primitive umbilical cord. Yolk sac AFP could also be shifted into the amniotic fluid via the vitelline duct and the embryonic gut when the anal membranes break down around 10 weeks after menstruation. By contrast, most AFP molecules of fetal liver origin are probably transferred from the embryonic circulation to the maternal circulation, mainly across the placental villous membrane.

In normal pregnancies, the concentration of human chorionic gonadotrophin (hCG) and its subunits is considerably higher in coelomic fluid than in amniotic fluid or maternal serum. It has been recently shown that the α-subunit is a major constituent of embryonic fluids. Except for one α-hCG-like immunoreactive band, immunoelectrotransfer analysis reveals a similar hCG pattern in coelomic fluid and maternal serum [7]. In contrast to maternal serum, coelomic levels of intact hCG and free α-hCG decrease progressively between 8 and 12 weeks of gestation; free β-hCG levels do not change significantly. These findings support the hypothesis that, in the first trimester, there is an excess of α over β subunit secretion by the villous trophoblast [7] and suggest that the hCG clearance rate is slower in the coelomic cavity than in maternal circulation. It is likely that maternal serum hCG levels are influenced by both villous and extravillous trophoblastic synthesis. The coelomic cavity, being completely surrounded by villous tissue, is only influenced by villous trophoblastic secretion. The decrease of coelomic levels of intact hCG and free α-hCG levels with advancing gestation may be secondary to a simultaneous decline in the number of differentiating cytotrophoblastic cells and/or to the disappearance of two-thirds of the original placental tissue occurring during the same period.

Coelocentesis for prenatal diagnosis

Coelocentesis has a success rate of more than 95% between 7 and 10 weeks of gestation and, in theory, it is a possible alternative to early amniocentesis and chorionic villous sampling because the risk of directly injuring the growing embryo or damaging its placenta is very small. Furthermore, the procedure is easy to learn, induces only minimal discomfort to the mother and is associated with a very low rate of contamination of the sample by maternal cells [8]. Although there are still no data about the relative risks of coelocentesis in ongoing pregnancies, the rate of fetal loss should be similar or lower than that associated with early amniocentesis. A study is in progress in our unit to investigate the short-term risks of coelocentesis.

Coelomic fluid contains cells that are mostly of haematopoietic origin, nucleated and predominantly erythroid lineage. The number of aspirated cells is very high in early pregnancy but then decreases with advancing gestation. More than 90% of cells are viable before 7 weeks' gestation, but between 8 and 10 weeks viability decreases to 30–50%. Morphological analysis has shown that after 8 weeks' gestation a high proportion of cells contains pycnotic nuclei typical of late normoblasts. Flow cytometry has also shown an increasing proportion of subdiploid cells later in gestation, which is consistent with apoptosis. The viability of the cells is the primary determinant of cell culture success. Our recent results show that the number of dividing cells in culture before 7 weeks' gestation may be sufficient for diagnostic purposes. However, most cultures fail later in pregnancy and very few analysable metaphase spreads can be obtained after 7 weeks.

In one of our early studies we attempted to determine fetal sex by analysing coelomic fluid and placental tissue. Polymerase chain reaction (PCR) with Y centromeric primers was carried out in 10 cases. In the other 10 cases, fluorescence *in situ* hybridization (FISH) was performed using the α-satellite repeat probes for X and Y chromosomes. In all cases FISH and PCR were successfully performed in samples from the placenta and coelomic fluid and in each case there was concordance in fetal sex prediction [8].

Another study investigated the feasibility of coelocentesis for the diagnosis of single-gene disorders in the fetus, using as a model inheritance of the mutation at codon 6 of the human β-globin gene. DNA was successfully amplified from all coelomic fluid samples. In 53 cases a normal fetal β-globin genotype was detected. In three out of five cases, where the maternal haemoglobin phenotype was HbAS, heterozygosity for the sickle mutation was demonstrated on analysis of coelomic fluid. In the remaining two cases a normal β-globin genotype was observed. Three further coelomic fluid samples were found to be heterozygous for the sickle mutation. In these instances the maternal haemoglobin phenotype was normal (HbAA), indicating paternal transmission of the sickle gene. The results of coelomic fluid analysis were compared with the fetal β-globin genotype determined by placental DNA analysis. In all cases there was complete concordance between coelomic fluid and placental DNA analysis [9].

The results of that study have established that the diagnosis of sickle cell anaemia and, potentially, other human single-gene disorders is feasible by analysis of coelomic fluid in early pregnancy. In recessive disorders such as sickle cell anaemia, the risk of diagnostic error due to maternal contamination is greatest where the putative fetal genotype is identical to that of the mother's, i.e. heterozygous. In our study this problem did not arise, but a larger study will be required to confirm this.

Coelocentesis constitutes a new invasive approach to prenatal diagnosis that can be performed with a high success rate from as early as 6 weeks' gestation. Our experience includes more than 600 procedures performed prior to elective termination of pregnancy. No significant intraoperative complications have been encountered in the mother or fetus. Specifically, there has been no evidence of bleeding inside the gestational sac or alterations in the embryonic heart rate.

At present we believe that coelocentesis may be successfully used for the diagnosis of genetic disorders in very early pregnancy. The feasibility of karyotyping by coelocentesis remains uncertain. By using FISH probes limited karyotypes may be obtained, but 30–40% of potentially significant chromosomal defects will be missed without a full karyotype. The most important issue is the safety of the procedure, which is currently being investigated. When its safety is proven the method may be used for prenatal detection of genetic disorders. At present it appears that karyotyping before 6 weeks may be possible. However, further work is necessary to improve culture success later in gestation.

References

1 Jauniaux E, Jurkovic D, Gulbis B, Gervy C, Ooms HA, Campbell S. Biochemical composition of exocoelomic fluid in early human pregnancy. *Obstet Gynecol* 1991;78:1124–1128.

2 Wathen NC, Cass PL, Kitau MJ, Chard T. Human chorionic gonadotrophin and alpha-fetoprotein levels in matched samples of amniotic fluid, extraembryonic exocoelomic fluid, and maternal serum in the first trimester of pregnancy. *Prenat Diagn* 1991;11:145–151.

3 Wathen NC, Cass PL, Campbell DJ, Kitau MJ, Chard T. Early amniocentesis: alpha-fetoprotein in amniotic fluid, extraembryonic colomic fluid and maternal serum between 8 and 13 weeks. *Br J Obstet Gynaecol* 1991;98:866–870.

4 Gulbis B, Jauniaux E, Jurkovic D, Thiry P, Campbell S, Ooms HA. Determination of protein pattern in embryonic cavities of early human pregnancies: a model to understand materno-embryonic exchanges. *Hum Reprod* 1992;7:886–889.

5 Jauniaux E, Gulbis B, Jurkovic D, Schaaps JP, Campbell S, Meuris S. Protein and steroid levels in embryonic cavities of early human pregnancy. *Hum Reprod* 1993;8:782–787.

6 Jauniaux E, Gulbis B, Jurkovic D, Campbell S, Collins WP, Ooms HA. Relationship between protein concentrations in embryological fluids and maternal serum and yolk sac size during human early pregnancy. *Hum Reprod* 1994;9:161–166.

7 Nagy A-M, Jauniaux E, Jurkovic D, Meuris S. Placental overproduction of human chorionic gonadotropin α subunit in early pregnancy as evidenced in exocoelomic fluid. *J Endocrinol* 1994;142:511–516.

8 Jurkovic D, Jauniaux E, Campbell S, Pandya P, Cardy DL, Nicolaides KH. Coelocentesis: a new technique for early prenatal diagnosis. *Lancet* 1993;341:1623–1624.

9 Jurkovic D, Jauniaux E, Campbell S, Mitchell M, Lees C, Layton M. Detection of sickle gene by coelocentesis in early pregnancy: a new approach to prenatal diagnosis of single gene disorders: *Hum Reprod* 1995;10:1287–1289.

Chapter 7/Chorionic villous sampling

RONALD J.WAPNER

Introduction

Amniocentesis has been available for over two decades as a second-trimester prenatal diagnostic technique. The safety, efficacy and accuracy of the procedure has been well documented, allowing it to become the major prenatal diagnostic tool. However, despite this excellent record, amniocentesis has been limited by the gestational age at which it is performed, leading to continued efforts to develop an equally safe alternative that could be utilized in the first trimester.

Initial attempts at first-trimester prenatal diagnosis involved the development of techniques to retrieve samples of chorionic villi by optically directed biopsy of the chorion frondosum. One approach used a modified cystoscopy that was inserted transcervically and then directed to the chorion frondosum [1–5]. While these attempts were somewhat successful, they were technically difficult, frequently complicated by inadvertent biopsy of the amnion and had an unacceptable risk of miscarriage. Alternatively, other investigators attempted to analyse the trophoblast cells spontaneously shed into the endocervical canal [6–8]. Unfortunately, there were not sufficient cells retrieved to be accurately analysed by the cytogenetic techniques available at that time. To improve the retrieval of appropriate cell types, Chinese investigators inserted a small catheter into the lower uterus [9]. Despite the blind nature of the procedure, they were able to retrieve adequate trophoblast to allow fetal sex determination and there was an exceptionally low risk of pregnancy loss.

Kazy was the first to suggest using ultrasound guidance to assist in biopsying the chorion frondosum [10]. Almost simultaneously, this approach was investigated and then modified by Humphrey Ward [11] in London and refined by Bruno Brambatti [12,13] in Milan. Brambatti demonstrated the advantage of using an ultrasound-guided catheter as opposed to either an unguided catheter or direct visualization. Following this, utilization of the technique spread rapidly throughout the world so that presently over 200 000 ultrasonically guided chorionic villous sampling (CVS) procedures have been performed.

This chapter discusses the standard techniques of CVS as well as its safety and efficacy. The present controversy concerning CVS and congenital abnormalities, specifically limb defects, is also discussed.

CVS: procedure-related anatomy and histology

Since anatomical relationships rapidly change with advancing gestational age, the performance of first-trimester prenatal diagnosis by CVS requires practical knowledge of developmental embryology. Figure 7.1 illustrates the anatomical arrangements at 9–12 weeks from the last menstrual period. At this time, the gestational sac does not completely fill the uterus and is composed of an outer chorionic membrane surrounding a smaller amniotic cavity. The extraembryonic coelom, which contains a tenacious mucoid-like substance, is readily evident and separates the thin, wispy, freely mobile amnion from the thick leathery chorion laeve. The villi over most of the chorionic membrane have degenerated, forming the chorion laeve, while those remaining begin to embed into the decidua basalis, forming the chorion frondosum, which will ultimately become the placenta. The individual chorionic villi float freely within the blood of the intervillous space and are only loosely anchored to the underlying decidua basalis.

As the pregnancy progresses beyond 12 weeks, the gestational sac expands to fill the entire intrauterine cavity and the extraembryonic coelom disappears as the amnion and chorion come into direct contact. The

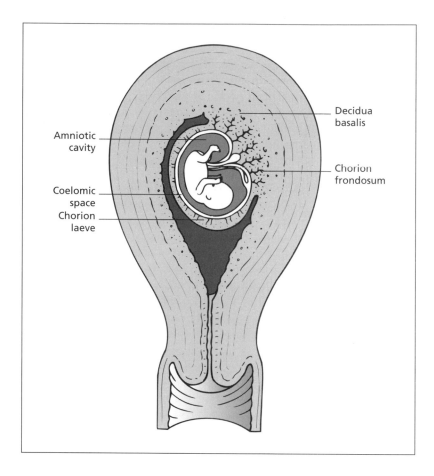

Amniotic
cavity

Coelomic
space
Chorion
laeve

Decidua
basalis

Chorion
frondosum

Fig. 7.1 Diagrammatic
representation of the first trimester
anatomy associated with chorionic
villous sampling. At this gestational
age the amnion and chorion have
not yet fused and are separated by
the extraembryonic coelom.
Beneath the developing chorion
frondosum is the vascular decidua
basilas.

chorion frondosum becomes anchored more deeply into the uterine wall and the individual villi interdigitate as the placenta takes on the appearance of a single organ.

The chorion frondosum contains the mitotically active villi and, therefore, is the preferred biopsy site. The individual villi have a distinctive branched appearance with an outer single cell layer, the syncytiotrophoblast, bordering the proliferative cytotrophoblast. The surface of the actively proliferating villi is punctuated by small buds consisting of an outer syncytial covering and a core of mitotically active cytotrophoblastic cells (Fig. 7.2b). Within the centre of the villous is the mesenchymal core, through which capillaries carrying fetal blood cells course (Fig. 7.2a). It is the cytotrophoblastic buds that provide the tissue for the direct preparation of karyotypes, while the embryologically distinct mesenchymal core serves as the source for tissue culture.

CVS procedure

Procedure preparation

All patients anticipating a CVS should have a cervical culture that specifically evaluates for the presence of *Neisseria gonorrhoeae* since this organism may cause chorioamnionitis after the procedure. Culture for other organisms, such as group B *Streptococcus*, *Ureaplasma* or *Chlamydia*, has not been shown to be of benefit [14] and is not routinely suggested.

Genetic counselling is mandatory prior to a CVS. The patient should be informed of the potential risks and complications of the procedure as well as the limitations of genetic diagnosis. In order to minimize patient anxiety, the practical aspects of the procedure should be explained in detail and the common complications

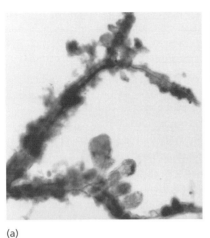
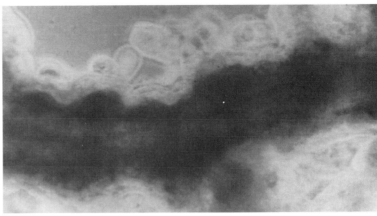

(a)   (b)

Fig. 7.2 (a) Low magnification image of a chorionic villus sampling demonstrating typical branched appearance. Buds are noted and fetal vessels containing fetal blood cells are seen coursing through the mesenchymal core. (b) Higher magnification view demonstrating the multiple buds and their syncytiotrophoblast shell with an inner cytotrophoblast.

that occur after the procedure, such as cramping and bleeding, should be outlined.

Prior to CVS, fetal viability and gestational age should be confirmed by ultrasound. We usually perform this initial evaluation 1–3 weeks prior to the anticipated sampling date. The presence of twins as well as other pregnancy-related pathology, such as a subchorionic haematoma or a co-existing blighted ovum, could potentially affect the procedure and its interpretation and must be identified. Most importantly, since CVS should not be performed prior to the 70th day after the last menstrual period, the initial screening ultrasound is used to accurately schedule the procedure.

The procedure is best performed between 70 and 91 days after the last menstrual period. On the day of the procedure a repeat ultrasound is performed immediately prior to sampling to confirm continued viability and appropriate growth of the embryo. At this gestational age the nuchal fold can frequently be seen and should be measured. A nuchal fold thickness greater than 3 mm has a 10-fold increased risk of being associated with a fetal chromosomal abnormality, most specifically trisomy 21 [15] and its presence should alert

the laboratory to perform rapid karyotyping by direct preparation.

On the ultrasound, the chorion frondosum appears as a hyperechoic homogeneous area and its location must be accurately determined prior to sampling. This is usually quickly accomplished by experienced operators. When uncertainty as to the exact location occurs, the umbilical cord insertion should be identified for confirmation. Colour flow Doppler may be helpful in rapidly accomplishing this.

Uterine contractions may be present prior to sampling and frequently alter the shape of the uterus and, most importantly, the appearance and location of the placenta. It has been our experience that these contractions pull the placental site into unusual locations, which can make sampling difficult. When contractions significantly alter a proposed sampling path, delaying the procedure for 15–30 min until they abate is suggested (Fig. 7.3). The presence of large placental lakes should also be noted, since sampling through these has been associated with increased bleeding after the procedure.

The bladder should be sufficiently filled to allow adequate visualization of the entire sampling path but overfilling should be avoided since it makes sampling more difficult. An overfilled bladder will push the uterus upwards into the abdomen, lengthen and stretch the cervix, and limit uterine mobility making transcervical sampling more difficult. If the bladder appears over-distended the patient should be asked to partially empty; we use small cups and specifically instruct the patient on how much urine to release.

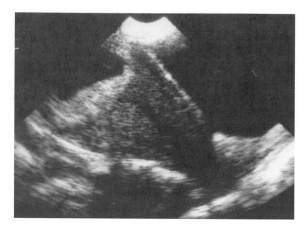

Fig. 7.3 Ultrasound demonstrating uterine contractions of the entire lower uterine segment that may alter the catheter path. Waiting 15–30 minutes will allow these to abate and will make sampling easier.

Sampling devices

TRANSCERVICAL CATHETERS

Transcervical sampling is performed with a polyethylene catheter through which a metal malleable stylet is inserted (Fig. 7.4). The most frequently used catheter (Portex) has a polyethylene outer sheath with an internal diameter of 0.89 mm. A stainless-steel stylet fits snugly through the catheter to add sufficient rigidity for adequate passage through the cervix and into the frondosum. The stylet has a rounded blunt end that protrudes slightly beyond the catheter and which prevents sharp edges from potentially perforating the membranes. The polyethylene catheter itself (Fig. 7.4) has a Luer-Lok end so that a syringe can be applied at the time of sampling. Other similar catheters are also available (Cook) and vary slightly in diameter and design.

A 20-ml syringe is used to apply suction once the catheter is in place; 5 ml of RPMI with heparin should be aspirated into the syringe so that the villi can be retrieved directly into this transport medium. The heparin prevents clotting of the small amount of blood that will be unavoidably retrieved.

TRANSABDOMINAL NEEDLES

Two techniques for transabdominal sampling are presently used. In the single-needle approach, a 20-gauge spinal needle is employed [16]. In general, a 9-cm needle is sufficient for most samples but a 13-cm or 15-cm needle should be available for very obese patients. Alternatively, the double-needle technique uses an outer guide needle, either an 18-gauge thin-wall needle or a 16–17-gauge standard spinal needle [17]. A smaller sampling needle, usually 20 gauge, is then used for the direct sampling. Once the needle is in place, a syringe

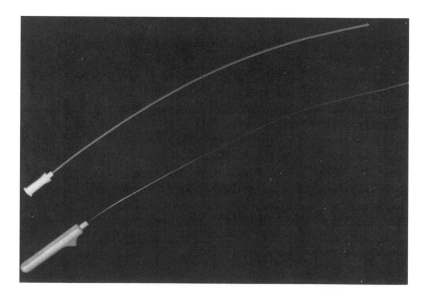

Fig. 7.4 Picture of a CVS sampling catheter. There is an outer polyethylene sheath and an inner metal stylet. Note the blunted tip to prevent penetration of the membranes.

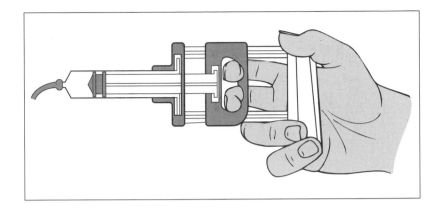

Fig. 7.5 Diagrammatic representation of hand grip used by some operators to facilitate transabdominal sampling.

with transport medium is attached to the biopsy needle to achieve adequate suction. Some operators attach a hand grip to the syringe to assist in applying appropriate pressure (Fig. 7.5).

Sampling techniques

Both transcervical and transabdominal CVS (Fig. 7.6) are best performed utilizing a two-person technique, with one individual performing the sampling and the other doing the ultrasound guidance. Communication between sonographer and sampler is imperative and the best results have come from centres in which the number of team members is limited.

TRANSCERVICAL SAMPLING (Fig. 7.6b)

The patient is placed in the lithotomy position and the vaginal area prepared with a povidone iodine solution. A sterile speculum is inserted and the cervix directly wiped with antiseptic. While the routine placement of a tenaculum on the anterior lip of the cervix was historically suggested, most patients find this exceedingly uncomfortable and it is usually unnecessary. A gentle bend is made in the distal 3–5 cm of the catheter to accommodate insertion through the cervical canal and into the frondosum. The catheter is then gently inserted through the cervix until the internal os is reached. There is usually a slight loss of resistance at this point. When the operator feels that the catheter has progressed through the os, he or she should delay further advancement until the sonographer is able to image the tip.

Once the catheter is through the os, the tip must be pointed in the correct direction. An anterior position can be approached by pulling the speculum downward, which will move the catheter tip upward and into the proper location. A posterior approach is facilitated by rotating the tip 180° downward and then lifting the speculum. Once the tip is in place, the catheter is then gently advanced into the chorion frondosum.

Under direct visualization, the catheter should continue to be passed parallel to the chorionic plate through the full length of the frondosum. Once in place, the stylet is removed, the medium-filled syringe attached and approximately 10–20 ml of pressure applied. The catheter is removed in one gentle motion while suction is continuously applied. When the catheter is in the appropriate tissue plane there is no resistance to further advancement. The catheter should only be advanced using minimal pressure, since if resistance is felt this indicates that the tip is either against the membrane or, more likely, within the decidua.

The chorionic villi can be easily identified in the syringe by holding it up to a light. The villi are seen as free-floating, white tissue with fluffy, filiform branches. In contrast, decidual tissue has a more amorphous shape and lacks branches. Experienced operators can easily confirm the presence of villous tissue by visual inspection. However, if visual identification is uncertain the presence of sufficient villi should be confirmed under a dissecting microscope prior to discharging the patient. Figure 7.7 demonstrates chorionic villi under direct inspection and under a dissecting microscope.

If sufficient villi are not obtained on the first pass, a second attempt should be made. Pregnancy loss rates

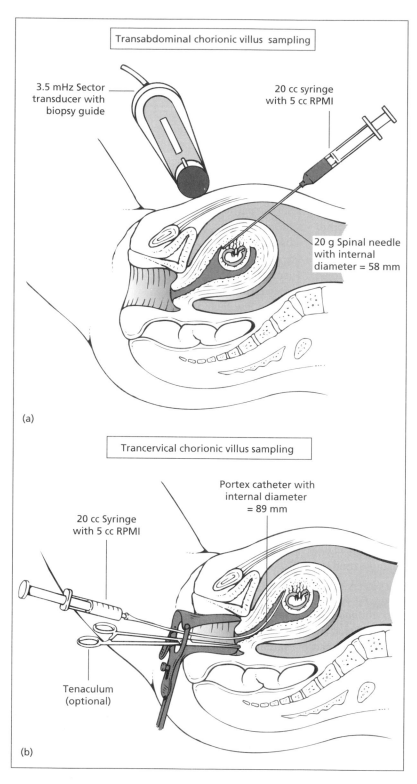

Fig. 7.6 Diagrammatic representations of (a) transabdominal and (b) transcervical chorionic villous sampling.

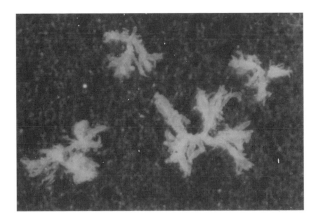

Fig. 7.7 Gross picture of chorionic villi. The branched appearance helps visually separate the villi from the more amorphous appearance of decidua.

increase significantly when more than two insertions are required, and may be as high as 10% if three attempts are made [18,19]. Therefore, a third transcervical pass should only be attempted when retrieval seems certain. Preferably, the cervical route should be abandoned and abdominal sampling considered.

TRANSABDOMINAL SAMPLING (Fig. 7.6a)

Single-needle technique

The abdomen is prepared with a povidone iodine solution as for amniocentesis. The anticipated sampling path should be chosen such that the needle will pass parallel to the chorion frondosum and will avoid any intervening bowel. A biopsy guide with a computer-generated needle path is quite helpful but its use is not mandatory. The sampling needle is then inserted through the abdominal wall and into the myometrium. Since the majority of discomfort occurs from the insertion of the needle into the myometrium rather than the skin, the use of local anaesthesia is not routinely required although some centres find it useful.

Once the needle is within the myometrium the angle is readjusted so that the tip will travel parallel to the chorionic plate and pass through the majority of the frondosum. Once within the placenta the stylet is removed and a medium-filled syringe or hand grip attached. To ensure that sufficient villi are collected, the needle should

be manoeuvred to and fro making three to four passes within the frondosum, while continuous suction is applied. The needle is then removed from the abdomen while suction is continued. This 'vacuuming' technique allows retrieval of sufficient villous tissue despite the slightly smaller diameter of the sampling needle compared with the catheter.

As with transcervical sampling, insertion of the needle tip in the appropriate tissue plane results in no resistance. A needle inserted into the decidua or myometrium will give a 'gripping' feeling and adjustment of the tip into the frondosum should be made.

Visual determination of the chorionic villi is made as with transcervical sampling. However, both the pieces of villi and the overall sample size will frequently be smaller than those retrieved with transcervical CVS [20,21].

Double-needle technique

The abdomen is prepared with povidone iodine and draped. The needle path is chosen as with the single-needle technique. The larger outer guide needle is inserted through the myometrium just to the edge of the chorion frondosum. After the stylet is removed, the thinner sampling needle is inserted through the guide needle and into the chorion frondosum. The inner needle is moved to and fro under continuous suction as with the single-needle technique and then removed. If insufficient villi are retrieved the sampling needle can be reinserted through the guide needle without the necessity for repuncture.

CHOOSING THE APPROPRIATE TECHNIQUE

Transabdominal and transcervical CVS have been shown to be equally safe [20]. While approximately 97% of patients can be sampled by either approach [20,21], CVS operators should be skilled in both techniques to allow all patients to be sampled by the technique most appropriate for them. In general, the best approach is the one in which the catheter or needle can be inserted parallel to the chorion frondosum with the smallest amount of uterine or placental manipulation. While experience is required to identify the ideal approach for an individual patient, certain general guidelines are helpful.

An anteverted or midposition uterus with a posterior placenta is most easily sampled by the transcervical route. Alternatively, an anteverted uterus with an anterior or fundal placenta may be more easily sampled by the transabdominal approach. An anterior placenta in a midposition uterus can usually be sampled by either approach.

A retroverted uterus with an anterior placenta can frequently be sampled by transcervical CVS. However, if the placenta is posterior, sampling by either route may be difficult. In these cases, some operators have suggested using either a transvesical needle approach through the abdominal wall or sampling through the vaginal fornix. We have found both of these to be markedly painful and we therefore prefer to manually antevert the uterus to allow easier sampling.

If a simple straightforward sampling approach is not initially present, waiting 15–20 min for a uterine contraction to develop may alter the anatomy and facilitate the CVS procedure. Filling or emptying the bladder can also be used to change the uterine position.

Certain anatomical or pathological conditions may dictate against one approach. For example, if the patient has large, necrotic, cervical polyps, transcervical CVS should be avoided if possible. Alternatively, bowel or bladder may intervene between the abdominal wall and the uterus and would contraindicate transabdominal sampling. In most cases, however, either approach can be performed and patient or physician preference will dictate. In general, although the discomfort with transabdominal CVS in usually well tolerated, patients find transcervical CVS almost painless.

CVS sampling in twin gestations

CVS can be successfully and safely performed in twin gestations [22–24]. However, a number of pitfalls not present with a singleton exist. For example, when performing an amniocentesis on twins, dye is usually instilled to allow confirmation that both fetal compartments have been entered separately. No such marker is available for CVS. Therefore, the operator must use meticulous ultrasound guidance to be certain that villi from each individual placental site is retrieved. To accomplish this we sample near the cord insertion sites which, in our experience, has consistently led to correct information about the fetal karyotypes. If

uncertainty exists that both fetuses have been sampled, an amniocentesis should be offered at 16–17 weeks. With experience this should occur very rarely.

Contamination of one sample with villi from the coexisting fetus can result in significant confusion and potential error. This is best avoided by choosing sampling routes that do not pass through both placental sites. A combination of abdominal and cervical sampling makes this possible. For biochemical testing, analysis of individual villi rather than combining them into one sample will also diminish the possibility of an error.

Discordant results and subsequent requests for selective pregnancy termination are inevitable when high-order gestations are sampled. Because of this, an accurate and detailed diagram of fetal and placental position should be drawn at the time of sampling so that an aneuploid fetus can be identified 1–2 weeks later. Even when this is done accurately, there will be cases in which subsequent identification of the affected fetus may be inconclusive. When this occurs, a repeat CVS should be performed immediately preceding the termination and a rapid direct chromosome preparation utilized to confirm the karyotype.

Recent prospective comparisons between CVS and amniocentesis in twin gestations have confirmed that CVS is equally safe and reliable [22]. Miscarriage of the entire pregnancy following a twin CVS occurs in approximately 2–3% of cases [22,23], which is similar to that for amniocentesis.

Since twins present unique difficulties in prenatal diagnosis, it is suggested that only very experienced operators sample these gestations. Multiple pregnancies of higher order, such as triplets and quadruplets, have also been successfully sampled but in these cases the patient must be completely informed of the potential risks of such a procedure.

Safety and complications of CVS

CVS has been used as a clinical tool for over 12 years with more than 200 000 procedures having been performed [25]. While early evaluation of CVS was limited to the experiences of single centres, there have now been three large prospective comparisons with second-trimester amniocentesis [19,26,27] that have demonstrated a low pregnancy loss rate and minimal complications. Recently, there has been sporadic controversy about whether under certain circumstances, such as sampling prior to 9 weeks' gestation, there may be an increased risk of fetal malformation [28,29].

Pregnancy loss

The desired advantage of an earlier diagnosis must be weighed against any increased risk of fetal loss that CVS may induce. However, determining the rate of procedure-induced pregnancy loss is complicated by relatively high background miscarriage rates. In addition, the background loss rates increase with maternal age and are highest precisely in the age range most likely to present for prenatal diagnosis [30–32].

The largest demonstration of data evaluating the relative safety of CVS comes from three recent collaborative reports. In early 1989, the Canadian Collaborative CVS/Amniocentesis Clinical Trial Group documented its experiences with a prospective randomized trial comparing CVS with second-trimester amniocentesis [26]. The results confirmed the safety of CVS as a first-trimester diagnostic procedure. There were 7.6% fetal losses (spontaneous abortions, induced abortions and late losses) in the CVS group and 7.0% in the amniocentesis group. Thus, in desired pregnancies an excess loss rate of 0.6% for CVS over amniocentesis was obtained, a difference that was not statistically significant.

Two months after the publication of the Canadian experience, the American collaborative report appeared. This was a prospective, though non-randomized, trial of over 2200 women who chose either transcervical CVS or second-trimester amniocentesis [19]. Patients in both groups were recruited in the first trimester of pregnancy. When the loss rates were adjusted for slight group differences in maternal and gestational ages, an excess pregnancy loss rate of 0.8% for CVS over amniocentesis was calculated, which again was not significant.

While both North American trials revealed no statistical difference in pregnancy loss when CVS was compared with amniocentesis, a prospective randomized collaborative comparison of over 3200 pregnancies sponsored by the European MRC Working Party on the Evaluation of CVS demonstrated a 4.6% greater pregnancy loss rate following CVS compared with amniocentesis (95% confidence interval (CI) 1.6–7.5%) [27]. This difference reflected more spontaneous deaths

before 28 weeks' gestation (2.9%), more terminations of pregnancy for chromosomal anomalies (1.0%) and more neonatal deaths (0.3%).

The factors contributing to the discrepant results between the European and North American studies remain uncertain. It is probable that operator experience accounts for a large part of this difference. While the US trial consisted of seven centres and the Canadian trial 11 centres, the European trial included 31 sampling sites. There were, on average, 325 cases per centre in the US study, 106 in the Canadian study and only 52 in the European trial. While no significant change in pregnancy loss rate was demonstrated during the course of the European trial, it appears that the learning curve for both transcervical and transabdominal CVS may exceed 400 or more cases [33,34]. Operators having performed less than 100 procedures may have two to three times the loss rate of operators who have performed more than 1000 procedures [34].

Multiple reports from individual centres have confirmed, and even improved upon, the results of these collaborative trials [35–39]. After adjustments for background loss, many of these studies have suggested that in experienced centres only minimal increases in pregnancy losses are attributable to CVS.

Randomized trials have recently compared the transcervical and transabdominal approaches [18,34,40–43]. With over 1000 patients randomized to each technique, our centre has demonstrated comparable loss rates with each approach [34,40]. In addition, equivalent numbers of patients required only one attempt to retrieve tissue (87%) or had unsuccessful procedures (<1%). Most recently, the US collaborative CVS project completed a randomized prospective study comparing transcervical and transabdominal CVS and also found no difference in the pregnancy loss rates between the two approaches (transcervical = 2.5%, transabdominal = 2.3%) [20]. Equally importantly, the overall spontaneous loss rate following CVS in this study (2.5%) was 0.8% lower than that in the initial US study comparing CVS with second-trimester amniocentesis. Since 0.8% was the quantitative difference in loss rates between amniocentesis and CVS in the original study, this suggests that when centres become equivalently experienced, amniocentesis and CVS may have the same risk of pregnancy loss. Smidt-Jensen [42] has confirmed this. In a prospective randomized study he found no difference in pregnancy loss between transabdominal CVS, the procedure with which his centre was most experienced, and second-trimester amniocentesis. It appears safe to speculate that fetal loss rates will be similar in most centres once equivalent expertise is gained with either approach. Integration of both methods into any single centre's programme will offer the most complete, practical and safe approach to first-trimester diagnosis [44].

Bleeding

All series have demonstrated an increased risk of vaginal bleeding following CVS. This may occur following 7–10% of transcervical CVS procedures but is rare following transabdominal procedures [19,22]. In the majority of cases, the bleeding is self-limited; while a small subchorionic haematoma may frequently be seen on ultrasound [45] (Fig. 7.8), these usually resorb prior to 16 weeks.

Failure to retrieve adequate tissue

Most centres are able to retrieve adequate tissue in over 99% of cases, with over 85% of procedures requiring only one pass [19,20]. Experienced operators require a third pass in less than 1% of cases. Utilizing a

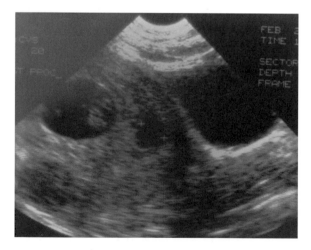

Fig. 7.8 Ultrasound appearance of a subchorionic hematoma identified following CVS sampling. These are almost always self-limited and will resolve in 3–5 weeks. This occurs more frequently following transcervical CVS.

combination of both transcervical and transabdominal procedures, we have performed over 13 000 consecutive procedures without a retrieval failure [34].

Contamination of a sample with maternal decidual tissue occurs in approximately 3% of cases [46,47] but is usually detectable and rarely leads to diagnostic errors. Small sample size is the most common contributing factor to clinically significant maternal cell contamination; as samplers become adept at retrieving adequate tissue, contamination becomes even less frequent [46]. In order to minimize the risk of maternal cell contamination and to allow the laboratory adequate, whole, typical material to analyse, a second pass of the catheter is preferred to risking inaccurate results.

Rupture of membranes

Spontaneous rupture of membranes occurring within 2 weeks of the CVS procedure is rare with either transcervical or transabdominal sampling [20,27]. The membranes in the first trimester are thick and buoyant and perforation by the blunt transcervical catheter is unlikely. While the sharper transabdominal needle may be more likely to pierce the chorionic membrane, this also is unlikely when direct ultrasound visualization is used.

Intentional penetration of the sac to transabdominally sample a posterior placenta should be avoided, since fluid leakage and subsequent oligohydramnios may follow [48]. In our experience of over 13 000 procedures this has never been required. Posterior placentas can usually be sampled transcervically or, in cases where this approach is unavailable or contraindicated, a sufficient portion of the frondosum is usually accessible, either in the fundus or lateral to the sac.

Oligohydramnios

The observation of severe second-trimester oligohydramnios has been seen following transcervical CVS. This usually is preceded by vaginal bleeding and is associated with a significantly elevated maternal serum α-fetoprotein (MSAFP) [49]. Once the oligohydramnios has been demonstrated, the prognosis is usually grim; however, in a few cases fluid has been seen to reaccumulate. Oligohydramnios, following CVS, occurs in approximately 4.5 of every 1000 transcervical procedures in experienced centres. However, inexperienced centres have seen this complication in as many as 2.7% of procedures [49]. The exact aetiology has not been definitively elucidated; however, it is theorized that haematoma formation is the aetiological stimulus. The haematoma can then either serve as a nidus for low-grade chronic infection leading to subtle rupture of membranes or, alternatively, may alter transmembrane diffusion and lead to the development of oligohydramnios by altering amniotic fluid production.

Infection

Infection is a rare complication following either transcervical or transabdominal CVS and occurs in less than 1–3 per 1000 procedures [19,26,50,51]. Most cases of infection have occurred in inexperienced centres or when a single catheter was used for more than one pass. While rare, chorioamnionitis following CVS can present with subtle signs including low-grade maternal fever and myalgia. These nondescript symptoms can frequently be confused with flu. If left unattended severe chorioamnionitis and uterine infections have developed and cases of sepsis have been reported [52,53]. Therefore, a high index of suspicion should be maintained when a patient presents within a week of a CVS procedure with febrile symptoms unexplained by other aetiologies. Although successful antibiotic treatment of mild uterine infection following CVS has been described, in most cases this is not sufficient and termination of the pregnancy is required.

Elevated MSAFP and Rh sensitization

An acute rise in MSAFP after CVS has been consistently reported, implying a detectable degree of fetal maternal bleeding [54,57]. The elevation is transient, occurs more frequently after transabdominal CVS and appears to be dependent upon the quantity of tissue aspirated [56,57]. Some studies have also demonstrated a correlation between the level of elevation and the incidence of pregnancy loss [57]. Levels will drop to normal ranges by 16–18 weeks, thus allowing serum screening for neural tube defect to proceed according to usual prenatal protocols.

In Rh-negative women, this otherwise negligible bleeding accrues special importance since Rh-positive cells in volumes as low as 0.1 ml have been shown to cause Rh sensitization. Since all women with even a single pass of a catheter or needle may show detectable rises in MSAFP, it seems prudent that all Rh-negative, non-sensitized women undergoing CVS receive Rh_0 (anti-D) immunoglobulin subsequent to the procedure.

The potential for a CVS-induced maternal fetal transfusion to worsen already existing Rh immunization has been described, suggesting that sampling previously sensitized patients represents a contraindication to the procedure [59]. The only exception to this would be red cell antigen incompatibility, in which CVS is specifically performed to evaluate the fetal blood type.

Perinatal complications

The incidence of perinatal complications, such as preterm labour, pre-eclampsia, abruptio placenta and intrauterine growth retardation, do not occur more frequently following CVS than in unsampled pregnancies [60].

Risk of fetal abnormalities following CVS

While initial reports demonstrated no increased risk of structural abnormalities following CVS, it has recently been suggested that CVS may be associated with specific fetal malformations. The first suggestion of this was reported by Firth *et al.* [28]. In their series of 539 CVS-exposed pregnancies, they identified five infants with severe limb abnormalities, all of which came from a cohort of 289 pregnancies sampled at 66 days' gestation or less. Four of these infants had the unusual and rare oromandibular–limb hypogenesis syndrome and the fifth had a terminal transverse limb reduction defect. Oromandibular–limb hypogenesis syndrome occurs with a prevalence of 1 per 175 000 live births [61]; limb reduction defects occur in 1 per 1690 births [62]. Therefore, the occurrence of these abnormalities in more than 1% of CVS-sampled cases raised strong suspicion of an association. In this initial report, all of the limb abnormalities followed transabdominal sampling performed between 55 and 66 days' gestation.

Subsequent to this initial report, others added supporting cases to this list. Using the Italian multicentre birth defects registry, Mastroiacovo *et al.* [63] reported, in a case–control study, an odds ratio of 11.3 (CI 5.6–21.3) for transverse limb abnormalities following first trimester CVS. When stratified by gestational age at sampling, it was demonstrated that pregnancies sampled prior to 70 days had a 19.7% increased risk of transverse limb reduction defects while patients sampled later did not demonstrate a significantly increased risk. Since that time, there have been additional reports of transverse limb defects following very early CVS. Most notably, Brambati *et al.* [64], an extremely experienced group with no increased risk of limb defects in patients sampled after the ninth week, reported a 1.6% incidence of severe limb reduction defects in a group of patients sampled at 6 and 7 weeks. This decreased to 0.1% for sampling at 8–9 weeks.

Using the extensive experience of the eight centres participating in the US collaborative evaluation of CVS, Mahoney [65] reported no cases of oromandibular–limb hypogenesis syndrome and no overall increase in the incidence of limb defects. CVS centres from Philadelphia and Milan have combined 10 000 CVS procedures and were unable to confirm the association when CVS was performed beyond the 10th week of gestation [66]. Alternatively, Burton *et al.* [29] reported a cluster of distal limb reduction defects occurring at their centre. Of 260 procedures, they had four babies with limb reduction defects. All were transverse distal defects involving hypoplasia or absence of fingers and toes. Sampling had been performed at 9.5, 10, 10.5 and 11.5 weeks. Unlike other clusters, three of the four abnormalities followed transcervical sampling. While this centre's report remains unique in that the patients were of more advanced gestational age, it raises the question of potential operator-specific contributing factors since this centre's spontaneous miscarriage rate following transcervical sampling was 10.9%.

The question remains whether CVS sampling after 10 weeks has the potential to cause more subtle defects, such as shortening of the distal phalanx or nail hypoplasia [67]. Presently, there are few data to substantiate this. On the contrary, most experienced centres performing CVS after 10 weeks have not seen an increase in limb defects [68].

At the present time, patients should be told of the controversy. However, the risk must be put into proper perspective and the patient should be counselled using outcome data that relates to the centre performing the procedure. Sampling prior to 10 weeks' gestation should be limited to exceptional cases.

Techniques for avoiding procedure-related complications

The incidence of miscarriage can be minimized by performing an atraumatic procedure. With transcervical CVS, this requires the insertion of the catheter directly into the chorion frondosum without penetration of the underlying vascular decidua basalis. Perforation of these large veins will lead to haematoma formation and bleeding that, if excessive, could cause miscarriage; this may also be an aetiological factor in certain cases of unexplained oligohydramnios. While ultrasound visualization is important in avoiding this complication, placement of the catheter into the appropriate tissue plane also requires tactile guidance that comes with experience. Advancement of the catheter through the more vascular decidual tissue will be met with resistance and a gripping sensation.

Spontaneous miscarriage can also be minimized by decreasing the number of catheter insertions, which can be accomplished in a number of ways. Waiting for contractions to abate when they interfere with the sampling path will make sampling easier and will decrease the need for a repeat insertion. The catheter must also be inserted parallel to the chorionic plate, whether transabdominal or transcervical CVS is performed. While insertion perpendicular to the membrane will only occasionally result in membrane injury, it will frequently limit the amount of tissue through which the instrument will pass and lead to smaller samples and more repeat attempts. Also, accurate demarcation of the placental location and boundaries is mandatory. Inserting the sampling instrument too lateral to the bulk of the villous tissue will lead to sampling failure. Scanning in a transverse plane in addition to the routine sagittal plane is helpful in avoiding this problem. Finally, the use of a tenaculum on the anterior lip of the cervix can be of help in difficult procedures. Specifically, an anteverted uterus with an anterior placenta can be straightened by gentle traction, hence allowing easier access.

Inadvertent injury of the membranes can also be avoided. It should be cautioned that the *tip* of the catheter/needle must be imaged rather than a portion of the shaft. This differentiation can be made by the operator watching the scan as the catheter is advanced. If the ultrasound image of the tip moves when the catheter is advanced this ensures a correct view. However, if a portion of the shaft is being imaged, no instantaneous movement will be seen. Only the operator, not the sonographer, can appreciate this and therefore constant communication is required. Additionally, the catheter should be held in the fingertips and only advanced slowly and gently; using this technique inadvertent advancement against the membrane can be detected as a buoyant feeling.

Chorioamnionitis following CVS can be avoided by adequate preparation of the cervix and attention to sterile technique. Is it likely that infection following CVS occurs very rarely unless a haematoma forms or significant tissue trauma occurs. Therefore, this complication can be minimized by atraumatic sampling. Cases of infection after transabdominal CVS have predominantly been secondary to bowel flora. To avoid this, attention must be paid to the sampling path and the operator must be certain that bowel has been removed from the sampling approach.

Avoiding haemorrhage is also possible with both transcervical and transabdominal CVS. With transcervical sampling, as stated above, the catheter must be in the appropriate sampling plane. With both sampling techniques, sampling should avoid perforation of visible placental lakes or areas of slow flow. Direct perforation of these lakes frequently leads to significant haemorrhage following the procedure.

Conclusions

CVS has dramatically improved women's reproductive options by providing a method for first-trimester prenatal diagnosis. As with any operative procedure, a learning curve is required, but operators experienced in ultrasound-guided procedures should be able to quickly add this technique to their armamentarium. Outcome following the procedure appears to be maximized in experienced centres in which a team consisting of a limited number of sonographers and operators perform the procedure on a regular basis. Centres in which the procedure is performed infrequently appear to have a higher miscarriage rate and increased risk of other untoward outcomes.

References

1 Mohr J. Foetal genetic diagnosis: development of techniques for early sampling of foetal cells. *Acta Pathol Microbiol Scand* 1968;73:7377.

2 Hahnemann N, Mohr J. Genetic diagnosis in the embryo by means of biopsy from extraembryonic membranes. *Bull Eur Soc Hum Genet* 1968;2:23.

3 Hahnemann N, Mohr J. Antenatal foetal diagnosis in genetic disease. *Bull Eur Soc Hum Genet* 1969;3:47.

4 Kullander S, Sandahl B. Fetal chromosome analysis after transcervical placental biopsies during early pregnancy. *Acta Obstet Gynecol Scand* 1979;52:355.

5 Hahnemann N. Early prenatal diagnosis: a study of biopsy techniques and cell culturing from extraembryonic membranes. *Clin Genet* 6:294.

6 Goldberg MF, Chen ATL, Ahn YW, Reidy JA. First trimester fetal chromosomal diagnosis using endocervical lavage: a negative evaluation. *Am J Obstet Gynecol* 1980;138:436.

7 Rhine SA, Cain JL, Cleary RE, Palmer CG, Thompson JF. Prenatal sex detection with endocervical smears: successful results utilizing Y-body fluorescense. *Am J Obstet Gynecol* 1975;122:155.

8 Rhine SA, Palmer CG, Thompson JF. A simple alternative to amniocentesis for first trimester prenatal diagnosis. *Birth Defects* 1977;12(3D):231.

9 Department of Obstetrics and Gynecology, Tietung Hospital of Anshan Iron and Steel Co., Anshan, China. Fetal sex prediction by sex chromatin of chorionic villi cells during early pregnancy. *Chin Med J* 1975;1:117.

10 Kazy Z, Rozovsky IS, Bakharev VA. Chorion biopsy in early pregnancy: a method of early prenatal diagnosis for inherited disorders. *Prenat Diagn* 1982;2:39.

11 Ward RHT, Modell B, Petrou M, Karagozlu F, Douratsos E. Method of sampling chorionic villi in first trimester of pregnancy under guidance of real time ultrasound. *Br Med J* 1983;286:1542.

12 Simoni G, Brambati B, Danesino C *et al.* Efficient direct chromosome analyses and enzyme determinations from chorionic villi samples in the first trimester of pregnancy. *Hum Genet* 1983;63:349.

13 Brambati B, Simoni G. Diagnosis of fetal trisomy 21 in first trimester. *Lancet* 1983;i:586.

14 Garden AS, Reid G, Benzie RJ. Chorionic villus sampling. *Lancet* 1985;i:1270.

15 Nicolaides KH, Azar G, Byrne D, Mansur C, Marks K. Fetal nuchal translucency: ultrasound screening for chromosomal defects in first trimester of pregnancy. *Br Med J* 1992;340:704–707.

16 Brambati B, Oldrini A, Lanzani A. Transabdominal chorionic villus sampling: a freehand ultrasound-guided technique. *Am J Obstet Gynecol* 1987;157:134.

17 Smidt-Jensen S, Hahnemann N. Transabdominal chorionic villus sampling for fetal genetic diagnosis. Technical and obstetric evaluation of 100 cases. *Prenat Diagn* 1988;8:7.

18 Jackson LG, Wapner RJ. Risks of chorionic villus sampling. *Clin Obstet Gynecol* 1987;1:513.

19 Rhoads GG, Jackson LG, Schlesselman SE *et al.* The safety and efficacy of chorionic villus sampling for early prenatal diagnosis of cytogenetic abnormalities. *N Engl J Med* 1989;320:609.

20 Jackson LG, Zachary JM. Randomized comparison of transcervical and transabdominal chorionic villus sampling. *N Engl J Med* 1992;327:594–598.

21 Wapner RJ, Davis GH, Johnson A *et al.* A prospective comparison between transcervical and transabdominal chorionic villus sampling. Abstract No. 8, Society of Perinatal Obstetricians Meeting, Houston.

22 Wapner RJ, Johnson A, Davis G *et al.* Prenatal diagnosis in twin gestations: a prospective comparison between second trimester amniocentesis and first trimester chorionic villus sampling. *Obstet Gynecol* 1993;82:49–60.

23 Pergament E, Schulman JD, Copeland K *et al.* The risk and efficacy of chorionic villus sampling in multiple gestations. *Prenat Diagn* 1992;12:377–384.

24 Brambati B, Tului L, Lanzani A *et al.* First trimester genetic diagnosis in multiple pregnancy: principles and potential pitfalls. *Prenat Diagn* 1991;11:767–774.

25 Jackson LG. *CVS Latest News, volume 32*, August 1994.

26 Canadian Collaborative CVS–Amniocentesis Clinical Trial Group. Multicentre randomized clinical trial of chorion villus sampling and amniocentesis. *Lancet* 1989;i:1.

27 MRC Working Party on the Evaluation of Chorionic Villus Sampling. Medical Research Council European trial of chorionic villus sampling. *Lancet* 1991;337:1491.

28 Firth HV, Boyd PA, Chamberlain P *et al.* Severe limb abnormalities after chorion villus sampling at 56–66 days gestation. *Lancet* 1991;337:726.

29 Burton BK, Schulz CJ, Burd LI. Limb anomalies associated with chorionic villus sampling. *Obstet Gynecol* 1992;79:726.

30 Wilson RD, Kendrick V, Witmann BK. Risks of spontaneous abortion in ultrasonographically normal pregnancies. *Lancet* 1984;ii:920.

31 Gilmore DH, McNay MB. Spontaneous fetal loss rate in early pregnancy. *Lancet* 1985;i:107.

32 Warburton D, Stein Z, Kline J *et al.* Chromosome abnormalities in spontaneous abortion: data from the New York City Study. In: Porter IH, Hook EB (eds) *Human Embryonic and Fetal Death*. New York: Academic Press, 1980:261.

33 Saura R, Gauthier B, Taine L *et al.* Operator experiences and fetal loss rate in transabdominal CVS. *Prenat Diagn* 1994;14:70.

34 Wapner RJ, Barr MA, Heeger S *et al.* Chorionic villus sampling: a 10 year, over 13 000 consecutive case experience. Abstract for the American College of Medical Genetics First Annual Meeting, Orlando, Florida, March 1994.

35 Young SR, Shipley CF, Wade RV *et al.* Single-center comparison of results of 1000 prenatal diagnoses with chorionic villus sampling and 1000 diagnoses with amniocentesis. *Am J Obstet Gynecol* 1991;165:255.

36 Green JE, Dorfman A, Jones SL *et al.* Chorionic villus sampling: experience with an initial 940 cases. *Obstet Gynecol* 1988;71:208.

37 Clark BA, Bissonnette JM, Olson SB *et al.* Pregnancy loss in a small chorionic villus sampling series. *Am J Obstet Gynecol* 1989;161:301.

38 Gustavii B, Claesson V, Kristoffersson U *et al.* Risk of miscarriage after chorionic biopsy is probably not higher than after amniocentesis. *Lakartidningen* 1989;86:4221.

39 Jahoda MGJ, Pijpers L, Reuss A *et al.* Evaluation of transcervical chorionic villus sampling with a completed follow-up of 1550 consecutive pregnancies. *Prenat Diagn* 1989;9:621.

40 Wapner RJ, Davis GH, Johnson A *et al.* A prospective comparison between transervical and transabdominal chorionic villus sampling. Abstract for Society of *Soc Perinat Obstet* Meg, Houston, Texas, 1990.

41 Brambati B, Lanzani A, Tului L. Transabdominal and transcervical chorionic villus sampling: efficacy and risk evaluation of 2411 cases. *Am J Hum Genet* 1990;35:160.

42 Smidt-Jensen S, Permin M, Philip J. Sampling success and risk by transabdominal chorionic villus sampling, transcervical chorionic villus sampling, and amniocentesis: a randomized study. *Ultrasound Obstet Gynecol* 1991;1:86.

43 Brambati B, Terzian E, Tognoni G. Randomized clinical trial of transabdominal versus transcervical chorionic villus sampling methods. *Prenat Diagn* 1991;11:285.

44 Copeland KL, Carpenter RJ, Fenolio KR *et al.* Integration of the transabdominal technique into an ongoing chorionic villus sampling program. *Am J Obstet Gynecol* 1989;161:1289.

45 Brambati B, Oldrini A, Ferrazzi E *et al.* Chorionic villus sampling: an analysis of the obstetric experience of 1000 cases. *Prenat Diagn* 1987;7:157–169.

46 Elles RG, Williamson R, Niazi D *et al.* Absence of maternal contamination of chorionic villi used for fetal gene analysis. *N Engl J Med* 1983;308:1433.

47 Ledbetter DH, Zachary JL, Simpson MS *et al.* Cytogenetic results from the US collaborative study on CVS. *Prenat Diagn* 1992;12:317.

48 Saura R, Taine L, Wen Q *et al.* Amnionic fluid leakage and miscarriage after TA CVS. *Prenat Diagn* 1994;14:897.

49 Cheng EY, Luth DA, Hickok D *et al.* Transcervical chorionic villus sampling and midtrimester oligohydramnios. *Am J Obstet Gynecol* 1991;**165**:1063.

50 Brambati B, Varotto F. Infection and chorionic villus sampling. *Lancet* 1985;ii:609.

51 Hogge WA, Schonberg SA, Golbus MS. Chorionic villus sampling: experience of the first 1000 cases. *Am J Obstet Gynecol* 1986;**154**:1249.

52 Barela A, Kleinman GE, Golditch IM *et al.* Septic shock with renal failure after chorionic villus sampling. *Am J Obstet Gynecol* 1986;**154**:1100.

53 Blakemore KJ, Mahoney MJ, Hobbins JC. Infection and chorionic villus sampling. *Lancet* 1985;ii:339.

54 Blakemore KJ, Baumgarten A, Schoenfeld-Dimaio M *et al.* Rise in maternal serum alpha-fetoprotein concentration after chorionic villus sampling. *Lancet* 1985;ii:339.

55 Brambati B, Guercilena S, Bonacchi I *et al.* Fetomaternal transfusion after chorionic villus sampling: clinical implications. *Hum Reprod* 1986;**37**.

56 Shulman LP, Meyers CM, Simpson JL, Anderson RN, Tolley EA, Elias S. Fetomaternal transfusion depends on amount of chorionic villi aspirated but not on method of chorionic villus sampling. *Am J Obstet Gynecol* 1990;**162**:1185.

57 Smidt-Jensen S, Philip J, Zachary J *et al.* Implications of maternal serum alpha-fetoprotein elevation caused by transabdominal and transcervical CVS. *Prenat Diagn* 1994;**14**:35–46.

58 Zipursky A, Israels LG. The pathogenesis and prevention of Rh immunization. *Can Med Assoc J* 1967;**97**:1245–1257.

59 Moise KJ, Carpenter RJ. Increased severity of fetal hemolytic disease with known Rhesus alloimmunization after first trimester transcervical chorionic villus biopsy. *Fetal Diagn Ther* 1990;**5**:76.

60 Williams J, Medearis AL, Bear MD, Kaback MM. Chorionic villus sampling is associated with normal fetal growth. *Am J Obstet Gynecol* 1987;**157**:708.

61 Hoyme F, Jones KL, Van Allen MI *et al.* Vascular pathogenesis of transverse limb reduction defects. *J Pediatr* 1982;**101**:839.

62 Foster-Iskenius U, Baird P. Limb reduction defects in over 1 000 000 consecutive livebirths. *Teratology* 1989;**39**:127.

63 Mastroiacovo P, Botto LD, Cavalcanti DP. Limb anomalies following chorionic villus sampling: a registry based case control study. *Am J Med Genet* 1992;**44**:856–863.

64 Brambati B, Simoni G, Traui M. Genetic diagnosis by chorionic villus sampling before 8 gestational weeks: efficiency, reliability, and risks on 317 completed pregnancies. *Prenat Diagn* 1992;**12**:784–799.

65 Mahoney MJ. Limb abnormalities and chorionic villus sampling. *Lancet* 1991;**337**:1422.

66 Jackson LG, Wapner RJ, Brambati B. Limb abnormalities and chorionic villus sampling. *Lancet* 1991;**337**:1422.

67 Burton BK, Schulz CJ, Burd LI. Spectrum of limb disruption defects associated with chorionic villus sampling. *Pediatrics* 1993;**91**:989–993.

68 Jackson L, Wapner R, Barr-Jackson M. Chorionic villus sampling (CVS) is not associated with an increased incidence of limb reduction defects. Abstract for the American Society of Human Genetics 43rd Meeting, New Orleans, LA, October 1993.

Chapter 8 / Amniocentesis

LUÍS F. GONÇALVES, ROBERTO ROMERO, HERNÁN MUNOZ,
RICARDO GOMEZ, MAURIZIO GALASSO, DAVID SHERER,
JOSÉ COHEN and FABIO GHEZZI

Introduction

Amniocentesis was introduced in clinical practice in the 19th century for the treatment of polyhydramnios [1–3]. The technique was subsequently used in the 1930s for amniography [4] and elective termination of the pregnancy [5,6], whereas the specific interest in obtaining amniotic fluid for prenatal diagnosis began in the 1950s with the management of pregnancies complicated by isoimmunization [7]. Following prenatal determination of fetal gender by Fuchs and Riis [8] in 1956, Jeffcoate et al. [9] reported the first prenatal diagnosis of a metabolic disorder, adrenogenital syndrome, in 1965, and in 1966 Steele and Breg [10] successfully determined the fetal karyotype from cultured amniotic fluid cells. The first prenatal diagnosis of a chromosomal anomaly, a balanced translocation, was reported by Jacobson and Barter [11] in 1967. Trisomy 21 was diagnosed prenatally for the first time by Valenti et al. in 1965 [12].

Real-time ultrasound added refinement and safety to the procedure, allowing continuous monitoring of the needle position inside the amniotic cavity [13,14]. The relative simplicity of the method and widespread availability of ultrasonographic equipment and expertise made amniocentesis the most widely used invasive method for prenatal diagnosis [15].

In this chapter we discuss the indications, technique and complications of amniocentesis, with special emphasis on early amniocentesis, isoimmunization, amniocentesis in twin pregnancies and the diagnosis of intrauterine infection.

Indications

The indications for amniocentesis are listed in Table 8.1. The most common indication is prenatal diagnosis, more specifically the diagnosis of chromosomal anomalies and neural tube defects in the early second trimester. In the third trimester, most of the procedures are performed to assess fetal lung maturity. The role of amniotic fluid analysis in the diagnosis of intrauterine infection has increased over the past few years and is discussed in more detail later in this chapter.

Amniocentesis for cytogenetic diagnosis

Cytogenetic diagnosis is routinely offered to women 35 years of age and older, to couples with chromosomal rearrangements, to women with a previous offspring affected by a chromosomal disorder, to women carrying an X-linked disease and to parents with a recessive gene for a metabolic disease or haemoglobinopathy [16]. When amniocentesis is used for cytogenetic diagnosis it is usually performed after 15 weeks, most commonly between 16 and 18 weeks. Cytogenetic studies are usually completed in 1–2 weeks, allowing timely interruption of the pregnancy in case of a positive diagnosis [17]. Although an amniocentesis may be performed at any time during gestation, cytogenetic studies of cord blood lymphocytes are usually preferred when rapid karyotyping is required since the results are available in approximately 48 hours [18]. The increased maternal risks involved in late second-trimester terminations and the psychological trauma of terminating a pregnancy that is both visible and felt led to the search for alternative procedures for earlier prenatal diagnosis, namely chorionic villous sampling (CVS) and early amniocentesis [15–17,19–49]. Early amniocentesis is discussed in detail below. For a discussion of CVS, see Chapter 7.

Table 8.1 Indications for amniocentesis.

Purpose	Indication
Late first and second trimester diagnosis	Cytogenetic diagnosis Diagnosis of neural tube defects Diagnosis of metabolic disorders
Late second and third trimester diagnosis	Evaluation of the severity of isoimmunization Evaluation of fetal lung maturity Diagnosis of intra-amniotic infection Confirmation of ruptured membranes
Therapeutic	Drainage of polyhydramnios Medical treatment of fetal disorders

Midtrimester amniocentesis

TECHNIQUE

Selecting a puncture site. Ultrasound is performed prior to amniocentesis to determine the number of fetuses, viability, placental location and the amount of amniotic fluid. The presence of uterine and fetal anomalies are specifically sought, since they may interfere with performance of the procedure. A site of puncture avoiding placental tissue or umbilical cord in the needle path is selected. Transplacental punctures are associated with an increased risk of pregnancy loss and maternal cell contamination and should only be performed as a last resource [50,51]. In case a transplacental puncture is necessary, the place with the least amount of placental tissue should be selected.

Selecting a needle. Needle selection is dependent upon the size of the patient and the amount of fluid to be retrieved. In the majority of cases we use a regular 20 to 22-gauge spinal needle with a standard length of 8.89 cm excluding the hub. Obese patients require longer needles. Smaller-bore needles prolong the time required to obtain amniotic fluid, whereas larger-bore needles have been associated with an increased fetal loss rate [52,53]. Needles with specially prepared tips designed to improve ultrasonographic visualization and side orifices to accelerate fluid withdrawal are commercially available. Although *in vitro* studies have shown that the flow rate during aspiration doubles with 22-gauge needles with side holes compared with standard spinal

needles of the same calibre, the use of these new needle types is strictly dependent upon personal preference until an adequate clinical trial is performed [54].

Monitoring the needle insertion and placement. Once a puncture site is selected, asepsis of the skin is performed with wide boundaries and the field is draped. Two approaches may then be used: (i) *ultrasonographic-guided amniocentesis* and (ii) *ultrasonographic-monitored amniocentesis.* Ultrasonographic-guided amniocentesis refers to the preselection of a puncture site with ultrasound before proceeding with blind insertion of the needle. Ultrasonographic-monitored amniocentesis refers to the continuous monitoring of needle insertion and fetal movements with real-time ultrasound. Monitoring the needle position with ultrasound reduces the frequency of bloody and dry taps and the risk of fetal injuries.

Convex, sector or linear-array transducers may be used to monitor the procedure with slight modifications of the technique. Irrespective of transducer selection, a non-sterile coupling agent is applied to the transducer surface before placing it inside a sterile glove or plastic bag. A sterile coupling agent is then applied to the patient's skin and the puncture site is re-evaluated.

When convex or sector transducers are used. Convex, and to a lesser extent sector, transducers have the advantage of allowing visualization of the entire needle, all the way from the patient's skin to the amniotic cavity. When these probes are used, the puncture site will be located in front and a few centimetres away from the transducer. The needle must enter the skin at an

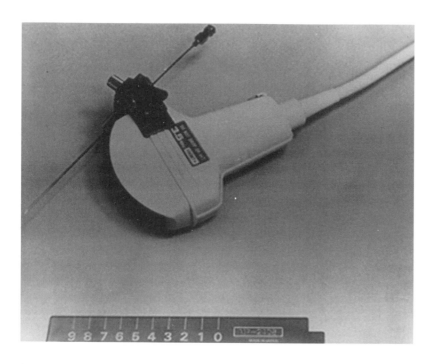

Fig. 8.1 Transducer with an attached needle guide device. (Reproduced with permission from Corometrics Medical Systems, Inc.)

angle so as to reach the amniotic fluid pocket underneath the transducer and, consequently, in the centre of the ultrasound image. Gentle pressure applied with the gloved finger to the selected puncture site produces a shadow in the ultrasound image that allows approximate identification of the needle path [55–56]. This technique requires expertise with needle–transducer spatial orientation since both of them must be aligned in the same plane in order for a successful procedure. Alternatively, a needle guide may be attached to the transducer (Fig. 8.1), thereby eliminating much of the 'guesswork' involved in proper alignment of transducer and needle [18]. Finally, the needle is inserted and directed to the selected pocket of amniotic fluid under direct ultrasonographic visualization.

When linear-array transducers are used. When a linear-array transducer is selected, a gloved finger is placed at the puncture site *directly under the transducer*, causing decoupling of the skin's surface and a shadow that allows identification of the needle path (Fig. 8.2). Then, under direct visualization, the needle is inserted along the side of the transducer and the tip, which appears as a bright echo, and is continuously monitored throughout the procedure (Fig. 8.3).

Amniotic fluid aspiration. Once the stylet is removed, an extension tube (which allows the needle to float free in the amniotic cavity, decreasing the likelihood of fetal injury) is attached to the hub of the needle and connected to the syringe. The first 0.5 ml of amniotic fluid is discarded in order to avoid maternal cell contamination. After obtaining the fluid, the stylet is relocated, the needle removed and fetal cardiac activity documented. The same technique is used for procedures performed during the late second and third trimesters.

Early amniocentesis

Early amniocentesis refers to procedures performed before 15 weeks of gestation. Early amniocentesis is, at present, a valid alternative to midtrimester amniocentesis, allowing the diagnosis of anomalies at a time when suction termination is still possible and before fetal movements are perceived [15–17,19–49]. Other potential advantages include the opportunity to screen for neural tube defects, by measurement of amniotic fluid α-fetoprotein (AFP) and acetylcholinesterase after 13 weeks, and the fact that there is no need for major changes in the operative technique, contrary to CVS [18,29,30,39]. In a study of 3325 pregnancies, Wald

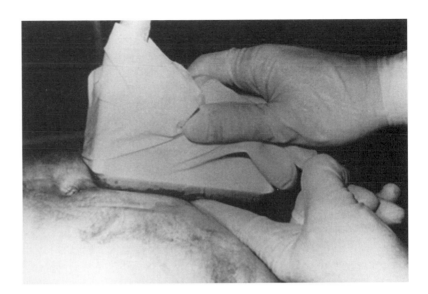

Fig. 8.2 Placing the gloved finger at the puncture site, underneath the linear transducer, produces a shadow in the ultrasound image that allows identification of the needle path.

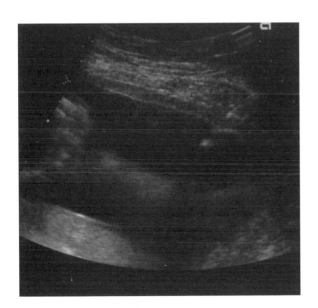

Fig. 8.3 Ultrasound guided amniocentesis procedure.

and Cuckle [57] demonstrated that amniotic fluid AFP obtained between 13 and 15 weeks had 100% sensitivity for the diagnosis of anencephaly and 96% sensitivity for the diagnosis of spina bifida using cut-off levels greater than 2.0 and 2.5 multiples of the normal median respectively. The question of whether amniocentesis is a valid alternative to CVS will only be answered by a randomized clinical trial comparing the two procedures. Preliminary results of the first 650 patients of such a trial do not provide evidence comparing the safety of both procedures with regard to the rate of spontaneous fetal loss [58]. There was no difference in the rates of successful cell cultures and chromosomal analysis when early amniocentesis was compared with CVS (98.1% [318/324] vs. 99.4% [321/323], NS). Cultures obtained by early amniocentesis had fewer mosaicisms than cultures obtained by CVS (0% [0/324] vs. 1.55% [5/323]), although this difference was not statistically significant.

GESTATIONAL AGE AT WHICH EARLY AMNIOCENTESIS MAY BE PERFORMED

Early amniocentesis has been performed as early as the seventh week of gestation [39]. However, Stripparo *et al.* [34] reported an increase in the spontaneous fetal loss rate for chromosomally normal fetuses within 2 weeks of the procedure and also before 28 weeks of gestation when the amniocentesis was performed before 13 weeks of gestation (11.1% [6/54] vs. 0.9% [3/330] within 2 weeks of the procedure, $P < 0.001$; 14.8% [8/54] vs. 2.1% [7/330] before 28 weeks of gestation, $P < 0.001$). The combined experience of seven centres for which data are available for comparison (Table 8.2) show an overall fetal loss rate of 1.32% (44/3296) within 2 weeks of the procedure, with a significant increase when amniocentesis is performed before 12 weeks (6.94% [5/72] vs. 1.21% [39/3224]; $P < 0.001$) [22,29,33,34,38,40,44,48]. Similarly, the combined spontaneous fetal loss rate before 28 weeks of gestation in four centres for which data are available for comparison is shown in Table 8.3. The overall fetal loss rate before 28 weeks of gestation was 1.44% (43/2982), increasing significantly when the amniocentesis was performed before 12 weeks of gestation (9.26% [5/49] vs. 1.30% [38/2928]; $P < 0.001$ [22,29,34,40,44].

From the point of view of cellular viability, Nelson and Emery [59] have demonstrated that the largest percentage of viable cells are present from 13 to 16 weeks of gestation.

TECHNIQUE

The technique for early amniocentesis is basically the same as for midtrimester amniocentesis, with minor modifications. Most authors recommend the use of a smaller-bore (22-gauge) spinal needle [15–41]. The recommended amount of fluid to be withdrawn is 1 ml per week of gestation [29]. The first 0.5–1 ml of fluid aspirated should be discarded in order to decrease the risk of maternal cell contamination or, as an alternative, the first 2 ml of amniotic fluid could be sent for AFP and acetylcholinesterase determinations [16]. The fluid should be aspirated slowly in order to prevent collapse of the amniotic sac [34]. Because the amniotic membrane may not be completely fused with the chorion at this stage in pregnancy, membrane tenting (separation of the chorioamniotic membrane from the anterior uterine wall during needle insertion) is a more frequent complication than with midtrimester amniocentesis. This difficulty may be overcome by a more vigorous thrust, twisting or redirecting the needle during perforation of the amniotic membrane. If these manoeuvres fail, the needle may be advanced into the posterior uterine wall, physically displacing the obstructing membrane down the shaft and away from the tip [18,30,40,60–63].

Transvaginal aspiration of amniotic fluid has been proposed as an alternative to the transabdominal approach for early amniocentesis [39,49]. Potential advantages would include the high resolution of the

transvaginal probe and easy access to the amniotic sac. Jorgensen *et al.* [39] attempted the procedure in 36 women between 7 and 12 weeks of gestation. Although amniotic fluid was obtained in all cases and the patients tolerated the procedure well, culture was unsuccessful in six cases (16.7%) because of bacterial or fungal overgrowth compared with culture success in all 96 control samples obtained via the transabdominal route. Shalev *et al.* [49] compared the clinical and laboratory results of first-trimester transvaginal amniocentesis with those of transcervical CVS and midtrimester amniocentesis. Transvaginal amniocentesis was performed in 355 women who voluntarily asked for the procedure between 10 and 12 weeks of gestation using a 20-cm, 22-gauge needle. The volume of amniotic fluid retrieved was 1 ml per week of gestation. The controls comprised 356 consecutive patients undergoing transcervical CVS and 356 consecutive patients undergoing midtrimester amniocentesis matched for maternal age and indication for the procedure. Amniotic fluid was successfully retrieved in 99.7% (355/356) of patients undergoing first-trimester amniocentesis and 100% (356/356) of patients undergoing midtrimester amniocentesis. In comparison CVS was successful in only 97.8% (346/356) of the cases ($P < 0.05$ compared with first-trimester and midtrimester amniocentesis respectively). No significant difference in culture success rates was observed between patients undergoing early transvaginal amniocentesis (96.9% [344/355]), midtrimester transabdominal amniocentesis (97.8% [348/356]) and CVS (96.5% [334/346]). However, the total pregnancy loss after excluding pregnancy terminations was significantly higher in patients submitted to early transvaginal amniocentesis compared with patients submitted to midtrimester transabdominal amniocentesis (3.2% [11/345] vs. 0.9% [3/350], $P < 0.05$). No differences in total pregnancy loss were observed between either group described above and patients submitted to CVS (2.9% [10/344]).

Amniotic fluid cell filtration (amnifiltration) has been proposed as a means to retrieve amniotic fluid cells in early amniocentesis without removing a relatively large proportion of amniotic fluid [15,37,64,65]. The basic principle is to interpose a filter membrane with appropriate pore size between the syringe and the needle, recirculate the amniotic fluid back to the amniotic cavity and retrieve the amniotic fluid cells directly from the filter membrane (Fig. 8.4). A three-way tap is interposed

Table 8.2 Early amniocentesis: fetal loss within 2 weeks of the procedure.

Reference	9 weeks		10 weeks		11 weeks		12 weeks		13 weeks		14 weeks		Total	
	n	Loss	n	Loss	n	Loss	n	Loss	n	Loss	n	Loss	n	Loss
Elias & Simpson [48]	1	0	3	0	4	0	12	0	47	0			67	0
Hanson et al. [22,44]							193	1	215	2	255	2	470	4
Henry & Miller [40]					14	0	193	1	426	3	1172	7	1805	11
Stripparo et al. [34]					13	3	41	3	154	3	110	1	318	10
Elejalde et al. [29]	3		6		18	2	77	2	98	0	121	14	323	18
Nevin et al. [33]	1	0	2	0	2	0	25	0	56	0	121	0	207	0
Hackett et al. [38]					5		24	1	42	1	35		106	1
Total	5	0	11	0	56	5	372	7	1038	8	1814	24	3296	44
Percentage loss	0.00		0.00		8.93		1.88		0.77		1.32		1.33	

Table 8.3 Early amniocentesis: fetal loss before 28 weeks of gestation.

Reference	9 weeks		10 weeks		11 weeks		12 weeks		13 weeks		14 weeks		Total	
	n	Loss	n	Loss	n	Loss	n	Loss	n	Loss	n	Loss	n	Loss
Hanson et al. [22,44]	1	0	3	0	4	0	12	0	215	4	255	5	470	9
Henry & Miller [40]					14	0	193	1	426	3	1172	7	1805	11
Stripparo et al. [34]					13	3	41	5	154	6	176	1	384	15
Elejalde et al. [29]	3		6		18	2	77	3	98	2	121	1	323	8
Total	3	0	6	0	45	5	311	9	893	15	1724	14	2982	43
Percentage loss	0.00		0.00		2.2		2.89		1.68		0.81		1.44	

between the syringe and the filter membrane and a second one between the filter membrane and the needle. Both three-way taps are connected through a bypassing T tube. Fluid is aspirated through the bypassing tube until air is drawn into the syringe; the three-way taps are then directed to allow aspiration of fluid through the filter membrane; once the desired amount of fluid is aspirated, the three-way taps are redirected to permit the amniotic fluid to bypass the membrane through the T tube back into the amniotic cavity. The process may be repeated as many times as necessary. Amniotic fluid cells are retrieved for culture by reverse flushing [37]. A 0.8-µm cellulose acetate membrane was compared with a 1.2-µm cellulose acetate membrane and a 1.2-µm polyamide membrane by Byrne *et al.* [37]. The 0.8-µm cellulose acetate membrane proved to be the most efficient filter in their experiment because it not only trapped all amniotic fluid cells but also allowed easy release of the trapped cells once the membrane was reverse flushed. Kennerknecht *et al.* [15] compared the prolongation in culture time for amniocytes obtained by amnifiltration using four different sets of filters: (i) 5.0-µm polyvinylidene difluoride filter (70% porosity); (ii) 0.45-µm polyvinylidene difluoride filter (75% porosity); (iii) 5.0-µm mixed cellulose ester filter (84% porosity); and (iv) 0.45-µm mixed cellulose ester filter (79% porosity). They used the culture time for amniocytes obtained directly from the amniotic fluid in 90 patients as a control group in their experiment.

The mixed cellulose ester and polyvinylidene difluoride filters with 5.0-µm pore size had the shortest mean prolongation in culture time for filtered amniocytes compared with amniocytes cultured directly from the amniotic fluid (2.4 and 3.0 days respectively vs. 6.5 and 6.3 days for the 0.45-µm mixed cellulose ester and polyvinylidene difluoride filters).

Byrne and Nicolaides [65] studied changes in amniotic fluid temperature during amnifiltration in 10 women undergoing surgical termination of pregnancy between 9 and 12 weeks of gestation. They observed a gradual decrease in temperature from a mean of 36.8°C before amnifiltration to 36.5°C after one fluid circuit (8 ml), 36.3°C after two fluid circuits (16 ml) and 36.2°C after three fluid circuits (24 ml). The authors speculate that although fetal cooling (unlike hyperthemia) has not been implicated in teratogenesis, measures to avoid a decrease in amniotic fluid temperature, such as increasing the room temperature or using isolated syringes and tubing, should probably be undertaken when performing amnifiltration.

Complications

FETAL LOSS

Fetal loss can be idiopathic or a result of direct fetal injury with subsequent exsanguination or infection. The term 'idiopathic' refers to unexplained fetal death

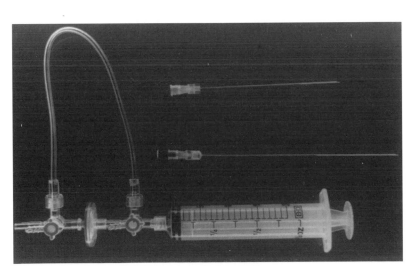

Fig. 8.4 Amniotic cell filtration apparatus.

that occurs during the procedure, with post-mortem examination yielding no demonstrable reason for the demise. In these cases, fetal heart activity is detected before but not after the amniocentesis. A neurogenic mechanism has been postulated; however, there is no evidence to support this mechanism.

Amniocentesis may lead to intra-amniotic infection by introducing microorganisms into the amniotic cavity (i.e. contaminated instruments, passage of the needle through contaminated skin or intra-abdominal viscera). Alternatively, if amniocentesis results in rupture of the membranes, ascending infection may occur. The midtrimester period seems particularly vulnerable to microbial invasion, as the antibacterial activity of amniotic fluid is at its nadir [66]. Antibiotic prophylaxis is not a routine practice. Blood cultures obtained around the time of the procedure were negative in a small study by Ager and Oliver [67].

The prevalence of intra-amniotic infection after midtrimester amniocentesis is unknown. The nature of the evidence implicating infection as an aetiological factor for pregnancy loss after midtrimester amniocentesis is anecdotal. There have been case reports in which there was a temporal association between the procedure and clinical chorioamnionitis. Positive microbial cultures of amniotic fluid obtained at the time of midtrimester amniocentesis in asymptomatic patients suggest that in some cases intra-amniotic infection may precede rather than follow the procedure [68,69]. In a series of 2641 second-trimester genetic amniocentesis procedures reported by Gray *et al.* [69], all of which were cultured for mycoplasmas (*Mycoplasma hominis* and *Ureaplasma urealyticum*), nine patients had a positive culture for *U. urealyticum*. One patient was excluded from the analysis because of a subsequent therapeutic abortion. The perinatal outcome of the other eight patients was compared with 86 patients with complete follow-up who had genetic amniocentesis during the same study period and negative cultures for mycoplasmas. Among the eight patients who cultured positive for *U. urealyticum*, 75% (6/8) had a spontaneous abortion within 4 weeks of the procedure compared with only 1.2% (1/86) of the patients with negative cultures. The other two patients in the positive culture group delivered prematurely at 24 and 30 weeks and only one of the infants survived. All eight placentas had evidence of chorioamnionitis on histological examination. Of the

samples obtained from *Ureaplasma*-positive patients 50% (4/8) were discoloured compared with 2.3% (2/86) of the samples obtained from *Ureaplasma*-negative patients. Discoloured amniotic fluid was significantly associated with the presence of *Ureaplasma* ($P < 0.001$) and an adverse perinatal outcome.

Fetal loss rates for midtrimester amniocentesis range from 0.3 to 2.8% [27]. A randomized clinical trial of genetic amniocentesis involving 4606 low-risk women provides the best fetal risk estimation available in the literature to date [70]. Patients were randomized to have either an amniocentesis or an ultrasound in midtrimester. All amniocentesis procedures were performed under ultrasound guidance by five physicians at the same institution using a 20-gauge needle. The study group had a higher rate of spontaneous abortion compared with the control group (1.7% vs. 0.7%; relative risk 2.3 [95% confidence limits 1.3–4.0]; $P < 0.01$). Also, a shorter interval between the procedure and spontaneous abortion was found for the study group compared with the control group (median time interval 21.5 days vs. 46.5 days). Risk factors for spontaneous abortion included a maternal serum AFP greater than two multiples of the median for gestational age, perforation of the placenta and discoloured amniotic fluid. The authors have pointed out that the 1% increased risk of spontaneous abortion after midtrimester amniocentesis may be an underestimation of the real risk. Pregnancy termination in fetuses affected with chromosomal abnormalities (identified in the study group and not in the control group) may have artificially reduced the rate of spontaneous abortion of the study group.

Multiple needle insertions and intra-amniotic bleeding have also been implicated as causes for an increased pregnancy loss rate [27,50–52]. The use of continuous ultrasonographic monitoring and increased operator experience have been shown to reduce the number of attempts needed to obtain amniotic fluid as well as the number of bloodstained taps [14,70,71]. A history of haemorrhage in the present pregnancy, a previous abortion or stillbirth and infertility have all been shown to predispose to spontaneous abortion regardless of the performance of an amniocentesis.

FETAL INJURY

A wide range of fetal injuries, from mild skin dimples to

fetal death due to exsanguination, have been attributed to amniocentesis [72–103]. Although fetal injuries are generally associated with bloody taps, they have also been reported after clear taps and even with the use of the sonographically monitored technique.

Several ocular injuries have been attributed to amniocentesis [76,80,91,95,99,101,103–105]. Typically, these are unilateral lesions detected after birth. In one case, the newborn had a small and cloudy eye, a coloboma of the upper lid and a hazy and oedematous cornea. The combination of lesions in the eyelid and cornea suggests that the injury occurred before separation of the eyelids. The mother had an amniocentesis at 19 weeks; the first 2 ml of fluid were bloody, but the subsequent 30 ml were clear [91]. In two cases, a red and photophobic eye in the newborn period was subsequently associated with the development of an enlarged cystic mass in the anterior chamber of the eye. The cystic lesion evolved over a period of several months and was lined by stratified squamous epithelium [76,80]. Similar findings have been recently reported for two children with unilateral and progressively large epithelial iris cysts occupying nearly half of the pupil. The lesions were diagnosed at 8 months and 5 years of age respectively and both mothers had an amniocentesis performed at 18 and 43 weeks. The children had no history of postnatal ocular trauma [103]. Five other children were reported with lesions attributed to ocular perforation during amniocentesis: the first child had an amniocentesis at 16 weeks and was found at birth to have a cystic lesion communicating with the right lateral ventricle, left homonymous hemianopia and possible damage to the right optic tract; the second child had an amniocentesis at 30 weeks and presented in the neonatal period with a distorted left pupil towards the 3 o'clock position and a small tag of iris drawn up towards a full-thickness corneal scar; the third child had an amniocentesis performed at 16 weeks and presented at birth with left esotropia, limitation of abduction and microphthalmia; the fourth child had an amniocentesis performed at 15 weeks and was noted at 3.5 years to have a small adherent leucoma near the limbus at 7 o'clock; the last child in this series had an amniocentesis performed during the second trimester and was found at 5 years of age to have a small chalazion on her right upper lid with a small full-thickness scar near the limbus at 9 o'clock [101].

A porencephalic cyst has been reported in a newborn with two subcutaneous nodules in the right and left occipital region (suggesting a needle tract) [92]; an amniocentesis had been performed at 18 weeks. *In utero* injection of contrast in the ventricular system during the course of amniograms has also been reported [74,75].

Thoracic lesions associated with amniocentesis include haemothorax [77,96], pneumothorax [74,77] and fetal cardiac tamponade [75]. In the abdomen, injuries have ranged from laceration of the liver, kidney and spleen to ileo-cutaneous fistula with ileal atresia [78,84,85,90,93]. In one case, a fragment of tissue retrieved during amniocentesis grew small bowel mucosa in culture, confirming intraoperative bowel injury [93].

Limb lesions have included disruption of the patellar tendon [89], gangrene of one arm (perforation of the subclavian artery) [81] and an arteriovenous fistula between the popliteal artery and vein [102]. Amniocentesis has been implicated by some authors in the aetiology of amniotic band syndrome [77,87,88,94]; however, there is no agreement regarding cause and effect between this syndrome and amniocentesis.

Two cases of umbilical cord haematoma have been reported [77,98]. Fetal exsanguination due to vascular puncture have also been reported [73,86].

The most frequent lesion associated with amniocentesis is skin puncture. Although cause and effect is difficult to establish, needle injuries should be suspected if the shape of the lesion resembles a needle tract or a depressed punctiform scar [82,83,89].

The British [104] and American [105] collaborative studies in amniocentesis reported an increased incidence of orthopaedic abnormalities (talipes equinovarus, congenital hip dislocation and metatarsus abductus) in fetuses submitted to midtrimester amniocentesis. A case–control study in which amniocentesis had not been performed more often in mothers of newborns with orthopaedic abnormalities than in a control group failed to demonstrate such an association [106]. This finding is supported by a randomized controlled trial of genetic amniocentesis in 4606 low-risk women by Tabor *et al.* [70].

PREVALENCE OF RESPIRATORY COMPLICATIONS

Experimental studies in monkeys (*Macaca fascicularis*) specifically designed to examine the effect of amniocentesis on lung development indicate that a reduction in the number of alveoli and lung volume can occur after amniocentesis at a period equivalent to 14–17 weeks of gestation in humans [107,108]. The British Collaborative Study [104] demonstrated an increased incidence of respiratory distress syndrome (RDS) (defined as respiratory difficulties requiring oxygen and lasting more than 24 hours) in neonates born to mothers who had an amniocentesis compared with those in the control group (1.27% [30/2370] vs. 0.38% [9/2402]). Tabor *et al.* [70] also observed a higher prevalence of RDS and pneumonia in neonates born to mothers who had an amniocentesis in the second trimester compared with women having an ultrasound in the midtrimester only (1.1% vs. 0.5% for RDS, $P < 0.05$; 0.7% vs. 0.3% for pneumonia, $P < 0.05$).

Thompson *et al.* [109] evaluated the prevalence of respiratory distress and lung growth by measuring the functional residual capacity (FRC) in 74 newborns of mothers who had an amniocentesis at 10–13 weeks and 86 newborns of mothers who had a CVS during the same gestational age interval. Six infants in the CVS group but none in the amniocentesis group required admission to the intensive care unit because of respiratory distress ($P < 0.005$). The FRC was not different between the two groups. However, the overall incidence of FRC values below the 2.5th centile for the normal range was higher than expected (9%), indicating that both amniocentesis and CVS performed in the first trimester of pregnancy may impair antenatal lung growth. This study is in agreement with the findings of Vyas *et al.* [110], who used the crying vital capacity as a measure of lung volume. In this study the crying vital capacity was lower than the normal range in 10 neonates of mothers who had a midtrimester amniocentesis compared with none in the control group [110].

AMNIOTIC FLUID LEAKAGE

Membrane rupture or amniotic fluid leakage are potential complications of amniocentesis. It has been suggested that the perinatal and maternal outcomes for membrane rupture and amniotic fluid leakage are better than the outcomes for patients who experience spontaneous rupture of the membrane in the second trimester of pregnancy. Although we lack enough data at the present time to support definitive conclusions, expectant

management was employed successfully in six of seven patients who experienced amniotic fluid leakage within 24 hours of a genetic amniocentesis in a series of 603 patients reported by Gold *et al.* [111]. All patients were placed on bed rest and had digital cervical examination prohibited, daily white blood cell counts with differential analysis and close maternal surveillance for clinical evidence of chorioamnionitis. Six patients delivered healthy neonates at term and one patient had an intrauterine fetal demise at 25 weeks. In this case, an unsuccessful amniocentesis was attempted 6 weeks before delivery.

BLOODY TAPS

Bloody amniotic fluid can be the result of contamination with maternal and/or fetal blood. As mentioned above, the prevalence of this complication also decreased with the use of ultrasonographic monitoring. Ron *et al.* [112] studied 706 women undergoing midtrimester amniocentesis in which the first 2 ml of fluid were examined for the presence of blood after centrifugation; 25% (180/706) of the samples were found to be contaminated with blood and in 84.4% of the cases the blood was of maternal origin. The incidence of spontaneous abortion was significantly higher for patients with bloody taps compared with women with clear taps (maternal blood contamination, 6.6%; fetal blood contamination, 14.3%; clear taps, 1.7%). The incidence of pregnancy loss when fetal blood contamination occurred was double that observed when maternal blood contamination was documented. However, this difference did not reach statistical significance.

FETOMATERNAL TRANSFUSION

Fetomaternal transfusion is important because it may lead to isoimmunization (see below) and an increased risk of pregnancy loss. Fetomaternal transfusion can be detected by performing a Kleihauer–Betke test after the amniocentesis or by determining maternal serum AFP before and after the procedure [113,114]. AFP determinations are more sensitive than the Kleihauer–Betke test [115].

Menutti *et al.* [114] reported a significant difference in the incidence of spontaneous abortion in patients with an elevated maternal serum AFP after amniocentesis compared with women with no elevation (14.2% vs. 0.98%).

DISCOLOURED AMNIOTIC FLUID

Brown- and green-stained amniotic fluids are occasionally obtained during midtrimester amniocentesis [116–127]. Although the possibility that some green-stained amniotic fluid could be due to meconium passage (the human fetus produces and can pass meconium before the 20th week of gestation) [128], compelling evidence suggests that green- and brown-stained amniotic fluids are the result of an intra-amniotic haemorrhage [84,128]. Green- and brown-stained amniotic fluids have a similar spectrophotometric pattern, consistent with the presence of oxyhaemoglobin and free haemoglobin. *In vitro* experiments, in which amniotic fluid was contaminated with blood, indicate a sequential colour change. Green-coloured fluid was seen after 3 days and brown-coloured fluid after 7 days of incubation [124]. This interpretation is consistent with the clinical observation that women with green or brown amniotic fluid have a positive history of vaginal bleeding. However, little is known about the aetiology of the bleeding episode. Cassel *et al.* [68] reported the recovery of *M. hominis* and *U. urealyticum* in 4 of 33 samples with discoloured second-trimester amniotic fluid. Similarly, Gray *et al.* [69] found the amniotic fluid to be discoloured in four of eight amniotic fluid samples positive for *U. urealyticum* (see above). It is possible that an intrauterine infection may lead to bleeding and clot formation, providing an adequate nidus for microbial growth. Although the evidence is not consistent, most studies that have examined the prognostic significance of dark-stained amniotic fluid suggest an increased risk of pregnancy loss. The relative risk of spontaneous abortion after retrieval of discoloured amniotic fluid has been reported to be 9.9% by Tabor *et al.* [70]. King *et al.* [119] have suggested that the prognosis is poorer if discoloured fluid is associated with elevated maternal serum AFP determined before the amniocentesis. These findings are at variance with those of Hankis *et al.* [124] who did not find an increased frequency of poor pregnancy outcome after examining data from 83 patients with dark or green fluid (77 green and 6 brown) from a total of 1227 women undergoing midtrimester amniocentesis.

DIFFICULTIES

The performance of early amniocentesis may pose extra difficulties compared with midtrimester amniocentesis. These difficulties are mainly related to the small amniotic cavity and the presence of the extracoelomic space. When the amniotic membrane is not totally adherent to the uterine wall, dry taps may occur since the amniotic membrane will be tented by the needle and not perforated (see above) [18,30,40,48]. An increased risk of amniotic fluid leakage has also been reported for early amniocentesis [42].

When chorioamniotic separation is noted during ultrasound, most of the authors recommend rescheduling the procedure. A small or retroverted uterus, the presence of overlying bladder or bowel, a decreased amniotic fluid volume, a history of recent bleeding or cramping, the presence of severe contractions prior to the procedure and obesity may all pose additional difficulties and are considered additional indications for rescheduling amniocentesis in some patients [40,42].

AMNIOTIC FLUID CULTURE

Success rates for amniotic fluid culture are similar for early and midtrimester amniocentesis. Depending on laboratory experience, the interval between amniocentesis and culture harvest ranges from 6.4 to 21 days [17,28,29,31–33,37,39–41].

Byrne *et al.* [129] studied 125 pregnancies at 8–18 weeks of gestation undergoing diagnostic amniocentesis. Live cells were identified by the vital stain trypan blue and counted using light microscopy. Although the number of total cells increased exponentially with gestational age, the number of viable cells remained the same, explaining why cell culture from early amniocentesis is as successful as traditional amniocentesis. The authors speculate that the increase in the number of dead cells is possibly due to exfoliated cells from the genitourinary tract, since this increase is coincident with the increasing contribution of fetal urine to the amniotic fluid volume.

Amniocentesis and isoimmunization

Fetal red blood cells contain the D antigen on their surface and are capable of immunizing the Rh-negative mother after a fetomaternal transfusion in the midtrimester. This event can occur spontaneously during pregnancy or after an amniocentesis. The World Health Organization (WHO) and the American College of Obstetrics and Gynecology (ACOG) have recommended the administration of anti-D IgG to women after midtrimester amniocentesis. There is no agreement on the dose; WHO recommends 50 µg, while the ACOG recommends 300 µg [130].

The basis for this recommendation is that midtrimester amniocentesis has been associated with an increased incidence of transplacental haemorrhage, a risk factor for isoimmunization. However, the precise risk of isoimmunization after midtrimester amniocentesis has not been well defined. The incidence of Rh isoimmunization in the randomized controlled clinical trial reported by Tabor *et al.* [70] was 0.3% (7/370) in the study group and 0.1% (3/347) in the control group (anti-D IgG was not administered to Rh-negative patients undergoing amniocentesis). Although this difference is not significant, the number of patients required to detect a difference of 1% between the amniocentesis and the control group would be 2896 in each group [70]. The analysis of previous reports suggest that midtrimester amniocentesis is associated with an increased risk of isoimmunization. The magnitude of the increased risk seems to be approximately 1% [67].

Murray *et al.* [131] have provided a comprehensive analysis of the pros and cons of anti-D IgG administration. The objections that have been raised against the routine use of anti-D IgG are unproven efficacy and unproven long-term safety. Isolated case reports indicate that sensitization can occur after anti-D IgG administration [132,133]. Anti-D IgG crosses the placenta and coats Rh-positive fetal red cells. It is unclear if this could have adverse effects. The theoretical risk of augmentation has been suggested. This phenomenon consists of an enhancement of the immune response in the context of small amounts of antibody. Furthermore, the long-term effects of exposing the immunologically 'naive' fetal immune system to human immunoglobulins are unknown [134].

Although there is no incontrovertible evidence to support the routine administration of anti-D IgG after midtrimester amniocentesis, this has become the standard of practice in the USA.

Amniocentesis in multiple gestation

Multiple pregnancy was once considered a contraindication for midtrimester amniocentesis; however, this is no longer the case. The prevalence of chromosomal anomalies is estimated to be higher in twins than in singleton pregnancies (for advanced maternal age indication) [135]. Similarly, the incidence of neural tube defects in patients with history of a previous child with a neural tube defect is higher in twin (as high as doubled) than in singleton gestations [67,135].

Before amniocentesis is carried out in a multiple gestation, the possible outcome, risks and management alternatives need to be discussed with the patient. The major problem to be considered is the possibility of discrepant results regarding cytogenetic diagnosis. If only one fetus is affected, the options available to the patient include abortion of both fetuses, continuation of the pregnancy or selective feticide of the affected fetus. Feticide is associated with potential complications, such as infection, disseminated intravascular coagulation and spontaneous abortion [136]. Under these circumstances, pregnancy termination implies the abortion of an unaffected fetus.

The technique for amniocentesis in multiple gestation is different from that in singleton pregnancies. The number of fetuses, location within the uterine cavity, presence of an intra-amniotic membrane, placentation, sex, fetal biometry and anatomy need to be documented. An important step is the topographic location of the fetus. This becomes critical in cases where discrepant results are reported and selective feticide is considered. Identification of the fetuses should be based upon their relationship to the maternal hemipelvis (left/right, anterior/posterior and superior/inferior). We recommend that a diagram of the procedure be drawn and kept in the medical record for reference.

Several techniques have been proposed to ensure that fluid is retrieved from each amniotic cavity [137–141]. In the majority of centres, after amniotic fluid is obtained from the first sac and before removing the needle, an indicator dye is injected into the cavity. Indigo carmine is presently the dye of choice [137,142–152]; alternatives are Congo red and Evan's blue. The use of a solution of maternal haemoglobin as a dye has also been reported [153]. The use of methylene blue is discouraged because of the risk of fetal haemolytic anaemia due to methaemoglobinaemia and a possible association with gastrointestinal obstruction. The association between the use of methylene blue and multiple ileal occlusions was first reported by Nicolini and Monni [152] in seven babies born to mothers who had a midtrimester amniocentesis and the injection of 10–30 mg of methylene blue into one of the amniotic sacs. Pruggmayer *et al.* [150] compared the incidence of gastrointestinal obstruction among 474 twin pregnancies who had either indigo carmine ($n = 351$) or methylene blue ($n = 123$) injected as a dye during midtrimester amniocentesis. Of the fetuses who had their sac injected with methylene blue 17% (21/123) required a postnatal operation to correct jejunal atresia compared with 0.3% (1/351) of the fetuses who had their sacs injected with indigo carmine and who presented with duodenal atresia in the neonatal period ($P < 0.0001$). Clear amniotic fluid should be obtained when the second sac is punctured. The same procedure is applicable to amniocentesis for a multiple gestation with more than two fetuses. The technique consists of sequential injections of dye into different sacs before removal of the needle. The number of clear amniotic fluid aspirations should equal the number of fetuses.

A technique for single-needle insertion in twin amniocentesis was described by Jeanty *et al.* [140]. Briefly, a puncture site clear of placental tissue demonstrating both gestational sacs and the interamniotic membrane is selected with real-time ultrasound. The most proximal sac is tapped first; the stylet is then replaced into the needle and advanced under ultrasound guidance through the interamniotic membrane into the second sac; finally, fluid is aspirated from the second sac. Amniotic fluid was successfully retrieved from both sacs in 17 of the 18 patients included in their study and no adverse perinatal outcomes were reported. Alternatively, two needle insertions may be performed simultaneously by two operators into two separate sacs under direct ultrasonographic guidance [141]. The procedure has been reported in a series of seven patients with successful retrieval of fluid in all cases and no perinatal complications [141]. A shortcoming of this technique is that it may not be used by a single operator. The overall success rate in obtaining fluid from both sacs is over 90%. A challenging situation occurs when one sac is behind the other. In this case we sample the second sac by advancing the needle to penetrate the intra-amniotic membrane under direct visualization as described above. The first 2 ml of amniotic fluid retrieved from the second sac are discarded to decrease the likelihood of contamination.

Another difficult situation arises when an intra-amniotic membrane cannot be identified. This can occur in the setting of polyhydramnios and in monoamniotic twins. A practical approach consists of sampling two sites in close proximity to each fetus but distant from each other. We have found it helpful to place a linear- or convex-array transducer along the transverse axis of the uterus and to monitor the turbulence created by the injection of the indicator dye. Before injection, the dye is diluted with 10 ml of amniotic fluid. The mixture is then injected into the amniotic cavity, producing a typical particulate image that identifies the boundaries of that sac. The operator must be ready to proceed with the second puncture because the image is short-lived. Another interesting approach was described by Tabsh [139]. After aspirating the amniotic fluid sample from the first sac, 0.1 ml of air and 0.5 ml of dye are drawn through a 15-μm filter into a 6-ml syringe. The syringe is then reattached to the needle hub and 5 ml of amniotic fluid is aspirated into the syringe. The mixture of dye, air and amniotic fluid is then reinjected into the amniotic sac with gentle pressure, enough to create microbubbles that will serve as an ultrasonographic contrast within the amniotic sac. If the microbubbles are seen around both fetuses, the diagnosis of monoamniotic twinning is made and no further attempts are necessary.

The risk of pregnancy loss in multiple gestations has been addressed in several reports [143,145,146,148–151,153–160] (Table 8.4). Anderson *et al.* [160] compared the risk of spontaneous abortion following midtrimester amniocentesis in 353 twin pregnancies and 687 singleton pregnancies matched for gestational age and indication for prenatal diagnosis (one preceding and one following each twin); 14 cases were excluded because of congenital anomalies, growth retardation, twin-to-twin transfusion or death of one twin at the time of the procedure, leaving 339 patients for subsequent analysis. The groups were not different with regard to maternal age or experience of the physician performing the procedure. Three pregnancies were terminated following the diagnosis of aneuploidy in one of the fetuses. After terminations for chromosomal abnormalities were excluded, the spontaneous fetal

Table 8.4 Perinatal outcome in multiple pregnancies undergoing midtrimester amniocentesis.

Reference	Period	Timing of amniocentesis	n	Loss of both twins <20 weeks		Loss of both twins <28 weeks		Loss of both twins >28 weeks		Loss of only one twin	
				n	%	n	%	n	%	n	%
Elias *et al.* [137]	Since 1979	>17 weeks	20	0	0.00	0	0.00	0	0.00	2	10.00
Bovicelli *et al.* [154]	1979–82	Midtrimester	13	0	0.00	1	7.69	0	0.00	—	—
Palle *et al.* [155]	1973–79	16–17 weeks	29	3	10.35	6	20.69	0	0.00	0	0.00
Goldstein & Stills [143]	1978–82	Midtrimester	22	0	0.00	1	4.55	1	4.55	0	0.00
Filkins *et al.* [145]	1976–82	17–18 weeks	31	2	6.45	1	3.23	0	0.00	0	0.00
Librach *et al.* [146]	1972–83	16–17 weeks	70	3	4.29	4	5.71	4	5.71	0	0.00
Tabsh *et al.* [148]	1972–83	Midtrimester	48	0	0.00	1	2.08	0	0.00	5	10.42
Kappel *et al.* [156]	1980–83	Midtrimester	48	—	—	6	12.5	0	0.00	0	0.00
Pijpers *et al.* [149]	1980–85	16–20 weeks	83	1	1.20	4	4.82	0	0.00	3	3.61
Anderson *et al.* [160]	1969–90	Midtrimester	336	—	—	12	3.57	6	1.79	1	0.30
Beekhuis *et al.* [153]	—	16 weeks	63	1	1.59	2	3.17	0	0.00	1	1.59
Pruggmayer *et al.* [150]	1985–91	14–19 weeks	529	12	2.27	20	3.78	11	2.08	31	5.86
Wapner *et al.* [151]	1984–90	16–18 weeks	70	1	1.43	2	2.86	1	1.43	7	10.00
Total			1362	17/949	1.79	60/1362	4.4	23/1362	1.69	48/1349	3.56

loss rate before 28 weeks was significantly higher for multiple pregnancies compared with singleton pregnancies (3.57% [12/336] vs. 0.6% [4/671]; $P < 0.001$). The perinatal mortality rate, however, was not different between the two groups (12.6/1000 [8/633] vs. 12.1/1000 [8/659]; NS). In another large series assessing the perinatal outcome of 529 twin pregnancies undergoing genetic amniocentesis, the combined fetal loss rate before 28 weeks was 3.7% (20/529) [150], comparable to the 3.57% rate reported by Anderson *et al.* [160]. Both studies concluded that although there is an increased risk of spontaneous pregnancy loss for twin pregnancies undergoing amniocentesis, it is unlikely that this increased risk exceeds the normal biological loss rate in twins. This conclusion is also supported by the analysis of the risks of midtrimester amniocentesis in twin gestations conducted by Ager and Oliver [67], although they used a different outcome measure, total fetal loss rate. Total fetal loss rate is defined as total spontaneous abortions plus stillbirths plus neonatal deaths. According to their analysis, the total fetal loss rate is 10.8% (range 3.6–22.2%), which is not different from the natural fetal loss rate for twin gestation after 17 weeks as estimated from 12 392 twin pregnancies collected in Japan [161].

Amniocentesis for the diagnosis of microbial invasion of the amniotic cavity

The amniotic cavity is normally sterile and isolation of any microorganisms from the amniotic fluid therefore constitutes evidence of microbial invasion. The traditional diagnosis of intra-amniotic infection relied on the recognition of chorioamnionitis, a clinical syndrome characterized by a combination of maternal fever, uterine tenderness, foul-smelling amniotic fluid, leucocytosis, and maternal and fetal tachycardia. However, microbial invasion of the amniotic cavity (MIAC) can exist even in the absence of clinical signs and symptoms of infection and has been implicated as a causative phenomenon for both preterm labour with intact membranes and premature rupture of the membranes (PROM) [162,163].

The combined experience in the diagnosis of MIAC with amniocentesis in women with preterm labour and intact membranes is presented in Table 8.5 [163,164–184]. Only 37.2% (51/214) of the women with a positive

amniotic fluid culture developed clinical chorioamnionitis. Likewise, combined data show that only 32.8% (42/298) of the patients with PROM and MIAC had clinical evidence of chorioamnionitis (Table 8.6) [180,182,185–191]. Early identification of MIAC is a desirable goal since neonates born to mothers with intra-amniotic infection are at higher risk for infectious complications [162,165–168,185]. Since it is clear that clinical chorioamnionitis is neither a sensitive nor specific criterion to identify MIAC, the modern diagnosis of intrauterine infection relies upon examination of the amniotic fluid [162,192].

The method of amniotic fluid collection for microbiological studies is critical. The two techniques that have been used are transabdominal amniocentesis and transcervical retrieval either by needle puncturing of the membranes or by aspiration through an intrauterine catheter. Transcervical amniotic fluid collection is associated with an unacceptable risk of contamination with vaginal flora and is contraindicated in patients with preterm labour and patients with PROM but not in labour [193]. Successful retrieval of amniotic fluid by ultrasonographically monitored amniocentesis is possible in virtually all patients with preterm labour with intact membranes and over 90% of patients with preterm PROM, making it the method of choice to obtain amniotic fluid from these patients.

Amniotic fluid culture

Amniotic fluid culture is the gold standard against which all other methods for the detection of microbial invasion of the amniotic cavity are tested. The prevalence of intra-amniotic infection, as assessed by positive amniotic fluid cultures obtained by amniocentesis, is presented in Tables 8.5 and 8.6 [163–191]. Infection is more prevalent among women with preterm PROM than with preterm labour and intact membranes (33.8% [298/882] vs. 12.8% (215/1675); $P < 0.001$). The reason why infection leads to PROM in some cases and to preterm labour in others remains to be answered, but probably lies in the regulation of the different components of the decidual inflammatory reaction. Decidual inflammation leads to the generation of proteases capable of degrading the extracellular matrix of the chorioamniotic membranes and to the formation of agents that induce myometrial contractility (i.e. prostaglandins). Differential

Table 8.5 Microbial invasion of the amniotic cavity in women with preterm labour and intact membranes as determined by amniotic fluid studies obtained by transabdominal amniocentesis.

Reference	Year	No. of patients	Positive culture*	Mycoplasma culture	Clinical chorioamnionitis*	Preterm delivery in patients with positive cultures*	Relative risk (95% confidence limits)
Miller et al. [169]	1980	23	11 (47.8)	No	8 (72.7)		
Bobitt et al. [170]	1981	31	8 (25.8)	No	6 (75.0)	7 (87.5)	
Wallace & Herrick [171]	1981	25	3 (12.0)	No	1 (33.3)		
Hammed et al. [172]	1984	37	4 (10.8)	No	3 (75.0)	3 (75.0)	0.27 (0.05–1.5)
Wahbeh et al. [173]	1984	33	7 (21.2)	No	2 (28.5)	5 (71.4)	
Wieble & Randall [174]	1985	35	1 (2.9)	No	1 (100)		
Leigh & Garite [175]	1986	59	7 (11.8)	No	4 (57.1)	7 (100.0)	
Gravett et al. [176]	1986	54	13 (24.0)	Yes	5 (38.5)	5 (38.5)	
Iams et al. [177]	1987	5	0 (0.0)	Yes			
Duff & Kopelman [166]	1987	24	1 (4.2)	No	0 (0)	0 (0)	
Romero et al. [178]	1988	41	4 (9.8)	Yes	1 (14.3)		
Skoll et al. [167]	1989	127	7 (5.5)	No	3 (12.5)	7 (100)	1.57 (1.2–1.9)
Romero et al. [163]	1989	264	24 (9.1)	Yes		24 (100)	2.75 (2.3–3.2)
Romero et al. [168]	1990	109	15/109 (13.8)	Yes		15 (100)	
Romero et al. [179]	1990	168	23/168 (13.6)	Yes	4 (17.4)		
Gauthier et al. [180]	1991	113	18/113 (16)	Yes			
Romero et al. [181]	1991	195	25/195 (12.8)	Yes	4 (16.0)	25 (100)	1.97 (1.6–2.3)
Coultrip et al. [182]	1992	107	12/107 (12.1)	Yes	7 (63.6)		
Watts et al. [183]	1992	105	20/105 (19.0)	Yes		17 (85)	
Romero et al. [184]	1993	120	11/120 (13.2)	Yes	2 (18.2)	11 (100)	
Total		1675	214/1675 (12.8)		51 (37.2)	101 (86.3)	2.00 (1.2–1.9)

* Numbers in parentheses are percentages.

Table 8.6 Microbial invasion of the amniotic cavity in women with preterm premature rupture of membranes as determined by amniotic fluid studies obtained by transabdominal amniocentesis.

Reference	Year	No. of patients	Positive culture*	Mycoplasma culture	Success rate (%)	Clinical chorioamnionitis*	Neonatal infection*
Garite et al. [185]	1979	59	9/30 (30.0)	No	51	6 (66.6)	2 (22.2)
Garite & Freeman [164]	1984	207	20/86 (23.2)	No	42	1 (55.0)	5 (25.0)
Cotton et al. [165]	1984	61	6/41 (14.6)	No	67	6/6 (100.0)	1 (16.6)
Broekhuizen et al. [186]	1985	79	15/53 (23.3)	No	67	3 (20.0)	8 (53.3)
Vintzileos et al. [187]	1986	54	12/54 (22.2)	No		2 (16.6)	4 (33.3)
Feinstein et al. [188]	1986	73	12/50 (20.0)	No	68	6 (50.0)	5 (41.6)
Romero et al. [189]	1988	230	65/221 (29.4)	Yes	95		5 (12.8)
Gauthier et al. [180]	1991	91	49/91 (53.8)	Yes			
Coultrip et al. [182]	1992	29	12/29 (41.4)	Yes		3 (25.0)	
Gauthier et al. [190]	1992	117	56/117 (47.9)	Yes			20 (47.6)
Romero et al. [191]	1993	110	42/110 (38.2)	Yes		5 (11.9)	
Total		1110	298/882 (33.8)		79	42/128 (32.8)	50/155 (32.2)

* Numbers in parentheses are percentages.

expression of these two distinct biological functions (protease and uterotonic activity) could result in either PROM or preterm labour. Preterm PROM without preterm labour associated with infection may occur when the main effect of inflammation is degradation of extracellular matrix components. Under these circumstances, prostaglandins or other uterotonic agents are not produced in sufficient quantities to simulate myometrial contractility or, alternatively, the myometrium does not respond to these agents. On the other hand, preterm labour with intact membranes in the setting of infection may be viewed as a condition in which the myometrium is the most responsive tissue to the inflammatory phenomenon. This may result from a preferential expression and bioavailability of uterotonic agents (i.e. prostaglandins) rather than proteolytic activity during the course of the intrauterine inflammatory reaction.

Once the amniotic fluid is obtained it should be immediately transported to the laboratory in a capped syringe. Keeping air from the specimen and plating as soon as possible maximizes the recovery of anaerobic microorganisms. The fluid should be cultured for aerobic and anaerobic bacteria as well as for *Mycoplasma* sp. Institutions that do not have a microbiology laboratory open 24 hours a day can use either an oxygen-free transport system or bedside plating with a portable anaerobic jar.

The most common microbial isolates from the amniotic cavity from women with preterm labour and intact membranes are *U. urealyticum*, *Fusobacterium* sp. and *M. hominis* [192,194,195]. Of patients with microbial invasion 50% have more than one microorganism isolated from the amniotic cavity. The inoculum size varies considerably and in 71% of the cases more than 10^5 colony-forming units (cfu)/ml are found [163]. It is noteworthy that the most common microorganisms responsible for neonatal sepsis are not frequently isolated from the amniotic fluid. The role of *Chlamydia trachomatis* as an intrauterine pathogen has not been clearly elucidated. This microorganism is an important cause of cervicitis and has been recently isolated from the amniotic fluid [196,197]. A case of congenital pneumonia caused by *C. trachomatis* suggests that this microorganism may be capable of causing ascending intra-amniotic infection [196]. The uncertainty about the role of *C. trachomatis* in the aetiology of microbial invasion and intrauterine infection may be related to difficulties in isolating the microorganism from amniotic fluid with standard culture techniques. The use of polymerase chain reaction to detect specific sequences of this microorganism should help resolve this question [198].

Rapid diagnosis of intra-amniotic infection

Although amniotic fluid culture is considered the gold standard for the diagnosis of intra-amniotic infection, the results take several days and are not immediately available for clinical management decisions. This has led investigators to search for alternative rapid methods to detect MIAC. Currently, Gram stain, white blood cell count and glucose concentration in the amniotic fluid are the most widely used tests for the rapid diagnosis of MIAC. Other tests, such as the acridine orange stain [199,200], *Limulus* amoebocyte lysate assay [201–204], gas–liquid chromatography of bacterial products [205–208] and evaluation of leucocyte esterase activity [209–213], have also been proposed as rapid diagnostic tests for the diagnosis of intra-amniotic infection. However, either they are more difficult to perform or they have a lower diagnostic accuracy compared with the other tests mentioned above and have been abandoned from clinical practice. Assessment of the concentration of cytokines in the amniotic fluid has recently emerged as a powerful indicator of MIAC, amniocentesis-to-delivery interval and neonatal complications in both preterm labour and PROM. These tests are discussed in detail below.

AMNIOTIC FLUID GRAM STAIN

Gram stain is an inexpensive test available in every medical institution. It is the most frequently used rapid diagnostic test for detecting intra-amniotic infection. The slide should be prepared with fluid obtained directly from the syringe because swabs absorb both fluid and cells, decreasing the likelihood of observing organisms in a smear or culture. Although centrifugation of amniotic fluid at low speed does not improve the detection of bacteria with Gram stain [180], the use of a cytocentrifuge increases the concentration of bacteria in the sediment and probably improves the sensitivity of the test [193].

Table 8.7 shows the accuracy of Gram stain as a diagnostic tool to detect microbial invasion of the amniotic cavity according to 20 published reports [163–167,169,170,172,178–182,184,185,188,190,191,214]. The overall sensitivity of the method was 48.5% (196/404), the specificity 97.6% (1526/1563), the positive predictive value 84.1% (196/233) and the negative predictive value 88.0% (1526/1734). In one report, the sensitivity increased from 44.8% to 80% with an increase in the inoculum size to more than 10^5 cfu/ml [178]. It is important to note that *Mycoplasma* organisms, which are frequently isolated in the amniotic fluid of patients in preterm labour with intact membranes or PROM, are not visible with Gram stain. In spite of the wide range of diagnostic accuracy indexes (see Table

8.7), Gram stain continues to be the standard against which other tests are compared [183].

AMNIOTIC FLUID WHITE BLOOD CELL COUNT

Neutrophils are not normally present in the amniotic fluid of women who are not in labour. Their presence in the amniotic fluid indicates the existence of an inflammatory reaction, usually caused by an intra-amniotic infection.

In a study of 195 patients in preterm labour and intact membranes who underwent amniocentesis for assessment of the microbiological status of the amniotic cavity, a white blood cell count $\geq 50/mm^3$ had a sensitivity of 80% (20/25) and a specificity of 87.6% (149/170) to

Table 8.7 Sensitivity, specificity, positive predictive value and negative predictive value of Gram stain in detecting microbial invasion of the amniotic cavity in patients with preterm labour and intact membranes and patients with premature rupture of membranes.

Reference	Year	No. of patients	Sensitivity (%)	Specificity (%)	Positive predictive value (%)	Negative predictive value (%)
Garite *et al.* [185]	1979	30	55.6	100.0	100.0	84.0
Miller *et al.* [169]	1980	37	84.6	87.5	78.6	91.3
Bobitt *et al.* [170]	1981	31	75.0	100.0	100.0	92.0
Garite & Freeman [164]	1984	86	70.0	97.0	87.5	91.4
Cotton *et al.* [165]	1984	41	83.3	97.1	83.3	97.1
Zlatnik *et al.* [214]	1984	29	25.0	95.2	66.7	76.7
Hammed *et al.* [172]	1984	37	50.0	100.0	100.0	94.2
Broekhuizen *et al.* [186]	1985	53	60.0	94.7	81.8	85.7
Feinstein *et al.* [188]	1986	50	75.0	92.1	75.0	92.1
Duff & Kopelman [166]	1987	18	0.0	100.0	0.0	94.4
Romero *et al.* [178]	1988	114	44.8	97.7	86.7	83.8
Skoll *et al.* [167]	1989	127	28.6	95.8	28.6	95.8
Romero *et al.* [163]	1989	264	79.2	99.6	95.0	98.0
Romero *et al.* [179]	1990	168	65.2	99.3	93.7	94.7
Gauthier *et al.* [180]	1991	204	29.9	97.8	87.0	74.0
Romero *et al.* [181]	1991	195	48.0	98.8	85.7	92.8
Coultrip & Grossman [182]	1992	136	84.6	93.8	65.0	90.5
Gauthier & Meyer [190]	1992	117	39.0	97.0	92.0	63.0
Romero *et al.* [184]	1993	120	63.6	99.8	87.5	96.4
Romero *et al.* [191]	1993	110	23.8	98.5	90.9	67.8
Total		1967	48.5 (196/404)	97.6 (1526/1563)	84.1 (196/233)	88.0 (1526/1734)

* The criteria for the diagnosis of intra-amniotic infection in this study included both a positive amniotic fluid culture and a placental pathological condition that revealed polymorphonuclear leucocytes that extended through the fetal membranes and/or the umbilical cord.

detect those patients with a positive amniotic fluid culture [181]. Although the sensitivity was higher than Gram stain (80% vs. 48%, $P < 0.05$), the trade-off was a lower specificity (87.6% vs. 98.8%, $P < 0.05$) and thus a high false-positive rate (12.4%). An important observation of this study was that 88% (15/17) of all patients with an amniotic fluid white blood cell count $\geq 50/mm^3$ and 66.3% (10/13) of patients with histological evidence of chorioamnionitis but a negative amniotic fluid culture had a spontaneous preterm delivery. Therefore, independently of the culture result, an elevated amniotic fluid white blood cell count identified a subset of patients at risk for failure to respond to tocolysis and impending preterm delivery. Possible explanations for this include microbiological invasion of the amniotic cavity undetected by the microbiological techniques employed in the study or neutrophil recruitment into the amniotic cavity driven by a non-infectious process. In spite of the high sensitivity of the test, its high false-positive rate may result in the withholding of tocolysis for fetuses who would benefit from the therapy. The visualization of white blood cells in conjunction with bacteria in a Gram stain reduces the possibility that a stain is false-positive because of contamination.

GLUCOSE CONCENTRATION IN THE
AMNIOTIC FLUID

Glucose determination is a rapid inexpensive test that does not require sophisticated interpretation by trained personnel and has been extensively used to diagnose infection in other body fluids (i.e. cerebrospinal fluid, pleural fluid and synovial fluid) [215,216]. Amniotic fluid glucose concentration is significantly lower in patients with intra-amniotic infection (identified by a positive amniotic fluid culture or clinical signs of infection) and in patients with PROM who develop clinical infection [182]. The mechanism involved in the decrease of amniotic fluid glucose concentration during infection is unclear but probably involves glucose metabolism by both microorganisms and polymorphonuclear leucocytes [182].

In a study of 168 patients with preterm labour and intact membranes we were able to demonstrate that patients with a positive amniotic fluid culture for microorganisms had significantly lower median amniotic fluid glucose concentrations than patients with negative amniotic fluid cultures (median 11 mg/dl, range 2–30 vs. median 28 mg/dl, range 3–74; $P < 0.001$) [179]. An amniotic fluid glucose concentration below 14 mg/dl had a sensitivity of 86.9% (20/23), a specificity of 91.7% (133/145), a positive predictive value of 62.5% (20/32) and a negative predictive value of 97.8% (133/136) for the detection of a positive amniotic fluid culture. Of interest, 75% (9/12) of the patients with a low amniotic fluid glucose concentration and a negative amniotic fluid culture delivered prematurely despite intravenous tocolysis and 85.7% (6/7) of the placentas examined in this group had histological evidence of inflammatory lesions in the placenta.

These results were independently confirmed by other investigators, although using different cut-off levels [180,182,217]. The efficacy of amniotic fluid glucose concentration in diagnosing intra-amniotic infection is displayed in Table 8.8. As in the case of white blood cell count, the false-positive rates with amniotic fluid glucose concentration were high. Again, the seriousness of a false-positive result is dependent on the action taken after an abnormal test result. If the course of action is to perform a Gram stain of the amniotic fluid, then a false-positive result is not clinically problematic. However, if the course of action is to deliver a preterm neonate that is believed to be infected, then there is the potential for serious consequences [180].

AMNIOTIC FLUID MACROPHAGE-DERIVED
CYTOKINES

A growing body of evidence indicates that preterm parturition in the setting of infection is associated with dramatic alterations in the amniotic fluid concentration of several cytokines. These cytokines are produced during the course of macrophage activation by microbial products and include interleukin (IL)-1 [218,219], tumour necrosis factor (TNF) [220,221], IL-6 [168,184,191,222] and IL-8 [223,224].

IL-6 has been studied as a rapid test for the detection of microbial invasion of the amniotic cavity [168,184,191,222]. In a group of 146 patients with preterm labour and intact membranes, patients with a positive amniotic fluid culture had a significantly higher median amniotic fluid IL-6 concentration than patients with a negative culture (median 91.2 ng/ml, range 0.9–

Table 8.8 Sensitivity, specificity, positive predictive value and negative predictive value of amniotic fluid glucose concentrations in predicting microbial invasion of the amniotic cavity as assessed by positive amniotic fluid culture.

Reference	No. of patients	Cut-off level (mg/dL)	Sensitivity* (%)	Specificity* (%)	Positive predictive value* (%)	Negative predictive value* (%)
Romero et al. [179]	168	<14	86.9 (20/23)	91.7 (133/145)	62.5 (20/32)	97.8 (133/136)
Gauthier et al. [180]	204	≤16	79 (53/67)	94.2 (129/137)	86.9 (53/61)	90.2 (129/143)
Kirshon et al. [217]	39	<10	75 (9/12)	100 (27/27)	100 (9/9)	90 (27/30)
Coultrip & Grossman [182]	107	≤10	85	90	57	97
Coultrip & Grossman [182]	107	≤15	92	75	36	98
Coultrip & Grossman [182]	29	≤10	85	90	57	97
Coultrip & Grossman [182]	29	≤15	92	75	36	98
Romero et al. [184]†	120	≤14	81.82 (9/11)	81.65 (89/109)	53.85 (7/13)	96.26 (103/107)
Romero et al. [191]‡	110	≤14	71.4 (30/42)	51.5 (35/68)	47.6 (30/63)	74.5 (35/47)
Romero et al. [191]‡	110	<10	57.1 (24/42)	73.5 (50/68)	57.1 (24/42)	73.5 (50/68)

* Figures in parentheses refer to actual numbers of samples.
† All patients enrolled were in preterm labour with intact membranes.
‡ All patients enrolled had premature rupture of the membranes.

437 vs. median 0.4 ng/ml, range <0.3–195; $P < 0.0001$) [222]. A cut-off level of ≥11.3 ng/ml had a sensitivity of 93.3% (14/15), specificity of 91.6% (120/131), positive predictive value of 56.0% (14/25) and negative predictive value of 99.1% (120/121) in the detection of MIAC. The sensitivity of amniotic fluid IL-6 determinations was higher than the amniotic fluid Gram stain but the difference did not reach statistical significance (93.3% [14/15] vs. 73.3% [11/15], $P = 0.33$). Also, a shorter amniocentesis-to-delivery interval was observed in patients with high amniotic fluid IL-6 concentrations. Finally, amniotic fluid IL-6 concentrations were found to be significantly higher among pregnancies ending in neonatal death compared with those with surviving neonates (median 19.7 ng/ml, range <0.3–437 vs. median 0.4 ng/ml, range <0.3–280; $P < 0.005$). Therefore, IL-6 has been proposed as a sensitive indicator of microbial invasion of the amniotic cavity, amniocentesis-to-delivery interval and neonatal complications in both preterm labour and PROM.

The diagnostic performance of amniotic fluid IL-6 in detecting microbial invasion of the amniotic cavity was compared to the amniotic fluid glucose concentration, white blood cell count and Gram stain in patients with preterm labour and intact membranes [184] and patients with PROM [191]. Figure 8.5 shows the receiver–operator characteristic (ROC) curves for amniotic fluid white blood cell count ≥50/mm³, glucose ≤14 mg/dl,

IL-6 ≥11.3 ng/ml and Gram stain in the detection of a positive amniotic fluid culture in patients with preterm labour and intact membranes. IL-6 was the most sensitive test for the detection of MIAC (100%), followed by glucose concentration (81.8%), white blood cell count (63.6%) and Gram stain (63.6%). The most specific test was Gram stain (99.1%), followed by white blood cell count (94.5%), IL-6 (82.6%) and glucose (81.6%). However, among the four tests evaluated, only IL-6 had a significant relationship with the amniocentesis-to-delivery interval and the development of neonatal complications as described above.

Figure 8.6 shows the ROC curves for amniotic fluid Gram stain, white blood cell count ≥50/mm³, glucose concentration ≤14 mg/dl and IL-6 ≥7.9 ng/ml in the detection of a positive amniotic fluid culture in patients with preterm PROM. Once again, IL-6 was the most sensitive test for the detection of microbial invasion of the amniotic cavity (80.9%), followed by white blood cell count (57.1%), glucose concentration (57.1%) and Gram stain (23.8%). The most specific test for the detection of microbial invasion of the amniotic cavity was Gram stain (98.5%) followed by white blood cell count (77.9%), IL-6 (75%) and glucose concentration (73.5%). IL-6 was the only test that had significant clinical value in the prediction of amniocentesis-to-delivery interval and neonatal complications in this series.

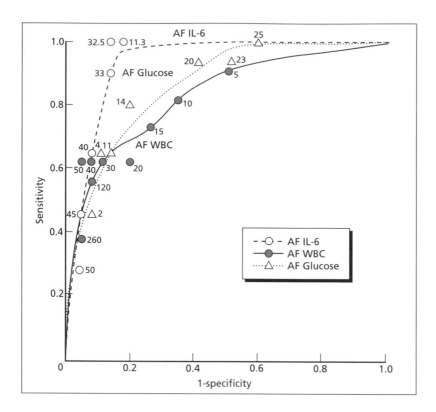

Fig. 8.5 Receiver–operator characteristic curves for amniotic fluid white blood cell count, glucose and IL-6 in the detection of a positive amniotic fluid culture in patients with preterm labour with intact membranes. Area under the curve: for amniotic fluid white blood cell count 0.846, SE 0.065, $P < 0.000001$; for amniotic fluid glucose concentration 0.873, SE 0.054, $P < 0.000001$; and for amniotic fluid IL-6 concentration 0.927, SE 0.024, $P < 0.000001$. (From Romero *et al.* [184] with permission.)

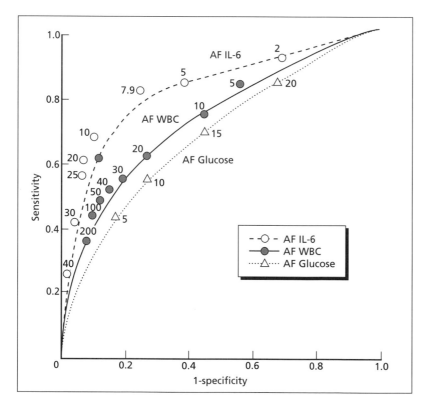

Fig. 8.6 Receiver–operator characteristic curves for amniotic fluid white blood cell count, glucose and IL-6 in the detection of a positive amniotic fluid culture in patients with preterm premature rupture of membranes. Area under the curve: for amniotic fluid white blood cell count 0.70, SE 0.05, $P < 0.000005$; for amniotic fluid glucose concentration 0.68, SE 0.05, $P < 0.000005$; and for amniotic fluid IL-6 concentration 0.80, SE 0.05, $P < 0.000001$. (From Romero *et al.* [191] with permission.)

Although, at the present time, the concentration of IL-6 in the amniotic fluid is the rapid test with the best diagnostic performance, Gram stain is currently the only rapid test upon which clinical decisions can be made while waiting for culture results. Whether administration of antibiotics to patients with a high index of suspicion for microbial invasion of the amniotic cavity would prolong the interval from amniocentesis to delivery is a question that awaits further evaluation.

References

1 Prochownick L. Beitrage zur lehre vorn fruchtwasser und seiner entstehung. *Arch Gynaekol* 1877;**11**:304.

2 Lambl D. Ein seltener fall van hydramnios. *Centralbl Gynaekol* 1881;**5**:329.

3 Von Shatz F. Eine besondre art von einseitiger polyhydramnie mit anderseitiger oligohydramnie bie eineiigen zweillingen. *Archiv Gynaekol* 1882;**19**:329.

4 Menees TO, Miller JD, Holly LE. Amniography: preliminary report. *Am J Roentgenol* 1930;**24**:363.

5 Boero E. Intra-amniotiques. *Semana Medica Buenos Aires*, 15 August 1935.

6 Aburel ME. Le declanchement du travail par injections intra-amniotiques du serum sale hypertonique. *Gynecologie et Obstetrique* 1937;**36**:393.

7 Bevis DCA. Composition of liquor amnii in haemolytic disease of newborn. *Lancet* 1950;**ii**:443.

8 Fuchs F, Riis P. Antenatal sex determination. *Nature* 1956;**177**:330.

9 Jeffcoate TNA, Fliegner JRH, Russel SH, Davis JC, Wade AP. Diagnosis of the adrenogenital syndrome before birth. *Lancet* 1965;**ii**:553.

10 Steele MW, Breg WR Jr. Chromosome analysis of human amniotic-fluid cells. *Lancet* 1966;**i**:383.

11 Jacobson CB, Barter RH. Intrauterine diagnosis and management of genetic defects. *Am J Obstet Gynecol* 1967;**99**:796.

12 Valenti C, Schutta EJ, Kehaty T. Prenatal diagnosis of Down's syndrome. *Lancet* 1965;**ii**:553.

13 Roger R. Mid trimester genetic amniocentesis with simultaneous ultrasound guidance. *J Clin Ultrasound* 1985;**13**:371.

14 Romero R. Sonographically monitored amniocentesis to decrease intraoperative complications. *Obstet Gynecol* 1985;**166**:427.

15 Kennerknecht I, Krämer S, Grab D, Terinde R. Evaluation of amniotic fluid cell filtration: an experimental approach to early amniocentesis. *Prenat Diagn* 1993;**13**:247.

16 Johnson A, Godmilow L. Genetic amniocentesis at 14 weeks or less. *Clin Obstet Gynecol* 1988;**31**:345.

17 Kerber S, Held KR. Early cytogenetic amniocentesis: 4 years experience. *Prenat Diagn* 1993;**13**:21.

18 Romero R, Pupkin M, Oyarzun E, Ávila C, Moretti M. Amniocentesis. In: Fleischer AF, Romero R, Manning FA, Jeanty P, James E (eds) *The Principles and Practice of Ultrasound in Obstetrics and Gynecology.* Appleton & Lange: Norwalk, Connecticut, 1991:439–453.

19 Henry G, Peakman DC, Winkler W, O'Connor K. Amniocentesis before 15 weeks instead of CVS for earlier prenatal cytogenetic diagnosis. *Am J Hum Genet* 1985;**37** (Suppl):abstract no. 650.

20 Luthardt FW, Luthy DA, Karp LE, Hickok DE, Resta RG. Prospective evaluation of early amniocentesis for prenatal diagnosis. *Am J Hum Genet* 1985;**37** (Suppl): abstract no. 659.

21 Luthy DA, Hickok DE, Luthardt FW, Resta RG. A prospective evaluation of early amniocentesis: an alternative to chorionic villus sampling for prenatal diagnosis. Abstract no. 268 presented at the 6th Annual Meeting of the Society of Perinatal Obstetricians in San Antonio, Texas, 30 January to 1 February 1986.

22 Hanson FW, Zorn EM, Tennant FR, Marianos S, Samuels S. Amniocentesis before 15 weeks' gestation: outcome, risks and technical problems. *Am J Obstet Gynecol* 1987;**157**:1524.

23 Miller WA, Davies RM, Thayer BA, Peakman D. Success, safety and accuracy of early amniocentesis (EA). *Am J Hum Genet* 1987;**41** (Suppl):abstract no. 835.

24 Weiner CP. Genetic amniocentesis at, or before, 14.0 weeks gestation. Abstract no. 63 presented at the 7th Annual Meeting of the Society of Perinatal Obstetricians in Lake Buena Vista, Florida, 5–7 February 1987.

25 Godmilow L, Weiner S, Dunn LK. Genetic amniocentesis performed between 12 and 14 weeks gestation. *Am J Hum Genet* 1987;**41** (Suppl):abstract no. 818.

26 Benacerraf BR, Greene MF, Saltzman DH *et al.* Early amniocentesis for prenatal cytogenetic evaluation. *Radiology* 1988;**169**:709.

27 Lowe CY, Alexander D, Bryla D, Seigel D. *The NICHD amniocentesis registry. The safety and accuracy of midtrimester amniocentesis.* US Department of Health, Education, and Welfare, DHEW Publication No. (NIH) 1978:78–190.

28 Evans MI, Drugan A, Koppitch FC, Zador IE, Sacks AJ, Sokol RJ. Genetic diagnosis in the first trimester: the norm for the 1990s. *Am J Obstet Gynecol* 1989;**160**:1332.

29 Elejalde BR, de Elejalde MM, Acuna JM, Thelen D, Trujillo C, Karrmann M. Prospective study of amniocentesis performed between weeks 9 and 16 of gestation: its feasibility, risks, complications and use in early genetic prenatal diagnosis. *Am J Med Genet* 1990;**35**:188–196.

30 Penso CA, Frigoletto FD Jr. Early amniocentesis. *Semin Perinatol* 1990;**14**:465.

31 Penso CA, Sandstrom MM, Garber MF, Ladoulis M, Stryker JM, Benacerraf BB. Early amniocentesis: report of 407 cases with neonatal follow-up. *Obstet Gynecol* 1990;**76**:1032.

32 Hanson FW, Happ RL, Tennant FR, Hune S, Peterson AG. Ultrasonography-guided early amniocentesis in singleton pregnancies. *Am J Obstet Gynecol* 1990;**162**: 1376–1383.

33 Nevin J, Nevin NC, Dornan JC, Sim D, Armstrong MJ. Early amniocentesis: experience of 222 consecutive patients, 1987–1988. *Prenat Diagn* 1990;**10**:79.

34 Stripparo L, Buscaglia M, Longatti L *et al*. Genetic amniocentesis: 505 cases performed before the sixteenth week of gestation. *Prenat Diagn* 1990;**10**:359.

35 Klapp J, Nicolaides KH, Hager HD *et al*. Early amniocentesis. *Geburtshilfe Frauenheilkd* 1990;**50**: 443.

36 Lindner C, Huneke B, Masson D, Schlotfeldt T, Kerber S, Held KR. Early amniocentesis for cytogenetic diagnosis. *Geburtshilfe Frauenheilkd* 1990;**50**:954.

37 Byrne DL, Marks K, Braude PR, Nicolaides KH. Amnifiltration in the first trimester: feasibility, technical aspects and cytological outcome. *Ultrasound Obstet Gynecol* 1991;**1**:320.

38 Hacket GA, Smith JH, Rebello MT *et al*. Early amniocentesis at 11–14 weeks' gestation for the prenatal diagnosis of fetal chromosomal abnormality: a clinical evaluation. *Prenat Diagn* 1991;**11**: 311–315.

39 Jorgensen FS, Bang J, Lind A, Christensen B, Lundsteen C, Philip J. Genetic amniocentesis at 7–14 weeks of gestation. *Prenat Diagn* 1992;**12**:277.

40 Henry GP, Miller WA. Early amniocentesis. *J Reprod Med* 1992;**37**:396.

41 Djalali M, Barbi G, Kennerknecht I, Terinde R. Introduction of early amniocentesis to routine prenatal diagnosis. *Prenat Diagn* 1992;**12**:661.

42 Assel BG, Lewis SM, Dickerman LH, Park VM, Jassani MN. Single-operator comparison of early and mid-second trimester amniocentesis. *Obstet Gynecol* 1992;**79**:940.

43 Bombard T, Rigson T. Prospective pilot evaluation of early (11–14 weeks' gestation) amniocentesis in 75 patients. *Milit Med* 1992;**158**:339.

44 Hanson FW, Tennant F, Hune S, Brookhyser K. Early amniocentesis: outcome, risks, and technical problems at ≤12.8 weeks. *Am J Obstet Gynecol* 1992;**166**: 1707.

45 Frydman R, Pons JC, Borghi E *et al*. Per-urethral transvesical first-trimester amniocentesis. *Eur J Obstet Gynecol Reprod Biol* 1993;**48**:99.

46 Eiben B, Goebel R, Rutt G, Jaspers KD, Hansen S, Hammans W. Early amniocentesis between the 12th–14th week of pregnancy. Clinical experiences with 1100 cases. *Geburtshilfe Frauenheilkd* 1993;**53**:554.

47 Gabriel R, Harika G, Carre-Pigeon F, Quereux C, Wahl P. Amniocentesis to study the fetal karyotype before 16 weeks of amenorrhea. Prospective study comparing it with conventional amniocentesis. *J Gynecol Obstet Biol Reprod* 1993;**22**:169.

48 Elias S, Simpson JL. Amniocentesis. In: Simpson JL, Elias S (eds) *Essentials of Prenatal Diagnosis*. New York: Churchill Livingstone, 1993:27–44.

49 Shalev E, Weiner E, Yanai N, Shneur Y, Cohen H. Comparison of first-trimester transvaginal amniocentesis with chorionic villus sampling and mid-trimester amniocentesis. *Prenat Diagn* 1994;**14**:279.

50 Andreasen E, Kristoffersen T. Incidence of spontaneous abortion after amniocentesis: influence of placental localization and past obstetric and gynecologic history. *Am J Perinatol* 1989;**6**:268.

51 Kappel B, Nielsen J, Brogaard Hansen K, Mikkelsen M, Therkelsen AAJ. Spontaneous abortion following mid-trimester amniocentesis. Clinical significance of placental perforation and blood-stained amniotic fluid. *Br J Obstet Gynaecol* 1987;**94**:50.

52 Simpson NE, Dallaire L, Miller JR *et al*. Prenatal diagnosis of genetic disease in Canada: report of a collaborative study. *Can Med Assoc J* 1976;**115**:739.

53 Lowe CU, Alexander D, Bryla D, Seigel D. *The NICHD amniocentesis registry. The safety and accuracy of mid-trimester amniocentesis*. US Department of Health, Education, and Welfare, DHEW Publication No. (NIH) 78–190, 1978.

54 Hurwitz SR, Nageotte MP. Amniocentesis needle with improved sonographic visualization. *Radiology* 1989; **171**:576.

55 Romero R, Jeanty P, Reece EA, Grannum P, Bracken M, Berkowitz R, Hobbins JC. Sonographically monitored amniocentesis to decrease intraoperative complications. *Obstet Gynecol* 1984;**65**:426.

56 Jeanty P, Rodesch F, Romero R, Venus I, Hobbins JC. How to improve your amniocentesis technique. *Am J Obstet Gynecol* 1983;**146**:593.

57 Wald NJ, Cuckle HS. Amniotic fluid alpha-fetoprotein measurement in antenatal diagnosis of anencephaly and open spina bifida in early pregnancy. *Lancet* 1979;ii: 651.

58 Byrne D, Marks K, Azar G, Nicolaides K. Randomized study of early amniocentesis versus chorionic villus sampling: a technical and cytogenetic comparison of 650 patients. *Ultrasound Obstet Gynecol* 1991;**1**:235.

59 Nelson MM, Emery AEH. Amniotic fluid cells: prenatal sex prediction and culture. *Br Med J* 1970;**1**:523.

60 Bowerman RA, Barclay ML. A new technique to overcome

failed second trimester amniocentesis due to membrane tenting. *Obstet Gynecol* 1987;70:806.

61 Platt LD, Manning FA, Lemay M. Real-time B-scan-directed amniocentesis. *Am J Obstet Gynecol* 1978;130: 700.

62 Benacerraf BR, Frigoletto FD. Amniocentesis under continuous ultrasound guidance: a series of 232 cases. *Obstet Gynecol* 1983;62:760.

63 McArdle CR, Cohen W, Nickerson C, Hann LE. The use of ultrasound in evaluating problems and complications of genetic amniocentesis. *J Clin Ultrasound* 1983;11: 427.

64 Sundberg K, Smidt-Jensen S, Philip J. Amniocentesis with increased cell yield, obtained by filtration and reinjection of the amniotic fluid. *Ultrasound Obstet Gynecol* 1991;1: 91–94.

65 Byrne DL, Nicolaides KH. Amniotic fluid temperature change during first trimester amnifiltration. *Br J Obstet Gynaecol* 1994;101:340.

66 Klein SA, Gobbo PN, Ristuccia PA, Epstein H, Cunha BA. Diagnostic amniocentesis and bacteremia. *J Hosp Infect* 1987;9:81.

67 Ager RP, Oliver RWA. *The Risks of Midtrimester Amniocentesis.* University of Salford, Lancashire, 1986.

68 Cassel GH, Davis RO, Waites KB *et al.* Isolation of *Mycoplasma hominis* and *Ureaplasma urealyticum* from amniotic fluid at 16–20 weeks of gestation: potential effect on outcome of pregnancy. *Sex Transm Dis* 1983;10: 294.

69 Gray DJ, Robinson H, Malone J, Thomson RB. Adverse outcome in pregnancy following amniotic fluid isolation of *Ureaplasma urealyticum. Prenat Diagn* 1992;12:111–117.

70 Tabor A, Madsen M, Obel EB, Philip J, Bang J, Norgaard-Pedersen B. Randomized controlled trial of genetic amniocentesis in 4606 low-risk women. *Lancet* 1986;i: 1287.

71 Williamson RA, Varner MW, Grant SS. Reduction in amniocentesis risks using a real-time needle guide procedure. *Obstet Gynecol* 1985;65:751.

72 Wiener JJ, Farrow A, Farrow SC. Audit of amniocentesis from a district general hospital: is it worth it? *Br Med J* 1990;300:1243.

73 Misenhimer HR. Fetal hemorrhage associated with amniocentesis. *Am J Obstet Gynecol* 1966;94:1133.

74 Creasman WT, Lawrence RA, Thiede HA. Fetal complications of amniocentesis. *JAMA* 1968;205:91.

75 Berner HW, Seisler EP, Barlow J. Fetal cardiac tamponade: a complication of amniocentesis. *Obstet Gynecol* 1972;40: 599.

76 Cross HE, Maumenee AE. Ocular trauma during amniocentesis. *Am J Obstet Gynecol* 1973;116:582.

77 Grove CS, Trombetta GC, Amstey MS. Fetal complications of amniocentesis. *Am J Obstet Gynecol* 1973;115: 1154.

78 Egley CC. Laceration of fetal spleen during amniocentesis. *Am J Obstet Gynecol* 1973;116:582.

79 Cook LN, Shott RJ, Andrews BF. Fetal complications of diagnostic amniocentesis: a review and report of a case with pneumothorax. *Pediatrics* 1974;53:421.

80 Fortin JG, Lemire J. Une complication oculaire de l'amniocentese. *Can J Ophthalmol* 1975;10:511.

81 Lamb MP. Gangrene of a fetal limb due to amniocentesis. *Br J Obstet Gynaecol* 1975;82:829.

82 Broome DL, Wilson MG, Weiss B, Kellogg B. Needle puncture of fetus: a complication of second-trimester amniocentesis. *Am J Obstet Gynecol* 1976;126:247.

83 Karp LE, Hayden PW. Fetal puncture during midtrimester amniocentesis. *Obstet Gynecol* 1977;49:115.

84 Rickwood AMK. A case of ileal atresia and ileo-cutaneous fistula caused by amniocentesis. *J Pediatr* 1977;92: 312.

85 Cromie WJ, Bates RD, Duckett JW Jr. Penetrating renal trauma in the neonate. *J Urol* 1978;119:259.

86 Young PE, Matson MR, Jones OW. Fetal exsanguination and other vascular injuries from midtrimester genetic amniocentesis. *Am J Obstet Gynecol* 1977;129:21.

87 Rehder H. Fetal limb deformities due to amniotic constrictions (a possible consequence of preceding amniocentesis). *Pathol Res Pract* 1978;162:316.

88 Rehder H, Weitzel H. Intrauterine amputations after amniocentesis. *Lancet* 1978;i:382.

89 Epley SL, Hanson JW, Cruikshank DP. Fetal injury with midtrimester diagnostic amniocentesis. *Obstet Gynecol* 1979;53:77.

90 Swift PGF, Driscoll IB, Vowles KDJ. Neonatal small-bowel obstruction associated with amniocentesis. *Br Med J* 1979;1:720.

91 Merin S, Beyth Y. Uniocular congenital blindness as a complication of midtrimester amniocentesis. *Am J Ophthalmol* 1980;89:299.

92 Youroukos S, Papedelis F, Matsaniotis N. Porencephalic cysts after amniocentesis. *Arch Dis Child* 1980;89: 299.

93 Therkelsen AJ, Rehder H. Intestinal atresia caused by second trimester amniocentesis. *Br J Obstet Gynaecol* 1981;88:559.

94 Moessinger AC, Blanc WA, Byrne J, Andrews D, Warburton D, Bloom A. Amniotic band syndrome associated with amniocentesis. *Am J Obstet Gynecol* 1981;141: 588.

95 Isenberg SJ, Heckenlively JR. Traumatized eye with retinal damage from amniocentesis. *J Pediatr Ophthamol Strabismus* 1985;22:65.

96 Achiron R, Zakut H. Fetal hemothorax complicating

amniocentesis: antenatal sonographic diagnosis. *Acta Obstet Gynecol Scand* 1986;**65**:869.

97 Kohn G. The amniotic band syndrome: a possible complication of amniocentesis. *Prenat Diagn* 1987;**7**:303.

98 Morin LRM, Bonan J, Vendrolini G, Bourgeois C. Sonography of umbilical cord hematoma following genetic amniocentesis. *Acta Obstet Gynecol Scand* 1987;**66**:669.

99 Admoni M, Ben Ezra D. Ocular trauma following amniocentesis as the cause of leukocoria. *J Pediatr Ophthalmol Strabismus* 1988;**25**:196.

100 Chong SKF, Levitt GA, Lawson J, Lloyd U, Newman CGH. Subarachnoid cyst with hydrocephalus: a complication of mid-trimester amniocentesis. *Prenat Diagn* 1989;**9**:677.

101 Naylor G, Roper JP, Willshaw HE. Ophthalmic complications of amniocentesis. *Eye* 1990;**4**:845.

102 Ledbetter DJ, Hall DG. Traumatic arteriovenous fistula: a complication of amniocentesis: *J Pediatr Surg* 1992;**27**:720.

103 Rummelt V, Rummelt C, Naumann GOH. Congenital nonpigmented epithelial iris cyst after amniocentesis: clinicopathologic report on two children. *Ophthalmology* 1993;**100**:776.

104 Chayen S (ed). An assessment of the hazards of amniocentesis. Report to the Medical Research Council by their Working Party on Amniocentesis. *Br J Obstet Gynaecol* 1978;**85** (Suppl 2):1.

105 NICHD National Registry for Amniocentesis Study Group. Midtrimester amniocentesis for prenatal diagnosis, safety and accuracy. *JAMA* 1976;**236**:1471.

106 Wald NJ, Terzian E, Vickers PA. Congenital talipes and hip malformation in relation to amniocentesis: a case–control study. *Lancet* 1983;**ii**:246.

107 Hislop A, Fairweather DVI. Amniocentesis and lung growth: an animal experiment with clinical implications. *Lancet* 1982;**ii**:1271.

108 Hislop A, Fairweather DVI, Blackwell RJ, Howard S. The effect of amniocentesis and drainage of amniotic fluid on lung development in *Macaca fascicularis*. *Br J Obstet Gynaecol* 1984;**91**:835.

109 Thompson PJ, Greenough A, Nicolaides KH. Lung volume measured by functional residual capacity in infants following first trimester amniocentesis or chorion villus sampling. *Br J Obstet Gynaecol* 1992;**99**:479.

110 Vyas H, Milner AD, Hopkin IE. Amniocentesis and fetal lung development. *Arch Dis Child* 1982;**57**:627.

111 Gold RB, Goyert GL, Schwartz DB, Evans MI, Seabolt LA. Conservative management of second-trimester post-amniocentesis fluid leakage. *Obstet Gynecol* 1989;**74**:745.

112 Ron M, Cohen T, Yaffe H, Beyth Y. The clinical significance of blood-contaminated midtrimester amniocentesis. *Acta Obstet Gynecol Scand* 1982;**61**:43.

113 Harwood LM. Detection of foetal cells in maternal circulation. *J Med Lab Technol* 1961;**19**:19.

114 Mennuti MT, Brummond W, Crombleholme WR, Schwarz RH, Arvan DA. Fetal–maternal bleeding associated with genetic amniocentesis. *Obstet Gynecol* 1980;**55**:48.

115 Lele AS, Carmody PJ, Hurd ME, O'Leary JA. Feto-maternal bleeding following diagnostic amniocentesis. *Obstet Gynecol* 1982;**60**:60.

116 Robinson A, Bowes W, Droegemueller W *et al*. Intrauterine diagnosis: potential complications. *Am J Obstet Gynecol* 1973;**116**:937.

117 Karp LE, Schiller HS. Meconium staining of amniotic fluid at midtrimester amniocentesis. *Obstet Gynecol* 1977;**50** (Suppl):47.

118 Seller M. Dark-brown amniotic fluid. *Lancet* 1977;**ii**:983.

119 King CR, Prescott G, Pernoll M. Significance of meconium in midtrimester diagnostic amniocentesis. *Am J Obstet Gynecol* 1978;**132**:667.

120 Bartsch FK, Lundberg J, Wahlstrom J. One thousand consecutive midtrimester amniocenteses. *Obstet Gynecol* 1980;**55**:305.

121 Crandal BF, Joward J, Lebhez TB, Rubinstein M, Sample WF, Sarti D. Follow-up of 2000 second-trimester amniocenteses. *Obstet Gynecol* 1980;**56**:625.

122 Svigos JM, Stewart-Rattray SF, Pridmore BR. Meconium-stained liquor at second trimester amniocentesis: is it significant? *Aust NZ J Obstet Gynaecol* 1981;**21**:5.

123 Cruikshank DP, Varner MW, Curikshank JE, Grant SS, Donnelly E. Midtrimester amniocentesis. *Am J Obstet Gynecol* 1983;**146**:204.

124 Hankis GDV, Rowe J, Quirk JG, Trubey R, Strickland DM. Significance of brown and/or green amniotic fluid at the time of second trimester genetic amniocentesis. *Obstet Gynecol* 1984;**64**:353.

125 Allen R. The significance of meconium in midtrimester genetic amniocentesis. *Am J Obstet Gynecol* 1985;**152**:413.

126 Hess LW, Anderson RL, Golbus MS. Significance of opaque discolored amniotic fluid at second-trimester amniocentesis. *Obstet Gynecol* 1986;**67**:44.

127 Zorn EM, Hanson FW, Greve LC, Phelps-Sandall B, Tennant FR. Analysis of the significance of discolored amniotic fluid detected at midtrimester amniocentesis. *Am J Obstet Gynecol* 1986;**154**:1234.

128 Abramovich DR, Gray ES. Physiologic fetal defecation in midpregnancy. *Obstet Gynecol* 1982;**60**:294.

129 Byrne D, Azar G, Nicolaides KH. Why cell culture is successful after early amniocentesis. *Fetal Diagn Ther* 1991;**6**:84.

130 American College of Obstetricians and Gynecologists. *Management of isoimmunization in pregnancy*. ACOG Technical Bulletin 80. Washington, DC: ACOG, 1984.

131 Murray JC, Karp LD, Williamson RA, Cheng EY, Luthy DA. Rh isoimmunization related to amniocentesis. *Am J Med Genet* 1983;**16**:527.

132 Henry G, Wexler P, Robinson A. Rh-immune globulin after amniocentesis for genetic diagnosis. *Obstet Gynecol* 1976;**48**:557.

133 Golbus MS, Stephens JD, Cann HM, Mann J, Hensleigh PA. Rh isoimmunization following genetic amniocentesis. *Prenat Diagn* 1982;**2**:149.

134 Frigoletto FD, Jewett JF, Konugres AA (eds). *Rh Hemolytic Disease: New Strategy for Eradication.* Boston: GK Hall, 1982.

135 Hunter AGW, Cox DM. Counseling problems when twins are discovered at genetic amniocentesis. *Clin Genet* 1979;**16**:34.

136 Rodeck CH, Mibashan RS, Campbell S. Selective feticide of the affected twin by fetoscopic air embolism. *Prenat Diagn* 1982;**2**:189.

137 Elias S, Gerbie AB, Simpson JL, Nadler HL, Sabbagha RE, Shkolnik A. Genetic amniocentesis in twin gestations. *Am J Obstet Gynecol* 1980;**138**:169.

138 Bang J, Niesel H, Philip J. Prenatal karyotyping of twins by ultrasonically guided amniocentesis. *Am J Obstet Gynecol* 1975;**123**:695.

139 Tabsh K. Genetic amniocentesis in multiple gestation: a new technique to diagnose monoamniotic twins. *Obstet Gynecol* 1990;**75**:296.

140 Jeanty P, Shah D, Roussis P. Single-needle insertion in twin amniocentesis. *J Ultrasound Med* 1990;**9**:511.

141 Bahado Singh R, Schmitt R, Hobbins JC. New technique for genetic amniocentesis in twins. *Obstet Gynecol* 1992;**79**:304.

142 Fribourg S. Safety of intraamniotic injection of indigo carmine. *Am J Obstet Gynecol* 1981;**140**:350.

143 Goldstein AI, Stills SM. Midtrimester amniocentesis in twin pregnancies. *Obstet Gynecol* 1983;**62**:659.

144 Wolf DA, Scheible FW, Young PE, Matson MR. Genetic amniocentesis in multiple pregnancy. *J Clin Ultrasound* 1979;**7**:208.

145 Filkins K, Russo J, Brown T, Schmerler S, Searle B. Genetic amniocentesis in multiple gestations. *Prenat Diagn* 1984;**4**:223.

146 Librach CL, Doran TA, Benzie RJ, Jones JM. Genetic amniocentesis in seventy twin pregnancies. *Am J Obstet Gynecol* 1984;**148**:585.

147 Di-Lin L, Zhi-Long Z. Double sacs amniocentesis in twin pregnancy. *Chin Med J* 1984;**97**:465.

148 Tabsh KMA, Crandall B, Lebherz TB, Howard J. Genetic amniocentesis in twin pregnancy. *Obstet Gynecol* 1985;**65**:843.

149 Pjipers L, Jahoda MGJ, Vosters RPL, Niermeijer MF, Sachs ES. Genetic amniocentesis in twin pregnancies. *Br J Obstet Gynaecol* 1988;**95**:323.

150 Pruggmayer MRK, Jahoda MGJ, Vand der Pol JG *et al.* Genetic amniocentesis in twin pregnancies: results of a multicenter study of 529 patients. *Ultrasound Obstet Gynecol* 1992;**2**:6.

151 Wapner RJ, Johnson A, Davis G, Urban A, Morgan P, Jackson L. Prenatal diagnosis in twin gestations: a comparison between second-trimester amniocentesis and first-trimester chorionic villus sampling. *Obstet Gynecol* 1993;**82**:49.

152 Nicolini U, Monni G. Intestinal obstruction in babies exposed *in utero* to methylene blue. *Lancet* 1990;**336**:1258.

153 Beekhuis JR, De Bruijn HWA, Van Lith JMM, Matingh A. Second trimester amniocentesis in twin pregnancies: maternal haemoglobin as a dye marker to differentiate diamniotic twins. *Br J Obstet Gynaecol* 1992;**99**:126.

154 Bovicelli L, Michelacci L, Rizzo N *et al.* Genetic amniocentesis in twin pregnancy. *Prenat Diagn* 1983;**3**:101.

155 Palle C, Andersen J, Tabor A, Lauritsen J, Bang I, Philip J. Increased risk of abortion after genetic amniocentesis in twin pregnancies. *Prenat Diagn* 1983;**3**:83.

156 Kappel B, Nielsen J, Hansen KB, Mikkelsen M, Therkelsen AAJ. Spontaneous abortion following mid-trimester amniocentesis. Clinical significance of placental perforation and blood-stained amniotic fluid. *Br J Obstet Gynaecol* 1987;**94**:50.

157 Grau P, Tabsh K, Crandall B. Genetic amniocentesis in twin gestation. *Am J Hum Genet* 1989;**xx**:A259.

158 Pruggmayer M, Bartels I, Rauskolb R, Osmers R. Abortrisiko nach genetischer Amniozentese im II. Trimenon be Zwillingsschwangerschaften. *Geburtshilfe Frauenheilkd* 1990;**50**:810.

159 Pruggmayer M, Baumann P, Schüttel H *et al.* Incidence of abortion after genetic amniocentesis in twin pregnancies. *Prenat Diagn* 1991;**11**:637.

160 Anderson RL, Goldberg JD, Golbus MS. Prenatal diagnosis in multiple gestation: 20 years' experience with amniocentesis. *Prenat Diagn* 1991;**11**:263.

161 Imaizumi Y, Asaka A, Inouye E. Analysis of multiple birth rates in Japan VII. Rates of spontaneous and induced terminations of pregnancy in twins. *Jpn J Hum Genet* 1982;**27**:235.

162 Romero R, Mazor M. Infection and preterm labor. *Clin Obstet Gynecol* 1988;**31**:554.

163 Romero R, Sirtori M, Oyarzun E *et al.* Infection and labor. V. Prevalence, microbiology, and clinical significance of intraamniotic infection in women with preterm labor and intact membranes. *Am J Obstet Gynecol* 1989;**161**:817–824.

164 Garite TJ, Freeman RK. Chorioamnionitis in the pre-term gestation. *Obstet Gynecol* 1984;**63**:38.

165 Cotton DB, Hill LM, Strassner HT *et al*. Use of amniocentesis in preterm gestation with ruptured membranes. *Obstet Gynecol* 1984;63:38.

166 Duff P, Kopelman JN. Subclinical intraamniotic infection in asymptomatic patients with refractory preterm labor. *Obstet Gynecol* 1987;69:756.

167 Skoll MA, Moretti ML, Sibai BM. The incidence of positive amniotic fluid cultures in patients in preterm labor with intact membranes. *Am J Obstet Gynecol* 1989;161:813.

168 Romero R, Avila C, Santhanam U, Sehgal PB. Amniotic fluid interleukin-6 in preterm labor. Association with infection. *J Clin Invest* 1990;85:1392.

169 Miller JM Jr, Hill GB, Welt SL *et al*. Bacterial colonization of amniotic fluid in the presence of ruptured membranes. *Am J Obstet Gynecol* 1980;137:151.

170 Bobitt JR, Hayslip CC, Damato JD. Amniotic fluid infection as determined by transabdominal amniocentesis in patients with intact membranes in premature labor. *Am J Obstet Gynecol* 1981;140:947.

171 Wallace RL, Herrick CN. Amniocentesis in the evaluation of premature labor. *Obstet Gynecol* 1981;57:483.

172 Hammed C, Tejani N, Verma UL *et al*. Silent chorioamnionitis as a cause of preterm labor refractory to tocolytic therapy. *Am J Obstet Gynecol* 1984;149:726.

173 Wahbeh CJ, Hill GB, Eden RD *et al*. Intra-amniotic bacterial colonization in premature labor. *Am J Obstet Gynecol* 1984;148:739.

174 Weible DR, Randall HW. Evaluation of amniotic fluid in preterm labor with intact membranes. *J Reprod Med* 1985;30:777.

175 Leigh J, Garite TJ. Amniocentesis and the management of premature labor. *Obstet Gynecol* 1986;67:500.

176 Gravett MG, Hummel D, Eschenbach DA *et al*. Preterm labor associated with subclinical amniotic fluid infection and with bacterial vaginosis. *Obstet Gynecol* 1986;67:229.

177 Iams JD, Clapp DH, Contos DA *et al*. Does extra-amniotic infection cause preterm labor? Gas–liquid chromatography studies of amniotic fluid in amnionitis, preterm labor, and normal controls. *Obstet Gynecol* 1987;70:365.

178 Romero R, Emamian M, Quintero R *et al*. The value and limitations of the Gram stain examination in the diagnosis of intraamniotic infection. *Am J Obstet Gynecol* 1988;159:114.

179 Romero R, Jimenez C, Lohda AK *et al*. Amniotic fluid glucose concentration: a rapid and simple method for the detection of intraamniotic infection in preterm labor. *Am J Obstet Gynecol* 1990;163:968.

180 Gauthier DW, Meyer WJ, Bieniarz A. Correlation of amniotic fluid glucose concentration and intraamniotic infection in patients with preterm labor or premature rupture of membranes. *Am J Obstet Gynecol* 1991;165:1105.

181 Romero R, Quintero R, Nores J *et al*. Amnniotic fluid white blood cell count: a rapid and simple test to diagnose microbial invasion of the amniotic cavity and predict preterm delivery. *Am J Obstet Gynecol* 1991;165:821.

182 Coultrip LL, Grossman JH. Evaluation of rapid diagnostic tests in the detection of microbial invasion of the amniotic cavity. *Am J Obstet Gynecol* 1992;167:1231.

183 Watts DH, Krohn MA, Hillier SL, Eschenbach DA. The association of occult amniotic fluid infection with gestational age and neonatal outcome among women in preterm labor. *Obstet Gynecol* 1992;79:351.

184 Romero R, Yoon BH, Mazor M *et al*. The diagnostic and prognostic value of amniotic fluid white blood cell count, glucose, interleukin-6 and Gram stain in patients with preterm labor and intact membranes. *Am J Obstet Gynecol* 1993;169:805–816.

185 Garite TJ, Freeman RK, Linzey EM *et al*. The use of amniocentesis in patients with premature rupture of membranes. *Obstet Gynecol* 1979;54:226.

186 Broekhuizen FF, Gilman M, Hamilton PR. Amniocentesis for Gram stain culture in preterm premature rupture of the membranes. *Obstet Gynecol* 1985;66:316.

187 Vintzileos AM, Campbell WA, Nochimson DJ *et al*. Qualitative amniotic fluid volume versus amniocentesis in predicting infection in preterm rupture of the membranes. *Obstet Gynecol* 1986;67:579.

188 Feinstein ST, Vintzileos AM, Lodeiro JG *et al*. Amniocentesis with premature rupture of membranes. *Obstet Gynecol* 1986;68:147.

189 Romero R, Quintero R, Oyarzyn E *et al*. Intraamniotic infection and the onset of labor in preterm premature rupture of membranes. *Am J Obstet Gynecol* 1988;159:661.

190 Gauthier DW, Meyer W. Comparison of Gram stain, leukocyte esterase activity and amniotic fluid glucose concentration in predicting amniotic fluid culture results in preterm premature rupture of membranes. *Am J Obstet Gynecol* 1992;167:1092.

191 Romero R, Yoon BH, Mazor M *et al*. A comparative study of the diagnostic performance of amniotic fluid glucose, white blood cell count, interleukin-6, and Gram stain in the detection of microbial invasion in patients with preterm premature rupture of membranes. *Am J Obstet Gynecol* 1993;169:839.

192 Romero R, Mazor M, Wu YK *et al*. Infection in the pathogenesis of preterm labor. *Semin Perinatol* 1988;12:262.

193 Romero R, Oyarzun E, Avila C, Mazor M. Diagnosis of intra-amniotic infection. *Contemp Obstet Gynecol* 1989;33:99.

194 Altshuler G, Hyde S. Clinicopathologic consideration of fusobacteria chorioamnionitis. *Acta Obstet Gynecol Scand* 1988;67:513.

195 Hillier SL, Martius J, Krohn M *et al*. A case–control study of chorioamnionic infection and histologic chorioamnionitis in prematurity. *N Engl J Med* 1988;319: 972.

196 Thorp JM Jr, Katz VL, Fowler LJ, Kurtzman JT, Bowes WA Jr. Fetal death from chlamydial infection across intact amniotic membranes. *Am J Obstet Gynecol* 1989;161: 1245–1246.

197 Thomas GB, Jones J, Sbarra A *et al*. Isolation of *Chlamydia trachomatis* from the amniotic fluid. *Obstet Gynecol* 1990;76:519.

198 Pao CC, Lao S-M, Whang H-C *et al*. Intraamniotic detection of *Chlamydia trachomatis* deoxyribonucleic acid sequences by polymerase chain reaction. *Am J Obstet Gynecol* 1991;164:1295.

199 Romero R, Emamian M, Quintero R *et al*. Diagnosis of intrauterine infection: the acridine orange stain. *Am J Perinatol* 1989;6:41.

200 Smaron MF, Boonlayangoor S, Zierdt CH. Detection of *Mycoplasma hominis* septicemia by radiometric blood culture. *J Clin Microbiol* 1985;21:198.

201 Romero R, Kadar N, Hobbins JC, Duff GW. Infection and labor: the detection of endotoxin in amniotic fluid. *Am J Obstet Gynecol* 1987;157:815.

202 Ten Cate JW, Buller HR, Sturk A *et al*. Editorial commentary in bacterial endotoxin: structure, biomedical significance and detection with the *Limulus* amebotyc lysate test. In: Ten Cate JW, Buller HR, Sturk A *et al*. (eds) *Progress in Clinical and Biological Research*. New York: Alan R Liss, 1985:15.

203 Wildfeuber A, Heymer B, Schleifer KH *et al*. Investigation on the specificity of the *Limulus* test for the detection of endotoxin. *Appl Microbiol* 1974;28:269.

204 Ray TL, Hanson A, Ray LF *et al*. Purification of mannan from *Candida albicans* which activates serum complement. *J Invest Dermatol* 1979;73:269.

205 Gorbach SL, Mayhew JW, Bartlett JG *et al*. Rapid diagnosis of anaerobic infections by direct gas–liquid chromatography of clinical specimens. *J Clin Invest* 1976;57:478.

206 Phillips KD, Tearle PV, Willis AT. Rapid diagnosis of anaerobic infections by gas–liquid chromatography of clinical material. *J Clin Pathol* 1976;29:428.

207 Wust J. Presumptive diagnosis of anaerobic bacteremia by gas–liquid chromatography of blood cultures. *J Clin Microbiol* 1977;6:586.

208 Romer R, Scharf K, Mazor M *et al*. The clinical value of gas–liquid chromatography in the detection of intra-amniotic microbial invasion. *Obstet Gynecol* 1988;72: 44.

209 Kusumi RK, Grover PJ, Kunin CM. Rapid detection of pyuria by leukocyte esterase activity. *JAMA* 1981;245: 1653.

210 Marquette GP, Dillard T, Bietla S *et al*. The validity of the leukocyte esterase reagent test strip in detecting significant leukocyturia. *Am J Obstet Gynecol* 1985;153: 888.

211 Whitehurst R, Clapp DH, Iams JD *et al*. Correlation of leukocyte esterase activity (LEA), nitrites, inflammatory exudates, and culture in amniotic fluid of patients with clinical chorioamnionitis. Abstract no. 25P presented at the 31st Annual Meeting of the Society of Gynecologic Investigation, San Francisco, California, 21–24 March 1984.

212 Egley CC, Katz VL, Herbert WNP. Leukocyte esterase: a simple bedside test for the detection of bacterial colonization of amniotic fluid. *Am J Obstet Gynecol* 1988;159:120.

213 Romero R, Emamian M, Wan M *et al*. The value of the leukocyte esterase test in diagnosing intra-amniotic infection. *Am J Perinatol* 1988;5:64.

214 Zlatnik FJ, Cruikshank DP, Petzold CR *et al*. Amniocentesis in the identification of inapparent infection in preterm patients with premature rupture of the membranes. *J Reprod Med* 1984;29:656.

215 Brody JS. Diseases of the pleura, mediastinum, diaphragm and chest wall. In: Wyngaarden JB, Smith LH Jr, (eds) *Cecil Textbook of Medicine*, 17th edn. Philadelphia: WB Saunders, 1985: 447–454.

216 Parker RH. Skeletal infections. In: Hoeprich PD, Jordan MC (eds) *Infectious Diseases*, 4th edn. Philadelphia: JB Lippincott, 1989:1376–1382.

217 Kirshon B, Rosenfeld B, Mari G, Belfort M. Amniotic fluid glucose and intraamniotic infection. *Am J Obstet Gynecol* 1991;164:818.

218 Romero R, Brody DT, Oyarzun E *et al*. Infection and labor. III. Interleukin-1: a signal for the onset of paturition. *Am J Obstet Gynecol* 1989;160:1117.

219 Romero R, Mazor M, Brandt F *et al*. Interleukin-1α and interleukin-1β in human preterm and term parturition. *Am J Reprod Immunol* 1992;27:117.

220 Romero R, Manogue KR, Mitchell MD *et al*. Infection and labor. IV. Cachectin–tumor necrosis factor in the amniotic fluid of women with intraamniotic infection and preterm and term labor. *Am J Obstet Gynecol* 1989.

221 W, Avila C, Copeland D, Williams J. Tumor necrosis factor in preterm and term labor. *Am J Obstet Gynecol* 1992;166:1576.

222 Romero R, Yoon BH, Kenney JS, Gomez R, Allison A, Sehgal P. Amniotic fluid IL-6 determinations are of diagnostic and prognostic value in preterm labor. *Am J Reprod Immunol* 1993;30:167.

223 Romero R, Ceska M, Avila C, Mazor M, Behnke E,

Lindley I. Neutrophil attractant/activating peptide-1/ interleukin-8 in term and preterm parturition. *Am J Obstet Gynecol* 1991;**165**:813.

224 Cherouny P, Pankuch G, Botti J, Appelbaum P. The presence of amniotic fluid leukoattractants accurately identifies histologic chorioamnionitis and predicts tocolytic efficacy in patients with idiopathic preterm labor. *Am J Obstet Gynecol* 1992;**167**:683.

Chapter 9/Ultrasound-guided fetal blood sampling

JOAQUIN SANTOLAYA-FORGAS, DANIEL GAUTHIER,
JEAN-ALAIN BOURNAZEAU and DIDIER LÉMERY

Throughout this book it is demonstrated that ultrasound is a principal diagnostic tool in the medical field of obstetrics and gynaecology. Also, by using ultrasound-guided procedures relatively safe diagnostic and surgical interventions can be performed. Within this field, fetal blood sampling has become important because it has expanded the spectrum of fetal diseases that can be diagnosed prenatally: it allows prenatal comparison of haematological determinations obtained from undisturbed appropriate-for-gestational age and metabolically normal fetuses and those obtained from fetuses affected with specific ultrasonographically determined pathological conditions. Access to the fetal circulation has also permitted the prenatal treatment of some of these fetal diseases and determination of the accuracy of non-invasive prenatal tests to diagnose fetal acidaemia. In this chapter we briefly review the history, indications, technical modalities and methods of monitoring the complications and failure rate of percutaneous ultrasound-guided fetal blood sampling techniques. We use the database of the fetal medicine unit in Clermont-Ferrand as well as published reports. At the fetal medicine unit in Clermont-Ferrand, 1000 percutaneous ultrasound-guided fetal blood sampling procedures were performed from 1984 to 1992 in 802 fetuses of 779 mothers (eight sets of twins and seven successive pregnancies). Mean gestational age at sampling was 28.5 weeks (SD 4.6, range 16–39). Chromosomal analysis (57.9%), prenatal diagnosis of congenital infection (25.2%) and maternal alloimmunization (12.5%) accounted for the majority of the indications in this series (D. Lémery, unpublished data). In addition, in this chapter we comment on alternative diagnostic techniques that have recently been developed and that are making an impact on the indications for percutaneous ultrasound-guided fetal blood sampling.

Historical review of percutaneous fetal blood sampling

Fetal blood sampling procedures were initially described in 1973, although fetoscopy made possible the withdrawal of pure fetal blood only in 1978 [1,2]. Fetoscopy was indicated for the diagnosis of haemoglobinopathies, coagulopathies and white cell disorders. It was performed using a 1.7-mm diameter endoscope that had a poor field of view and was associated with a 5–7% rate of pregnancy wastage. In 1982, the sharper axial and lateral resolution of ultrasound equipment made possible the catheterization of the fetal left ventricle and the intra-abdominal part of the umbilical vein through an ultrasound-guided trocar [3]. In 1983, Daffos et al. [4] described the technique of ultrasound-guided percutaneous umbilical blood sampling (PUBS or cordocentesis) using a 20-gauge needle and this led to a new era in the field of fetal medicine. Intracardiac fetal blood sampling and blood transfusions are no longer considered as initial approaches to the fetal circulation due to their unacceptably high mortality and the damage that may be caused to the cardiac valves and coronary arteries [5]. However, the intracardiac approach should be considered in desperate situations in which intrauterine fetal resuscitation may be required.

Indications for PUBS

Chromosomal analysis and detection of Mendelian genetic diseases

Both amniocentesis and chorionic villous sampling (CVS) may not allow a karyotype report until 7–14 days after tissue sampling. A rapid karyotype result, available within 48–72 hours after sampling, may be provided from fetal lymphocytes obtained by PUBS. PUBS may be indicated in order to provide quick genetic information to patients referred for evaluation of fetal malformations or to confirm or refute mosaicism seen after CVS or amniocentesis. This may be particularly important near the gestational age where elective pregnancy termination is no longer an option. Approximately one of four fetuses in which mosaicism is detected on CVS has two cell lines on their white blood cells. Confirmation of mosaicism confined to the extraembryonic tissue is therefore important for counselling patients with regard to the significance of the CVS result [6]. Fetal blood sampling may also be indicated later in pregnancy, in situations in which a clinical decision must be made with regard to the time and mode of delivery of a severely growth-retarded or malformed fetus. In a study of 936 fetuses with structural anomalies, the overall incidence of chromosomal aberrations was reported to be 12.1% if the anomaly was isolated and 29.2% in cases with multiple anomalies [7]. Trisomies 21, 18 and 13, monosomy X and triploidy accounted for 84% of all chromosomal abnormalities. In this same study, the prevalence of structural chromosomal abnormalities in 108 patients with isolated fetal growth restriction was 6.7%. This increased to 27% if growth restriction was accompanied by polyhydramnios, 31.5% when associated with structural anomalies, and 47% if associated with both polyhydramnios and congenital anomalies. Once again, the most frequent anomalies were trisomies 21, 18 and 13 and triploidy. Similar results have been reported by other authors and have been summarized elsewhere [8]. Knowledge of the fetal karyotype may alter management decisions, both intrapartum and throughout the neonatal period, since the majority of the associated chromosomal abnormalities in viable growth-restricted or malformed fetuses are semi-lethal or carry with them a significant burden to the newborn, family and society.

At the University of Illinois at Chicago, in addition to PUBS we offer patients confronted with these clinical situations an amniocentesis and fluorescence *in situ* hybridization (FISH) for evaluation of the number of chromosomes 21, 18, 13, X and Y. The chromosomal abnormality rate has been 31.8% (7/22 fetuses with structural anomalies). We are finding that the acceptance rate, both for patients and referring physicians, of

this alternative diagnostic technique is progressively increasing, the reasons being that the results can be provided within a similar time range as PUBS, the test is less expensive and the technical complication rate is significantly lower (J. Santolaya-Forgas, unpublished data).

Inherited haematological disorders, such as haemoglobinopathies, coagulopathies and certain congenital immunodeficiencies, can be diagnosed by analysing DNA obtained from chorionic villi or amniocytes [9]. Direct fetal haematological studies may still be the technique of choice for those haematological disorders in which DNA studies on family members are not available or are non-informative. For example, the severe combined immunodeficiency (SCID) syndrome includes a wide range of disorders that can have autosomal recessive or X-linked inheritance. Prenatal diagnosis relies on:
1 enzymatic activity in CVS cells to diagnose those autosomal recessive disorders where there is deficient enzymatic activity [10];
2 nitroblue tetrazolium dye reduction test using fetal neutrophils for the diagnosis of chronic granulomatous disease [11]; and
3 counting specific fetal lymphocyte subpopulations and functional assays for the majority of the remaining disorders [12].
Deficiency of factors V, VII and XIII are associated with a risk of intrauterine or early postnatal haemorrhage. Normal values for the activity of these coagulation factors provide the framework for prenatal diagnosis [13,14].

Diagnosis of congenital viral and parasitic infections

Infections occur in 5–15% of pregnancies and structural damage as a consequence of congenital infection may occur in up to 1–2% of exposed fetuses. Most non-bacterial infections are diagnosed either by isolating the infectious organism or by documenting seroconversion with acquisition of specific antibodies suggestive of recent infection. Intrauterine viral infections usually have more severe consequences when they occur early in gestation and at the time of organogenesis. A study of 103 pregnant women with evidence of rubella infection has shown intrauterine infection rates of 10, 11.8, 2.9 and 6.5% after maternal infection at 1–10, 11–14,

15–19 and 20–29 weeks gestation respectively [15]. Therefore, the risk of congenital viral infection in seropositive pregnant women is relatively low and dependent on gestational age. However, once a viral infection is established little can be done to alter its clinical course and this may be significant. During the second and third trimester, the major concern is disruption of the normal development of the neurological system. Currently, one exception to the lack of opportunity to alter the course of a viral infection is infection with human parvovirus B19, which causes a transitory aplastic crisis that may lead to fetal anaemia, myocarditis, hepatic fibrosis, fetal hydrops and intra-uterine demise. Although spontaneous resolution of non-immune hydrops caused by parvovirus has been observed, fetal blood transfusions can be used to support the fetus during the aplastic crisis [8,16].

Antimicrobial therapy is beneficial in some parasitic diseases. Congenital infection will occur in 5% of pregnancies exposed to *Toxoplasma gondii* and prenatal diagnosis of this infection is possible. Furthermore, if the fetus is infected treatment with pyrimethamine and sulphadiazine has been shown to reduce the incidence of the severe sequelae of the disorder [17].

Direct isolation of organisms from fetal blood or amniotic fluid is still used to diagnose congenital infection. Until recently, indirect ultrasonographic markers were followed throughout pregnancy in an attempt to assess the severity of congenital infections. These indirect markers included growth restriction, cerebral calcifications, hydrocephaly, microcephaly, limb hypoplasia and cardiac defects. Beyond the 20th week of pregnancy, evidence of fetal infection may be supported by quicker but also indirect methods such as the presence of specific IgM antibodies in fetal blood, changes in fetal blood cell count (e.g. thrombocytopenia, erythroblastosis, leucocytosis and eosinophilia) or elevated serum levels of lactic dehydrogenase, γ-glutamyl transferase or interferon [8,17–21]. For example, the combination of these tests can identify 92% of cases of congenital toxoplasmosis. Currently, and in the future, the diagnosis of fetal exposure to an organism will rely on molecular techniques because they are faster and more sensitive. Polymerase chain reaction studies on amniotic fluid have been shown to be highly reliable in detecting certain antenatal viral (e.g. cytomegalovirus, parvovirus) and parasitic (e.g. *T. gondii*) infections

[22,23]. Using hybridization, rubella virus-specific antigens and RNA sequences have also been detected in CVS material [24,25]. However, the rate of false-positives and of actual clinical fetal infection after exposure has not yet been determined. Thus in the diagnosis of fetal infection PUBS is used to assess the severity of fetal involvement, which is important for counselling the patient with regard to the prognosis.

Red blood cell alloimmunization

In Rh(D) alloimmunized mothers, fetal red blood cell D antigenic status can be determined very early in pregnancy by DNA analysis of amniocytes. When amniocentesis is performed for this purpose care should be taken to avoid the placenta since this would greatly increase the risk of fetomaternal haemorrhage, which is known to aggravate the disease process [26–28]. Knowledge of fetal antigenic status before any indirect signs of fetal haemolysis are present allows the preparation of a strategy for clinical management based on the particular obstetrical history and changes of maternal indirect Coombs' titre. At the University of Illinois we perform amniocentesis for determination of Rh(D) status from the 14th week of gestation and offer PUBS for complex alloimmunizations or in the presence of any of the reported indirect signs of fetal haemolysis, since fetal anaemia is the ultimate test of which fetus requires treatment [29] (see Chapters 7 & 9).

Evaluation for fetal thrombocytopenia

Amegakaryocytic thrombocytopenia [30], thrombocytopenia with absent radii (TAR syndrome) [31] and Wiskott–Aldrich syndrome have all been diagnosed using PUBS. Prior to the onset of labour PUBS may also be offered to patients with a positive antiplatelet antibody test and idiopathic thrombocytopenia with normal Ivy bleeding time. Knowledge of the fetal platelet count in this condition may be useful in determining the optimal route of delivery: elective Caesarean section has been recommended for fetuses with a platelet count $< 50\,000/mm^3$ [32]. However, this management plan is not accepted by all authors because the probability of the fetus being severely thrombocytopenic ($< 50\,000/mm^3$) is only about 10%, and also because there is a risk of fetal exsanguination during PUBS if the fetus happens to be severely affected. The latter situation would certainly lead to either pregnancy loss or an emergency, instead of elective, Caesarean delivery with a higher risk of traumatic haemorrhage [33,34]. PUBS should always be used to assess fetal platelet antigenic status and count in those cases in which the mother is alloimmunized to fetal platelet antigens. Usually, the mother is PLA1 antigen negative and HLA-B8,DR3 positive with the father being PLA1 positive [35]. If the fetus is PLA1 positive there is a high risk for fetal thrombocytopenia, with intracranial haemorrhage occurring in up to 10% of cases during pregnancy.

Currently two management strategies have been advocated for alloimmune thrombocytopenia.
1 Diagnostic PUBS is performed at 28 weeks' gestation and serial fetal platelet transfusions at approximately weekly intervals until fetal maturity [36].
2 Diagnostic PUBS and platelet transfusion if necessary at 20 weeks and weekly maternal intravenous γ-globulin administration (1 mg/kg) with or without prednisone. In this plan a second PUBS is repeated at 24 weeks and a third prior to delivery to assess fetal response to the maternal treatment [37].

The controversy is due to the fact that thrombocytopenic fetuses are at higher risk of exsanguination from the cord puncture and therefore the patient should be aware of the increased risk of the procedure in these circumstances.

Evaluation of non-immune hydrops

Ultrasonically, both immune and non-immune hydrops fetalis are similar and characterized by extensive accumulation of fluids in fetal tissues or body cavities, reflecting a massive disturbance of fetal water balance. Because the condition is multifactorial, clinical outcome can be predicted only if the correct aetiology is identified [16,38]. Most cases of non-immune fetal hydrops are due to fetal abnormalities also detected by ultrasound. However, PUBS can help in determining the overall fetal status and its karyotype or possible infectious aetiology. If some understanding of the pathogenic mechanism involved in the development of hydrops is obtained, individualized management plans for the hydropic fetus may be implemented.

Perinatal fetal assessment

Without a doubt PUBS has allowed a better understanding of the types and pathophysiology of intrauterine growth retardation (IUGR). The value of non-invasive testing for the evaluation of antenatal acidaemia and fetal well-being has also been demonstrated.

In fetal life, different tissues of the body grow during periods of rapid cell division. The timing of these periods differs for different tissues. Fetal growth depends on nutrients, hormones, growth factors and oxygen. The main adaptation of the fetus to lack of these is to slow the rate of cell division, especially in those tissues undergoing rapid cell division.

Growth-restricted fetuses have higher serum erythropoietin concentrations than adequate-for-gestational age fetuses [39], and can be hypoxaemic, hypercapnic, hyperlacticaemic and acidotic [40]. A significant correlation has been demonstrated between fetal Po_2 and both maternofetal gradient of glucose and fetal glucose [41,42]. In hypoxaemic growth-restricted fetuses, this suggests an intrinsic limitation of placental transfer over the entire range of maternal glucose concentrations. Low fetal insulin concentrations and blunted insulin response to intravenous glucose loading has been described in growth-restricted fetuses [43]. The hyperglucagonaemia found in growth-restricted fetuses is probably due to chronic activation of pancreatic A cells by long-term hypoglycaemia since it is inversely correlated with glucose, a finding not seen in normal fetuses [44]. Pregnancies complicated with IUGR and hypoxaemia also present a disturbance in both maternal and fetal plasma amino acid profile. Fetal plasma concentration and the fetomaternal ratio of essential amino acids are decreased because of reduced umbilical uptake or perhaps increased fetoplacental consumption, as suggested by increased lactate production. In hypoxaemic growth-restricted fetuses the ratio of non-essential to essential amino acids is increased, suggesting intrauterine starvation [45]. Blood cell membrane fluidity is lower in control fetal cells than in adults and lower in IUGR than control. The mechanism may involve a low cholesterol concentration and a low unsaturated/saturated free fatty acid ratio in fetal blood cell membranes and plasma, in part reflecting nutritional status [46].

Antepartum fetal heart rate monitoring can be performed from the 20th week of pregnancy. Approximately

45% of hypoxaemic 20–26-week fetuses have tachycardia, a baseline fetal heart rate variability of < 5 beats/min and prolonged fetal heart rate decelerations. The biophysical profile score significantly correlates with prenatal acidaemia and we know that fetal heart rate reactivity and fetal breathing movements are the first biophysical activities to disappear in the presence of acidaemia. Lack of fetal tone or gross body movements may identify the most severely acidaemic fetuses [47]. In response to fetal hypoxaemia there is redistribution of fetal blood flow, which may be reflected by decreased urine production and oligohydramnios [48].

Not all ultrasonographically diagnosed growth-restricted fetuses have abnormal umbilical artery blood velocity waveforms. However, we know that IUGR is a significant factor for increasing umbilical artery Doppler indices, and that Doppler indices can predict which of the growth-restricted fetuses are at higher risk of perinatal distress and adverse outcome [49]. Doppler evaluations can help in the identification of growth-restricted fetuses with antepartum hypoxia, acidosis and thrombocytopenia, and therefore those that need close perinatal surveillance [50–53].

Despite all this information, there is no available evidence demonstrating that the biochemical identification of the acidotic fetus by cordocentesis reduces the perinatal mortality and/or morbidity of these growth-restricted fetuses. The decision to deliver such a fetus is still based on protocols that depend on gestational age, fetal weight and non-invasive evaluations of fetal well-being.

Recently, the role of PUBS in the diagnosis of fetal infection in patients with preterm premature rupture of membranes has been investigated and in the majority of cases with positive fetal blood and/or amniotic fluid cultures there is fetal leucocytosis, which indicates active fetal infection that could perhaps be treated with antibiotics [54].

Evaluation and treatment of twin-to-twin transfusion syndrome and twin-reversed arterial perfusion sequence

When severe discordant fetal growth with abnormal amounts of amniotic fluid are detected too early in a multiple pregnancy to allow a safe delivery, the survival is poor [55–57]. Evaluation of discordant growth in multiple pregnancies is reviewed in Chapter 14; however, the authors have reported that when ultrasound and Doppler cannot determine the presence of blood shunting within a monochorionic placenta, a single PUBS determination of serum erythropoietin concentration in the large co-twin may be sufficient to allow the differentiation of discordant twins with placental vascular communications and those with growth discordance due to other causes [58]. Expectant management, amnioreduction, selective feticide and laser ablation of superficial placental vessels in cases with classical signs of twin-to-twin transfusion syndrome are very controversial and selection of the option will depend on gestational age, degree of polyhydramnios, fetal health status and location of the placenta [59].

Twin-reversed perfusion syndrome is a rare anomaly developing during the early stages of pregnancy, with a perinatal mortality in the normal twin as high as 55% [60]. Once again management options are currently controversial, ranging from expectant management to obliteration of the umbilical artery or removal of the acardiac fetus [61].

Technical modalities of PUBS

PUBS is usually performed from the 18th week of pregnancy. PUBS should be performed in referral centres experienced with the technique and in a room prepared for ultrasound-guided interventional procedures. In patients with a viable fetus, the authors perform PUBS in an area with access to an operating room so that a rapid caesarean delivery can be accomplished if fetal distress necessitating delivery occurs. The physician performing the PUBS should (i) be familiar with the patient and her medical history; (ii) have previously performed an ultrasound examination of the patient; (iii) have determined the appropriate diagnostic tests to be performed; and (iv) have counselled the patient on the risks and benefits of PUBS. The ultrasound equipment may vary from centre to centre, although both 5-MHz and 3.5-MHz probes should be available and used according to the characteristics of the patient to allow the optimal visualization of the sampling target. We prefer curvilinear transducers because of their manoeuvrability. Selection of the sampling site basically depends on optimal target visualization, which in turn depends on the patient's body habitus, placental location, fetal position and amniotic fluid volume. PUBS can be performed where the umbilical vein inserts in the placenta, at the intrahepatic portion of the umbilical vein, or in a free loop of umbilical cord. If the placenta is anterior or lateral and the cord insertion is clearly seen and accessible, we prefer sampling the umbilical vein at its placental insertion (Fig. 9.1). If the cord insertion into the placenta is not well seen, operator preference will determine if the alternative target will be the intrahepatic portion of the umbilical vein or a free loop of umbilical cord. At the University of Illinois at Chicago, we use the intrahepatic portion of the umbilical vein because it has the advantages of ensuring a pure fetal blood sample without additional testing, and because in the case of haemorrhage this will occur intraperitoneally and therefore will behave as an autologous transfusion. The intrahepatic portion of the umbilical vein may be used electively in multiple pregnancies to avoid confusion with regard to the origin of the sample [62]. The success rate of sampling the intrahepatic portion of the umbilical vein has been reported to be 91% [63]. On the other hand, while traditional thinking has been that there are many difficulties in sampling a loop of cord, this has not been the experience at the University of Clermont-Ferrand. In our series of 1000 cases, PUBS was performed in a

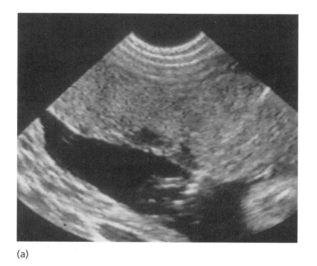

(a)

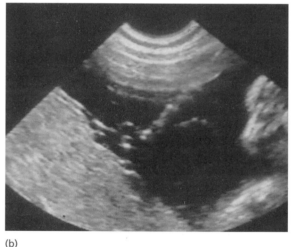

(b)

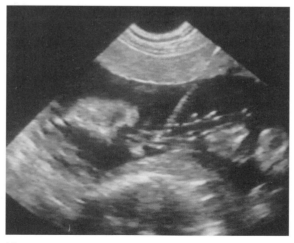

(c)

Fig. 9.1 (a) Anterior placenta, direct access into the umbilical root. (b) Posterior placenta, access to the cord insertion. (c) Free loop puncture.

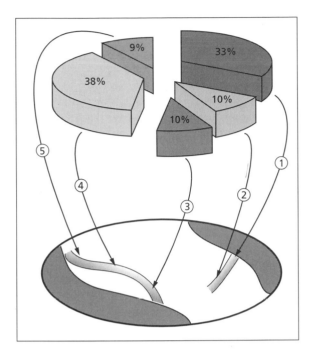

Fig. 9.2 Puncture sites used at the Maternal Fetal Medicine Division, Clermont-Ferrand. 1, Anterior placenta, direct transplacental access to the insertion; 2, anterior placenta, transplacentoamniotic access to the insertion; 3, posterior placenta, access to the insertion; 4, any placental location, free loop access; 5, any placental location, immobilization of a loop.

free loop of cord in 38% of cases, with a failure rate similar to that of the direct anterior approach. To achieve good results the cord must be immobilized between the bevel of the needle and any fetal part, placenta or uterine wall (Fig. 9.2).

Different types of needle guides fixed to the transducers can be used and are optional [64]. Needle guides provide easier access to the sampling site according to some authors [65]; however, others feel that this is true only if the sampling site remains fixed, ideally when PUBS is done through the placenta [66]. In conditions where the target is not fixed, or a transamniotic approach to the cord root is attempted, fetal movements may dislodge the needle. A free-hand technique has the advantage of providing greater flexibility to move the needle and keep the needle path within the ultrasound beam, allowing reinsertion or correction of the path. Also, we prefer the free-hand technique because it allows the operator to move the transducer independently from the needle and therefore monitor the fetal heart during the procedure. Another advantage with the free-hand technique is that the ultrasound probe may be held by a second operator. Of course, this technique works best if the team has experience in working together with ultrasonographic-guided procedures. If not, the single-operator technique is preferable, since perception of three dimensions and coordination of adjustment will be better. If fetal blood sampling ultrasound guidance are performed by the same operator, a trained assistant should aspirate the blood. The two-operator technique may be preferred when PUBS is foreseen to be difficult or for more prolonged procedures such as intrauterine transfusions.

The fetus can be temporarily immobilized by intramuscular or intravenous injection of curare or pancuronium [67,68]. If the fetus is very active, we prefer the intravascular route since it avoids an additional needle insertion. However, this may not always be possible given the position of the fetus and placenta.

For PUBS, the patient should be placed on the examination table in the wedge supine position under no or mild (diazepam) sedation. We do not routinely give prophylactic antibiotics for an anticipated short diagnostic procedure but consider a broad-spectrum antibiotic, such as a second- or third-generation cephalosporin, when a more prolonged procedure is expected. A careful ultrasonographic examination is then performed to confirm the ideal sampling site. The authors would like to stress the importance of this step: taking adequate time to ensure that the target is optimally visualized will usually simplify the procedure greatly and reduce its risk. Colour Doppler may aid in accurately visualizing the cord insertion into the placenta or intrahepatic portion of the umbilical vein and in differentiating the umbilical arteries and vein. Once the operator has determined the target, entrance site and needle path, the maternal abdomen is cleansed with a povidone iodine solution in the same manner as for a laparotomy. A sterile field is prepared and the ultrasound transducer inserted in a sterile plastic sheath. A local anaesthetic may be administered in the selected site for puncture and a small skin incision may be made at the entrance site with a scalpel. Finally, the needle is advanced under continuous ultrasound guidance to the selected target. Most PUBS can be done using a

20- or 22-gauge spinal needle (8.89 cm long). In cases complicated by maternal obesity or polyhydramnios, a longer 20-gauge needle may be needed.

At the time of fetal blood sampling, the venous or arterial origin of the blood can be determined by the direction of the turbulence that is generated after a small infusion of saline. The umbilical vein should be the sampling site, thus avoiding the risk of arterial vasospasm; 2–5 ml of fetal blood are then aspirated using dry or heparinized disposable 1-ml syringes, depending on the tests to be performed. If fetal blood sampling is performed at the placental cord insertion or in a free loop of cord, the fetal origin of the sample must be immediately assessed by evaluating the mean corpuscular volume (MCV) of the fetal sample and comparing this with the MCV of a previously obtained maternal blood sample [69]. Contaminated fetomaternal blood cannot be used for genetic or other diagnostic purposes and dilution with amniotic fluid will clearly alter some of the fetal haematological parameters. Therefore, depending on the indication, determination of white blood cell differential, blood and Rh grouping, anti-I and anti-i antigen, Kleihauer–Betke test, concentration of β-human chorionic gonadotrophin, factors IX and VIIC, and α-fetoprotein levels in maternal and fetal blood may be necessary [8,70]. Sampling from the intrahepatic portion of the umbilical vein avoids the necessity of checking the origin of the sample. Once the purity of the fetal blood sample has been established, the blood should be immediately placed in the appropriate microcontainers for diagnostic and perhaps storage purposes.

Monitoring complications and failure rate of PUBS

It is important to obtain a diagnosis when fetal blood sampling is indicated but it is also important for physicians to evaluate their technical success. An attempt of PUBS should be defined as a single transuterine needle insertion. For technical evaluation, the failure rate should be defined with regard to each attempt rather than with regard to each fetus. Success rate at the first attempt in the 1000 cases presented in the Clermont-Ferrand series (1986–92) was 92.5%. Only two cases were complete failures after two PUBS sessions. Failure includes the inability to obtain fetal blood or

the aspiration of contaminated blood. In 6.7% of the cases performed for rapid karyotyping, there was failure of lymphocyte culture requiring a repeat PUBS or amniocentesis. The PUBS procedure lasted < 5 min in 74% of cases, and > 20 min in only six cases (0.76%). Interestingly, the mean duration of PUBS in patients with subsequent preterm premature rupture of membranes was 17 min while in those cases in which pregnancy continued normally it was 4.8 min (P < 0.001). The 1991 North American PUBS registry [71], which contained data from 7462 diagnostic procedures performed on 6023 patients, reported a mean rate of PUBS failure of 5.7% (range per centre 2–9.4%). The procedure is more difficult early in pregnancy. Boulot et al. [72] have reported a 50% failure rate before 20 weeks, which decreases to 9% after 30 weeks. A failure rate per attempt below 10% may therefore be acceptable depending on maternal characteristics, gestational age at sampling and indications. As reported by others, we feel that experience is one of the main parameters of success, helping to shorten the procedure and to decrease the risks to the pregnancy. In the Clermont-Ferrand series, and analysing data from a single operator, pregnancy loss rate and preterm premature rupture of membranes occurred in 8% and 5% of cases during the first 100 procedures and in 1.5% and 1% of cases during the subsequent 333 procedures (P < 0.01 for both parameters analysed). In case of PUBS failure, the patient should be offered a repeat PUBS attempt within the next 2–7 days depending on gestational age and indication. We would recommend avoidance of immediate serial needling insertions because they may be associated with a higher risk to the pregnancy.

The procedure-related risk of fetal death after PUBS has been estimated at 2% [73]. In the Clermont-Ferrand series, the overall fetal loss rate was 4.34% (range 1.43–9.3% depending on indication: 1.7% for the combination of genetic/infection; 6.2% in IUGR and 9.3% in hydropic fetuses). Elective termination of pregnancy occurred in 15.5% of the cases referred for prenatal diagnosis. The North American PUBS registry reported in 1991 an overall pregnancy loss rate of 1.13% per procedure (range of losses in participating centres 1–6.7%). Maxwell et al. [74] in 1991, also reported that pregnancy loss related to fetal blood sampling differed depending on the indication: (i) prenatal diagnosis in fetuses with normal ultrasound findings,

1%; (ii) prenatal diagnosis in fetuses with structural abnormalities, 7%; (iii) fetal metabolic status assessment, 14%; and (iv) fetuses with non-immune hydrops, 25%. The presumed causes of pregnancy losses following PUBS are chorioamnionitis, premature rupture of membranes, fetal exsanguination, severe bradycardia and thrombosis. Indeed, fetal blood sampling has been associated with risks of fetal bradycardia, amnionitis, premature onset of labour, acute or subacute fetal distress or death due to haematoma of the cord producing tamponade, fetomaternal haemorrhage, abruptio, air embolism and exsanguination into the amniotic cavity [75–80]. Once again, strict asepsis and duration of the procedure are dependent on the experience of the operator and are significant factors for pregnancy loss. In addition, the gestational age at which fetal blood sampling is performed will determine not only the success rate but also the pregnancy loss rate, since a viable fetus may survive premature labour or an emergency Caesarean section if fetal distress is detected during the PUBS procedure or immediately after. In the series reported here, fetal bradycardia was observed by ultrasound in 12.38% of cases and resolved by placing the mother in lateral decubitus and/or administration of oxygen and occasionally maternal intravenous injection of 0.5 mg of atropine sulphate. After an uncomplicated PUBS has been completed, the needle should be gently removed from the sampling site. If a free loop of cord was used, this can be done slowly to try to obtain a little clot in the Wharton's jelly in order to limit the amount of bleeding into the amniotic fluid. If bleeding occurs after PUBS, the type and duration should be recorded noting that bleeding longer than 1 min is abnormal and pulsatile bleeding is of arterial origin. In the Clermont-Ferrand series, bleeding was not observed in 36.8% of cases and lasted < 1 min in 61.8% of cases. Fetal heart rate should be monitored for at least 1 hour. In this series the recording was reactive in 85.66% of cases, bradycardia below 100 beats/min was present in 12.38% of cases and tachycardia above 180 beats/min in 1.96% of cases. Intrauterine fetal demise following an abnormal heart rate recording occurred in 10% of cases, while this occurred in 2.6% of cases with reactive non-stress tests ($P < 0.001$). If the recording is normal the patient may be discharged, with a return visit scheduled within a week either at the same centre or the referring centre. The patient should be able to contact the unit where the PUBS was performed at any time after the procedure in order to discuss possible complications. If the recording is abnormal the patient should remain in hospital, have continuous fetal monitoring and be counselled with regard to the likelihood of an emergency Caesarean section. Anti-D immunoglobulin should be administered when a Rh(D)-positive fetal blood phenotype is diagnosed in a non-alloimmunized Rh(D)-negative mother.

Conclusions

The risk to the fetus of a PUBS procedure can be anticipated by taking note of the circumstances and indications. After complete information is obtained, patients should be offered several sampling procedures comparing the benefit–risk ratio of each.

References

1 Valenti C. Antenatal detection of hemoglobinopathies: a preliminary report. *Am J Obstet Gynecol* 1973;115:851.

2 Rodeck C, Campbell S. Sampling pure fetal blood by fetoscopy in second trimester of pregnancy. *Br Med J* 1978;ii:728.

3 Bang J, Bock J, Trolle D. Ultrasound-guided fetal intravenous transfusion for severe rhesus haemolytic disease. *Br Med J* 1982;284:373.

4 Daffos F, Cappella-Pavlovksy M, Forestier F. A new procedure for fetal blood sampling *in utero*: preliminary results of 53 cases. *Am J Obstet Gynecol* 1983;146:985.

5 Westgren M, Selbing A, Strangenberg M. Fetal intracardiac transfusions in patients with severe rhesus isoimmunization. *Br Med J* 1988;296:885.

6 Ledbetter DH, Martin AO, Verlinsky Y *et al.* Cytogenetic results of chorionic villus sampling: high success rate and diagnostic accuracy in the United States collaborative study. *Am J Obstet Gynecol* 1990;162:495.

7 Eydoux P, Choiset A, Le Porrier N *et al.* Chromosomal prenatal diagnosis: study of 936 cases of intrauterine abnormalities after ultrasound assessment. *Prenat Diagn* 1989;9:255.

8 Romero R, Ghidini A, Santolaya J. Fetal blood sampling. In: Milunsky A (ed) *Genetic Disorders and the Fetus*, 3rd edn. Baltimore: Johns Hopkins University Press, 1995:649.

9 Phillips III J, Vnencak-Jones C. Molecular genetic techniques for prenatal diagnosis. In: Milunsky A (ed) *Genetic Disorders and the Fetus*, 3rd edn. Baltimore: Johns Hopkins University Press, 1994:257.

10 Perignon JL, Durandy A, Peter MO *et al.* Early prenatal

diagnosis of inherited severe immunodeficiencies linked to enzyme deficiencies. *J Pediatr* 1987;**111**:595.

11 Newburger PE, Cohen HJ, Rothchild SB *et al.* Prenatal diagnosis of granulomatous disease. *N Engl J Med* 1979;**300**:178.

12 Lau YL, Levinsky RJ. Prenatal diagnosis and carrier detection in primary immunodeficiency disorders. *Arch Dis Child* 1988;**63**:758.

13 Forestier F, Daffos F, Rainaut M *et al.* Blood chemistry of normal human fetuses at midtrimester of pregnancy. *Pediatr Res* 1987;**21**:579.

14 Daffos F, Forestier F, Kaplan C *et al.* Prenatal diagnosis and management of bleeding disorders with fetal blood sampling. *Am J Obstet Gynecol* 1988;**158**:939.

15 Hsiao-Lin HWA, Ming-Kwang S, Chien-Nan L *et al.* Prenatal diagnosis of congenital rubella infection from maternal rubella in Taiwan. *Obstet Gynecol* 1994;**84**:415.

16 Santolaya J, Warsof SL. Hydrops and associated anomalies. In: Brock, Rodeck, Fergusson-Smith, (eds) *Prenatal Diagnosis and Screening*. Edinburgh: Churchill Livingstone, 1992:329.

17 Daffos F, Forestier F, Capella-Pavlovsky M *et al.* Prenatal management of 746 pregnancies at risk for congenital toxoplasmosis. *N Engl J Med* 1988;**318**:271.

18 Daffos F, Forestier F, Grangeot-Keros L *et al.* Prenatal diagnosis of congenital rubella. *Lancet* 1984;**ii**:1.

19 Lebon P, Daffos F, Checoury A *et al.* Presence of an acid-labile alpha-interferon in sera from fetuses and children with congenital rubella. *J Clin Microbiol* 1985;**21**:775.

20 Desmonts G, Couvreur J. Toxoplasmose congenitale: etude prospective de l'issue de la grossesse chez 542 femmes atteintes de toxoplasmose acquise en cours de gestation. *Ann Pediatr* 1984;**31**:805.

21 Raymond J, Poissonnier MH, Thulliez PH *et al.* Presence of gamma interferon in human acute and congenital toxoplasmosis. *J Clin Microbiol* 1990;**28**:1434.

22 Lynch L, Daffos F, Emanuel D *et al.* Prenatal diagnosis of fetal cytomegalovirus infection. *Am J Obstet Gynecol* 1991;**165**:714.

23 Grover CM, Thulliez O, Remington JS, Boothroyd JC. Rapid prenatal diagnosis of congenital toxoplasma infection by using polymerase chain reaction in amniotic fluid. *J Clin Microbiol* 1990;**28**:2297.

24 Ho-Terry L, Terry GM, Londesborough P *et al.* Diagnosis of fetal rubella infection by nucleic acid hybridization. *J Med Virol* 1988;**24**:175.

25 Ho-Terry L, Terry GM, Londesborough P. Diagnosis of fetal rubella virus infection by polymerase chain reaction. *J Gen Virol* 1990;**71**:1607.

26 Golbus MS, Stephens JD, Cann HM *et al.* Rh isoimmunization following genetic amniocentesis. *Prenat Diagn* 1982;**2**:149.

27 Nicolini U, Kochenour NK, Greco P *et al.* Consequences of fetomaternal haemorrhage after intrauterine transufsion. *Br Med J* 1988;**297**:1379.

28 Bowman JM, Pollock JM, Petereson LE *et al.* Fetomaternal hemorrhage following funipuncture: increase in severity of maternal red-cell alloimmunization. *Obstet Gynecol* 1994;**84**:839.

29 Rodeck CH, Santolaya J, Nicolini U. Management of the fetus with immune hydrops. In: Harrison MR, Golbus MS, Filly RA (eds) *The Unborn Patient: Prenatal Diagnosis and Treatment*, 2nd edn. Philadelphia: Harcourt Brace Jovanovich, WB Saunders, 1990:215.

30 Kaplan C, Daffos F, Forestier F *et al.* Management of alloimmune thrombocytopenia: antenatal diagnosis and *in utero* transfusion of maternal platelets. *Blood* 1988;**72**: 340.

31 Donnenfield AE, Wiseman B, Lavi E *et al.* Prenatal diagnosis of thrombocytopenia absent radius syndrome by ultrasound and cordocentesis. *Prenat Diagn* 1990;**10**:29.

32 Scioscia AL, Grannum PA, Copel JA *et al.* The use of percutaneous umbilical blood sampling in immune thrombocytopenic purpura. *Am J Obstet Gynecol* 1988;**159**:1066.

33 Samuels P, Bussel JB, Braitman LE *et al.* Estimation of the risk of thrombocytopenia in the offspring of prenatal women with presumed immune thrombocytopenic purpura. *N Engl J Med* 1990;**323**:229.

34 Kaplan C, Daffos F, Forestier F *et al.* Fetal platelet counts in thrombocytopenic pregnancy. *Lancet* 1990;**ii**:979.

35 Daffos F. The fetus at risk for thrombocytopenia. In: Harrison MR, Golbus MS, Filly RA (eds) *The Unborn Patient: Prenatal Diagnosis and Treatment*, 2nd edn. Philadelphia: Harcourt Brace Jovanovich, WB Saunders, 1990:210.

36 Nicolini U, Rodeck CH, Kochenour NK *et al. In-utero* platelet transfusion for alloimmune thrombocytopenia. *Lancet* 1988;**ii**:506.

37 Lynch L, Bussel JB, McFarland JG *et al.* Antenatal treatment of alloimmune thrombocytopenia. *Obstet Gynecol* 1992;**80**:67.

38 Santolaya J, Alley D, Jaffe R *et al.* Antenatal classification of hydrops fetalis. *Obstet Gynecol* 1992;**79**:256.

39 Lémery D, Santolaya J, Serre A-F, *et al.* Serum erythropoietin in small-for-gestational age fetuses. *Biol Neonate* 1994;**65**:89–93.

40 Soothill PW, Nicolaides KH, Campbell S. Prenatal asphyxia, hyperlacticaemia, hypoglycaemia, and erythroblastosis in growth retarded fetuses. *Br Med J* **294**:1051–1053.

41 Nicolini U, Hubinont C, Santolaya J *et al.* Maternal–fetal glucose gradient in normal pregnancies and in pregnancies complicated by alloimmunization and fetal growth retardation. *Am J Obstet Gynecol* 1989;**161**:924–927.

42 Economides DL, Proudler A, Nicolaides KH. Blood glucose and oxygen tension levels in small-for-gestational-age fetuses. *Am J Obstet Gynecol* 1989;**160**:385.

43 Nicolini U, Hubinont C, Santolaya J *et al.* Effects of fetal intravenous glucose challenge in normal and growth retarded fetuses. *Horm Metab Res* 1990;22:426.

44 Hubinont C, Nicolini U, Fisk NM *et al.* Endocrine pancreatic function in growth-retarded fetuses. *Obstet Gynecol* 1991;77:541.

45 Economides DL, Nicolaides KH, Gahl WA *et al.* Plasma amino acids in appropriate and small-for-gestational-age fetuses. *Am J Obstet Gynecol* 1989;161:1219.

46 Lemery DJ, Beal V, Vanlieferinghen P, Motta C. Fetal blood cell membrane fluidity in small for gestational age fetuses. *Biol Neonate* 1993;64:7–12.

47 Ribbert LS, Snijders RJM, Nicolaides KH, Visser GHA. Relationship of fetal biophysical profile and blood gas values at cordocentesis in severely growth-retarded fetuses. *Am J Obstet Gynecol* 1990;163:569–571.

48 Nicolaides KH, Peters MT, Vyas S *et al.* Relation of rate of urine production to oxygen tension in small-for-gestational-age fetuses. *Am J Obstet Gynecol* 1990;162:387–391.

49 Santolaya J. Evaluation of the cord and utero-placental circulation. In: Jaffe R, Warsof SL (eds) *Color Doppler Imaging in Obstetrics and Gynecology.* Pergamon Press, 1992.

50 Soothill PW, Nicolaides KH, Bilardo K *et al.* Uteroplacental blood velocity resistance index and umbilicalvenous pO_2, pCO_2, pH, lactate and erythroblast count in growth-related fetuses. *Fetal Ther* 1986;1:176–179.

51 Nicolaides KH, Bilardo CM, Soothill PW, Campbell S. Absence of end diastolic frequencies in umbilical artery: a sign of fetal hypoxia and acidosis. *Br Med J* 1988;297:1026–1027.

52 Ferrazzi E, Pardi G, Buscaglia M *et al.* The correlation of biochemical monitoring versus umbilical flow velocity measurements of the human fetus. *Am J Obstet Gynecol* 1988;159:1081–1087.

53 Nicolini U, Nicolaidis P, Fisk N *et al.* Limited role of fetal blood sampling in prediction of outcome in intrauterine growth retardation. *Lancet* 1990;336:768–772.

54 Carroll SG, Nicolaides KH. Fetal haematological response to intra-uterine infection in preterm prelabour amniorrhexis. *Fetal Diagn Ther* 1995;10:279.

55 Fisk NM, Borrel A, Hubinont C *et al.* Feto fetal transfusion syndrome: do the neonatal criteria apply *in utero? Arch Dis Child* 1990;65:657.

56 Brunner JP, Rosemond RL. Twin to twin transfusion syndrome: a subset of the twin oligohydramnios–polyhydramnios sequence. *Am J Obstet Gynecol* 1993;169:925.

57 Tanaka M, Natori M, Ishimoto H *et al.* Intravascular pancuronium bromide infusion for prenatal diagnosis of twin–twin transfusion syndrome. *Fetal Diagn Ther* 1992;7:36.

58 Lemery D, Santolaya J, Serre A *et al.* Fetal serum erythropoietin in twin pregnancies with discordant growth. *Fetal Diagn Ther* 1995;10:86.

59 Lemery DJ, Vanlieferinghen P, Gasq M *et al.* Fetal umbilical cord ligation under ultrasound guidance. *Ultrasound Obstet Gynecol* 1994;4:399.

60 Moore T, Gale S, Benirschke K. Perinatal outcome of forty-nine pregnancies complicated by acardiac twinning. *Am J Obstet Gynecol* 1990;163:907–912.

61 Quintero RA, Romero R, Reich H *et al.* In utero percutaneous umbilical cord ligation in the management of complicated monochorionic multiple gestations. *Ultrasound Obstet Gynecol* 1996;8:16–22.

62 Santolaya J, Warsof SL. Combined intravascular–intraperitoneal transfusion in hydropic twins due to Rh (D) alloimmunization. *Fetal Diagn Ther* 1990;5:70.

63 Nicolini U, Santolaya J, Ojo OE *et al.* The fetal intrahepatic umbilical vein as an alternative to cord needling for prenatal diagnosis and therapy. *Prenat Diagn* 1988;8:665.

64 Sonek J, Nicolaides K, Sadowski G *et al.* Instruments and methods. Articulated needle guide: report on the first 30 cases. *Obstet Gynecol* 1989;74:821.

65 Weiner CP. Cordocentesis for diagnostic indications: two years' experience. *Obstet Gynecol* 1987;70:664.

66 Miller RC, Seeds JW. Ultrasonographically monitored procedures and therapies in obstetrics. *The Female Patient* 1992;17:121.

67 De Crespigny LC, Robinson HP, Quinn M *et al.* Ultrasound-guided fetal blood transfusion for severe Rhesus isoimmunization. *Obstet Gynecol* 1985;66:529.

68 Moise JK, Deter RL, Kirshon B *et al.* Intravenous pancuronium bromide for the fetal neuromuscular blockade during intrauterine transfusion for red-cell alloimmunization. *Obstet Gynecol* 1989;74:905.

69 Fisk NM, Tannirandorn Y, Santolaya J *et al.* Fetal macrocytosis in association with chromosomal abnormalities. *Obstet Gynecol* 1989;74:611.

70 Forestier F, Cox W, Daffos F, Rainaut M. The assessment of fetal blood samples. *Am J Obstet Gynecol* 1988;158:1184.

71 Ludomirsky A. Data presented at the Sixth International Conference on Cordocentesis, Philadelphia, October 1991.

72 Boulot P, Deschamps F, Lefort G *et al.* Pure fetal blood samples obtained by cordocentesis: technical aspects of 322 cases. *Prenat Diagn* 1990;10:93.

73 Daffos F, Capella-Pavlovski M, Forestier F. Fetal blood sampling during pregnancy with use of a needle guided by ultrasound: a study of 606 consecutive cases. *Am J Obstet Gynecol* 1985;153:655.

74 Maxwell DJ, Johnson P, Hurley P *et al.* Fetal blood sampling and pregnancy loss in relation to indication. *Br J Obstet Gynaecol* 1991;98:892.

75 McColgin SW, Hess LW, Martin RW *et al.* Group B

streptococcal sepsis and death *in utero* following funipuncture. *Obstet Gynecol* 1989;74:464.

76 Seeds JW, Chescheir NC, Bowes WA, Owl-Smith FA. Fetal death as a complication of intrauterine intravascular transfusion. *Obstet Gynecol* 1989;74:461.

77 Moise KJ, Carpenter RJ, Huhta JC *et al*. Umbilical cord hematoma secondary to *in utero* intravascular transfusion for Rh isoimmunization. *Fetal Ther* 1987;2:65.

78 Chénard E, Bastide A, Fraser WD. Umbilical cord hematoma following diagnostic funipuncture. *Obstet Gynecol* 1990; 76:994.

79 Feinkind L, Nanda D, Delke I, Minkoff H. Abruptio placentae after percutaneous umbilical cord sampling: a case report. *Am J Obstet Gynecol* 1990;162:1203.

80 Wilkins I, Mezrow G, Lynch L *et al*. Amnionitis and life-threatening respiratory distress after percutaneous umbilical blood sampling. *Am J Obstet Gynecol* 1989;160: 427.

Chapter 10/Intrauterine fetal transfusion

MARIE HÉLÈNE POISSONNIER

The purpose of transfusing fetuses or adults is to correct deficits in blood components. Fetal transfusion carries two major difficulties: the first relates to the transfusion itself and necessitates perfect preparation of the blood products to ensure haemato-immunological safety; the second relates to fetal accessibility. Liley proposed the X-ray-guided approach to perform fetal peritoneal transfusions. Charles Rodeck then performed fetal intravascular transfusions using a fetoscope. In 1983 Daffos reported a new alternative, puncturing the fetal cord under ultrasound control.

Indications for fetal transfusions (see ref. 1)

Fetal anaemia

The most common reason for fetal anaemia is alloimmunization. Prophylactic use of specific Rh(D) immunoglobulins has decreased the number of alloimmunizations due to the Rh(D) antigen. In our centre, maternal antibody titres, obstetrical history and concentration of bilirubin dictates the indication and timing of percutaneous umbilical blood sampling (PUBS) and fetal transfusion.

Fetomaternal bleeding has been reported as another indication for fetal transfusions [2]. The diagnosis is made by demonstrating the presence of hydrops fetalis, a sinusoidal fetal heart rate pattern and a positive Kleihauer–Betke smear or high α-fetoprotein concentration in maternal blood.

Parvovirus B19 infection represents the third indication; 50% of pregnant women are parvovirus B19 seronegative and 2% of them will be infected during pregnancy. Fetal infection by parvovirus B19 may generate an aplastic crisis, leading to severe fetal anaemia, myocardial lesions and hydrops. Spontaneous recovery is exceptional in such cases. In a multicentre study of the French fetal medicine group, including 25 fetuses of 24 pregnancies (one set of twins), the infection was clinically not apparent in 14 patients. However, hydrops fetalis was found during an ultrasonographic evaluation in 24 of the fetuses and polyhydramnios in one. These ultrasonographic diagnoses were made between 18 and 28 weeks' gestation. In 22 cases, a fetal blood sample was obtained and in 21 of these the presence of B19 was demonstrated by polymerase chain reaction (haemoglobin concentration ranged from 1.2 to 10 g/dl).

Fetal thrombocytopenia

Fetal thrombocytopenia may be associated with greater perinatal morbidity and mortality if fetal intraventricular haemorrhage develops. Fetal thrombocytopenia may be due to autoimmune antibodies or to alloimmunization. In the latter case, the antigen most commonly incriminated is PLA1. In such cases, the diagnosis is made after a first perinatal complication; during the second pregnancy, PUBS is performed at 24 weeks for platelet typing and count. Serial platelet transfusions or corticotherapy are then proposed if the fetus is PLA1 positive. However, most centres try to avoid serial invasive procedures during pregnancy and only repeat PUBS at 37 weeks' gestation in order to perform a platelet transfusion, to increase the fetal platelet count to $\geq 150\,000/mm^3$, and then induce labour. In cases of autoimmune thrombocytopenia, platelet transfusions are not indicated since transfused platelets will be destroyed.

Other indications

Other blood products that have been infused include immunoglobulin and albumin [3,4]. Erythropoietic stem cells have also been transfused intraperitoneally [5] for correction of immunodeficiencies.

Technique

In this section the route for fetal access and the technique of transfusion will be reviewed.

Fetal access

As previously mentioned donor blood may be infused into the fetal peritoneal cavity or intravascularly.

INTRAPERITONEAL TRANSFUSIONS (IPT)

An IPT may be performed from 14 weeks' gestation. The path of entry in the fetal abdomen depends on fetal position, limb interposition and placental location. If possible, a transplacental route must be avoided. The needle (20-gauge, spinal) is introduced into the peritoneal cavity under continuous ultrasonic control. We recommend insertion of the needle in the pelvic area in order to avoid liver injury. Infusion of saline after the abdominal wall puncture will confirm the correct location of the needle tip in the peritoneal cavity ('ascites-like aspect'). The blood is then infused in variable quantity depending on gestational age. This procedure can be repeated once a week until term. Although the efficiency of this technique is limited in cases of hydrops fetalis, it should be considered a good alternative for early management of fetal anaemia.

INTRAVASCULAR TRANSFUSIONS (IVT)

An IVT may be given via three main sites of puncture: umbilical cord, intra-abdominal portion of the umbilical vein and, exceptionally, the left cardiac ventricle. Access to the first two sites have been described in Chapter 9. Umbilical cord catheterization has also been proposed in certain circumstances (see Chapter 12). Intracardiac access is indicated in desperate situations. A transverse section of the fetal thorax, showing the four chambers of the heart, is the only acceptable plane in which the needle should be introduced. The site of entry of the needle through the maternal abdomen must be selected to permit a direct path into the left ventricle.

Technique of transfusion

Both a bolus transfusion or an intra-uterine exchange transfusion (IUET) can be performed intravascularly. When the needle is in the lumen of the vessel, the first step is to determine the purity of the fetal blood sample (mean cell corpuscular volume, 'i'-antigen determination) and the severity of the deficit that indicated the fetal blood sampling procedure. During a bolus transfusion a single infusion of donor blood is given. For IUET, successive aspirations and infusions of equal volumes of blood are performed.

Potential risks of fetal transfusions and preventive operating guidelines

Invasive procedure-related risks

Difficulties while accessing the fetal targets may lead to fetal death. As in other procedures described in this book, a good training in interventional ultrasound is required as well as perfect cooperation between the ultrasonographer and the operator. The site of entry must be chosen carefully prior to the intervention. The patient and the operator's positioning are conditioned by this choice [6].

All techniques share certain risks, which include premature onset of labour, premature rupture of membranes, chorioamnionitis and fetal bradycardia. It is mandatory to perform fetal transfusions in an operating room and under aseptic surgical conditions. Fetal heart rate should be monitored throughout the procedure. Fetal well-being as well as uterine activity are checked before and after the procedure by the non-stress test. Since these risks remain the same in each procedure performed during the pregnancy, it is important to perform the minimum number of transfusions. IUET may extend the interval between procedures because it replaces fetal cells that are immunologically sensitive to donor cells that are immunologically similar to maternal cells. There are other complications which are specific to the previously described transfusion techniques. For example, bowel injuries may occur during intraperitoneal transfusion or after accessing the intrahepatic portion of the umbilical vein; all vascular access routes carry a risk of laceration of the umbilical vein or of creating a Wharton's jelly haematoma and cord tamponade [7–9]. One of the reasons for umbilical vein laceration is complete or partial dislodgement of the needle due to fetal movements. This can be prevented by fetal intravascular or intramuscular injection of pancuronium bromide or by the fetal umbilical cord catheterization procedure (see Chapter 12). Fetal bleeding into the amniotic cavity may also occur secondary to chorionic plate vessel puncture or after removing the needle, especially in presence of thrombocytopenia. Bleeding after intra-abdominal intravascular transfusions may be of less concern because the blood can be reabsorbed through the peritoneum.

Transfusion risks

The preventive attitude should focus on the risks related to blood products and those related to potential overload. The use of blood products carries a risk of infection with cytomegalovirus, HIV or hepatitis [10]. Therefore, cautious preparation and testing regarding these viruses is mandatory. The bacteriological risk must also be considered and may be diagnosed by fetal and donor blood cultures. Immunological problems such as graft-versus-host disease will be prevented by 25-Gy irradiation of the blood and, if possible, by separating the white cells in order to infuse red cells or platelets only. The cells to be transfused must be compatible and cross-matched with the mother. If possible, these cells are obtained from compatible donor pools; if this is not possible, it is recommended to transfuse the fetus with maternal cells.

The risks due to overloading the fetal intravascular compartment are dramatically increased in cases of hydrops fetalis due to red cell alloimmunization. Anaemic hydropic fetuses may be haemodynamically unstable most likely due to myocardial ischaemia and caution must be taken to avoid the overload. Fetal bradycardia or tachycardia, as alterations of cardiac function, have been observed during intravascular transfusions and have been related to the increase in fetal blood volume [11]. Tolerance to intravascular transfusions may be achieved by transfusing smaller volumes of blood concentrated to 70–80% haematocrit. Alternatively, to avoid the problem of overload, intravascular injection of furosemide in these solutions has been considered. However, this may also lead to an increase in fetal blood viscosity and abnormal myocardial contractility. No matter what transfusion technique is used it is therefore important to have permanent control of the fetal heart rate during the procedure. This can be done by ultrasound, non-stress test or pulsed Doppler. IUET has also been used to avoid overload problems because it theoretically keeps a constant fetal volaemia since similar quantities of blood are infused and aspirated.

The determination of the volume of donor blood to infuse is based on gestational age, which correlates with fetoplacental blood volume, and on fetal haemoglobin concentration:

$$V = \frac{V_f (H_2 - H_1)}{H_t}$$

where V is volume to transfuse, V_f fetal blood volume, H_1 fetal haemoglobin concentration at beginning (g/dl), H_2 fetal haemoglobin concentration expected (g/dl) and H_t haemoglobin concentration in transfused blood.

The final haemoglobin concentration should be 14 g/dl in the presence of hydrops fetalis and 16 g/dl in the absence of hydrops. However, this rapid correction of fetal anaemia in the presence of hydrops remains a matter of discussion and some centres prefer to repeatedly transfuse small volumes until the hydropic signs resolve.

Alloimmunization risk

Any fetal invasive procedure has a risk of fetomaternal haemorrhage which may further activate the immunization, increasing the maternal antibody titre as well as occasionally inducing sensitization to another antigen. For example, platelet alloimmunization has been reported after fetal transfusion [12]. The only way to reduce this risk is to limit the number of fetal transfusions. Knowledge of the previous perinatal history and current maternal antibody titre will help in the decision of when to perform the first amniocentesis, PUBS or transfusion. A severe history of alloimmunization involves perinatal death or neonatal and/or fetal exchange transfusions. In such circumstances, a fetal transfusion may be indicated before 24 weeks unless the fetal Rh(D) positive genotype has been determined through chorionic villous or amniotic fluid sampling. When the previous history is less severe, it is preferable to follow the antibody titre every other week and not to be invasive until it reaches 1 μg. The presence of the ultrasonic signs of fetal anaemia is currently an important finding in the flow chart of decision-making. Finally, in certain cases, the use of the mother as donor may prevent the risk of further maternal immunization [10].

In summary, intrauterine fetal demise may be secondary to the severity of the immunization or due to a complication of the transfusion procedure.

Results and follow-up of red cell transfusions

Red cell alloimmunization (see ref. 13)

In our institution, 817 IUETs have been performed in 338 fetuses between 1985 and 1994. It must be noticed that fetal status (i.e. hydropic or not hydropic) prior to the first procedure influences the outcome during both intrauterine life and the neonatal period. In cases of twin pregnancies each fetus must be considered a single patient except when placental anastomosis is suspected and the transfusion is given via one of the twins. In such a situation, we transfuse alternately into each of the cords.

Fetomaternal haemorrhage

Prenatal treatment of fetomaternal haemorrhages have been reported in the literature. Success in the management of such a complication of pregnancy is more related to the ability in making the diagnosis than to the transfusion procedure itself.

Fetal anaemia secondary to parvovirus B19 infection

As previously discussed, in the French fetal medicine group collaborative study (1994) 24 patients had a parvovirus B19 infection during pregnancy; 13 of these fetuses received *in utero* exchange transfusions, all of them except one having severe anaemia (haemoglobin ≤6 g/dl). Sixteen of these 25 fetuses died *in utero* or in the neonatal period: one died before PUBS, three before transfusion and nine after invasive procedures; three patients elected to terminate the pregnancy. Seven fetuses survived, five after IUET and four spontaneous regressions (including the set of twins). These results suggest

that only symptomatic fetuses should undergo active and invasive management in the presence of maternal parvovirus B19 infection. The potential risk of myocardial lesions should lead to consideration of maintaining a constant blood volume (i.e. IUET) rather than bolus transfusions in cases of severe anaemia. Not to transfuse may be a good alternative in cases of mild fetal anaemia since spontaneous recovery from the aplastic crisis may occur.

Follow-up after fetal transfusion should include fetal growth [14] and complete neonatal evaluation; Musemeche and Reynolds [15] have reported a case of necrotizing enterocolitis after fetal transfusion.

Conclusions

Ultrasound-guided fetal blood sampling has made possible diagnosis and treatment of fetal anaemia and thrombocytopenia. In the future, this technique may allow treatment of genetic disorders. However, the maternal and fetal risks described need to be presented to the parents during the counselling session and prior to any intervention.

References

1 Moise KJ Jr. Intrauterine transfusion with red cells and platelets. *West J Med* 1993;**159**:318–324.

2 Thorp JA, Cohen GR, Yeast JD *et al.* Nonimmune hydrops caused by massive fetomaternal hemorrhage and treated by intravascular transfusion. *Am J Perinatol* 1992;**9**:22–24.

3 Bowman J, Harman C, Mentigolou S, Pollock J. Intravenous fetal transfusion of immunoglobulin for alloimmune thrombocytopenia. *Lancet* 1992;**340**:1034–1035.

4 Marianowski L, Debski R, Rokicki T, Lukaszewicz E, Gromadzki J. Albumin and packed red blood cells in the treatment of severely isoimmunised pregnancies. *Materia Med Polona* 1992;**24**:260–261.

5 Touraine JL, Raudrant D, Rebaud A *et al. In utero* transplantation of stem cells in humans: immunological aspects and clinical follow-up of patients. *Bone Marrow Transplant* 1992;**9** (Suppl 1):121–126.

6 Weiner CP, Wenstrom KD, Sipes SL, Williamson RA. Risk factors for cordocentesis and fetal intravascular transfusion. *Am J Obstet Gynecol* 1991;**165**:1020–1025.

7 Doyle LW, de Crespigny L, Kelly EA. Haematoma complicating fetal intravascular transfusions. *Aust NZ J Obstet Gynaecol* 1993;**33**:208–209.

8 Jauniaux E, Nicolaides KH, Campbell S, Hustin J. Hematoma of the umbilical cord secondary to cordocentesis

for intrauterine fetal transfusion. *Prenat Diagn* 1990;10: 477–478.

9 Keckstein G, Tschurtz S, Schneider V, Hutter W, Terinde R, Jonatha WD. Umbilical cord haematoma as a complication of intrauterine intravascular blood transfusion. *Prenat Diagn* 1990;10:59–65.

10 Evans DG, Lyon AJ. Fatal congenital cytomegalovirus infection acquired by an intra-uterine transfusion. *Eur J Pediatr* 1991;150:780–781.

11 Moise KJ Jr, Mari G, Fisher DJ, Huhta JC, Cano LE, Carpenter RJ Jr. Acute fetal hemodynamic alterations after intrauterine transfusion for treatment of severe red blood cell alloimmunization. *Am J Obstet Gynecol* 1990;163: 776–784.

12 Gibble JW, Ness PM. Maternal immunity to red cell antigens and fetal transfusion. *Clin Lab Med* 1992;12:553–576.

13 Weiner CP, Williamson RA, Wenstrom KD *et al.* Management of fetal hemolytic disease by cordocentesis. II. Outcome of treatment. *Am J Obstet Gynecol* 1991;165: 1302–1307.

14 Roberts A, Grannum P, Belanger K, Pattison N, Hobbis J. Fetal growth and birthweight in isoimmunized pregnancies *Fetal Diagn Ther* 1993;8:407–411.

15 Musemeche CA, Reynolds M. Necrotizing enterocolitis following intrauterine blood transfusion. *J Pediatr Surg* 1991;26:1411–1412.

Chapter 11/Fetal Shunts

CLIVE ALDRICH and CHARLES RODECK

Introduction

Together with the widespread use of obstetric ultrasound, the significant advances in technology and clinical expertise that have occurred over the past decade have allowed a rapid increase in the antenatal detection and management of fetal structural abnormalities. A number of non-invasive and invasive treatments have been developed; of the latter, percutaneous introduction of a catheter or shunt has been applied to a number of conditions [1–5]. Fetal shunting should only be contemplated for conditions frequently associated with significant neonatal morbidity or mortality and if there is sufficient evidence, from both animal and human studies, that the natural history of the anomaly can be altered by the procedure. Furthermore, reliable antenatal predictors are needed in selecting cases for intervention, so that fetal surgery is withheld from those who would otherwise have a satisfactory outcome and from those in whom the pathology is irreversible and the prognosis poor. The principles governing invasive fetal therapy are summarized in Table 11.1.

Fetal shunting has been performed for a variety of problems, such as obstructive uropathy, pleural effusions, pulmonary cysts, ventriculomegaly and fetal ascites (Table 11.2). These attempts at improving fetal outcome have met with variable success: to date the results of vesico-amniotic and pleuro-amniotic shunting procedures suggest that in carefully selected cases it is an effective and safe method for the chronic drainage of fetal fluid collections [3,4]. This is quite unlike the intrauterine treatment of fetal ventriculomegaly, which was abandoned a number of years ago [2,5].

Pathophysiology

In certain cases, an uncorrected fetal malformation may result in progressive damage *in utero*. Increased pressure caused by pathological fluid collections can cause damage to adjacent organs or tissues and interfere with fetal development. The pressure within the abnormal fluid collection almost always exceeds that of the amniotic fluid and insertion of a fetal–amniotic shunt allows drainage into a sterile environment, at the same time relieving the pressure within the fetal cavity. This can arrest the destructive or deleterious consequences of the underlying defect and allow normal development to continue [1].

Urinary tract

In cases of lower urinary tract obstruction (i.e. posterior urethral valves or urethral atresia) the bladder is enlarged and its wall is often thickened, although this may not be obvious on ultrasound scans until after bladder decompression. Other ultrasound features include dilatation of the upper urethra and a variable degree of hydroureter with or without hydonephrosis, which is often asymmetrical. There may also be vesico-ureteric reflux, which frequently accompanies gross obstruction. The rationale for vesico-amniotic shunting is to prevent progressive renal damage and correct the associated oligohydramnios, which in turn may prevent pulmonary hypoplasia [6–9].

Pleura and lungs

Pleural effusions and pulmonary cysts (i.e. cystic adenomatoid malformation (CAM) type 1) can result in fetal lung and mediastinal compression and lead to the development of fetal hydrops and polyhydramnios, which are associated with a high risk of premature delivery and intrauterine or neonatal death. Polyhydramnios is frequently observed and this may be a consequence of

Table 11.1 Principles of invasive fetal therapy.

The natural history of the condition should be known
The condition should be severe enough to interfere with
　normal development and cause death or disability
The treatment should be capable of improving the natural
　history of the condition
Evidence from an animal model should support this
Other fetal abnormalities must be excluded as far as possible
Reliable prognostic tests should be available, to detect
　appropriate cases for treatment
The fetus should be too immature for delivery and postnatal
　treatment
The benefits to the fetus should outweigh the risks to the
　mother and fetus
The parents must be counselled and informed
After treatment antenatal monitoring must continue
Postnatal follow-up is essential
The treatment should be evaluated scientifically

Table 11.2 Fetal shunting.

Pathology	Type of shunt
Obstructive uropathy	
Posterior urethral valves	Vesico-amniotic
Hydronephrosis	Pyelo-amniotic
Hydrothorax or chylothorax	Pleuro-amniotic
Pulmonary cyst (CAM type 1)	Cysto-amniotic
Ascites	Peritoneo-amniotic
Cerebral ventriculomegaly	Ventriculo-amniotic

CAM, cystic adenomatoid malformation.

a reduction in fetal swallowing due to oesophageal compression and/or an increase in fluid production by abnormal lung tissue. When there is compression of the heart and major blood vessels in the thorax, fetal hydrops may develop [10,11]. Thoraco-amniotic shunting may be effective in relieving lung compression and any coexisting mediastinal shift. This too may prevent pulmonary hypoplasia and in addition reverse fetal hydrops and polyhydramnios, thereby reducing the risk of fetal death or preterm delivery [4,12].

Cerebral ventricles

The rationale for chronic cerebral ventricular decompression was to reduce ventricular pressure and size, thus preserving cerebral tissue [2,5,13]. Ventriculomegaly develops when there is an imbalance of cerebrospinal fluid production and drainage and the most frequent causes of obstructive hydrocephalus include spina bifida, aqueduct stenosis, Dandy–Walker syndrome, chromosomal abnormalities, viral infections and isolated (idiopathic) cases [14]. Postnatal shunting improves survival and reduces mortality in these infants, although data reported to the International Fetal Medicine and Surgery Society (IFMSS) registry indicate that only fetal survival is improved with *in utero* therapy; they do not indicate any obvious improvement in survivor morbidity and indeed shunting may have increased the survival of severely handicapped infants [15]. Furthermore, animal models cannot answer the critical question of whether prenatal therapy can preserve intact intellectual development among survivors and the procedure has been abandoned by most centres.

Ascites

This can cause gross distension of the abdominal wall, leading to a 'prune-belly' appearance, and pressure on the diaphragm may reduce space in the chest, leading to pulmonary hypoplasia. It may be part of a generalized hydrops or secondary to increased pressure in the thorax, or rarely due to escape of urine from the urinary tract [1]. Shunting has only been rarely used.

Case selection

Recognition of fetuses who will not benefit from *in utero* therapy is the most important step in case selection. This is determined mainly by the detection of other anomalies and of evidence for severe compromise of organ function. Consequently, those selected for treatment have had other defects excluded as far as possible and show evidence of at least reasonably healthy organ function. They are also unlikely to be beyond 34 weeks' gestation since postnatal treatment is then the better option. These decisions are best made in collaboration with the relevant paediatric specialists. The criteria for shunting are included in Table 11.1.

Detailed high-resolution sonographic examination for the exclusion of other anatomical defects is essential, as up to 50% of these fetuses may have cardiovascular, gastrointestinal, skeletal and central nervous system abnormalities [16]. An assessment of the degree of associated abnormalities, such as oligohydramnios in fetal uropathy and skin oedema or ascites in cases of fetal hydrops with pleural effusions, is also useful in determining the severity and prognosis of the condition. A diagnostic amnio-infusion may improve the image quality in cases of oligohydramnios [17]. There is also a high incidence of chromosomal abnormalities and the fetal karyotype should be obtained by fetal blood sampling, amniocentesis, chorionic villous sampling or aspiration of urine/cyst fluid prior to shunt insertion [15,18]. Additional tests, such as infection screen and haematological, biochemical and acid–base blood analysis, should also be considered. This enables a more accurate diagnosis and hence prognosis to be given to the parents, who may then wish to consider termination of pregnancy. It could also provide valuable information about the risks in any future pregnancies. This assessment should not be confined to the second trimester, as the results will influence decisions regarding shunt placement and the timing of delivery and may avoid unnecessary interventions both antepartum or intrapartum. Multiple pregnancies require special consideration, especially if only one of the fetuses is affected. If treatment is considered, the prognosis for the affected fetus must be fully assessed and the potential benefits of shunting weighed against the harmful effects on the unaffected fetus [19]. Contraindications to shunt insertion are shown in Table 11.3.

Obstructive uropathy

Posterior urethral valves (PUV) are the most frequent

Table 11.3 Contraindications to shunt insertion.

There are associated ultrasonically detectable lethal abnormalities or aneuploidy
The parents wish a termination of pregnancy
The pregnancy is early (< 16–17 weeks) and the fetus is physically too small for the shunt
The fetus is mature and postnatal treatment is a better option

cause of lower urinary tract obstruction in the fetus and occur almost exclusively in males [20]. Obstruction can result in bladder enlargement (megacystis), which may be detectable as early as 11 weeks [21]. The differential diagnosis should be considered, especially in a female fetus, and includes cloacal anomalies, urethral atresia, vesico-ureteric reflux, megacystis–microcolon–intestinal hypoperistalsis syndrome (MMIH) and the prune-belly syndrome [3]. Most of these are unlikely to benefit from any type of prenatal decompression and shunting is usually not indicated. The sonographic recognition of the typically dilated posterior urethra in PUV is of crucial importance and is illustrated in Fig. 11.1.

Fetal intervention is not usually required either for bilateral hydronephrosis or unilateral disease, unless hydronephrosis is present in a solitary kidney in conjunction with oligohydramnios. The presence of a normal amount of amniotic fluid has previously been

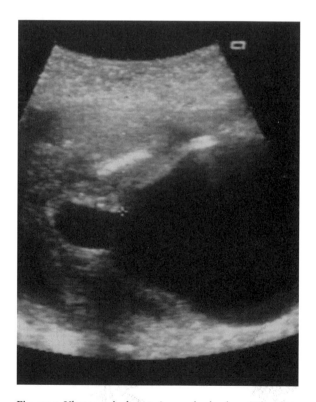

Fig. 11.1 Ultrasound of posterior urethral valves. Dilated bladder and proximal urethra in a fetus with posterior urethral valves demonstrating the 'keyhole sign'.

regarded as a contraindication, although this may change in the future. Poor selection and shunting of hopeless cases is probably the most important factor for the poor results in the literature and if intrauterine intervention is to be advocated as a method of preventing further deterioration of renal function in a fetus with obstruction, it is vital that fetal kidney function is assessed accurately. Ultrasound findings of renal cysts are visualized in only 44% of dysplastic kidneys, and hyperechogenicity of the renal parenchyma only predicts dysplasia with a sensitivity and specificity of 73% and 80% respectively [22]. In view of this inaccuracy, biochemical analysis of urine obtained from the fetal bladder [23] and/or from each renal pelvis [24] has been recommended and become an accepted predictive parameter [25]. However, some values are dependent upon gestational age and this must be taken into account during assessment of renal function [26] (Fig. 11.2). At gestations below 20 weeks, fetal urine normally has a high sodium concentration, making prediction more difficult. Sodium, calcium, phosphate and sodium/creatine levels show a significant correlation with the degree of renal impairment, with the best sensitivity achieved by calcium and the highest specificity by sodium [26]. Another parameter, β_2-microglobulin, has

been suggested to be highly predictive of renal dysplasia [27].

A single evaluation of fetal urine may not accurately reflect current or long-term renal function and serial sampling at 1–2 weekly intervals may give a better idea of the degree of renal damage [24]. This should precede the decision about whether or not to offer prenatal shunting. Rarely, simple percutaneous bladder aspiration with a 22-gauge spinal needle may be enough to open up a urethral obstruction. Renal function may also appear to improve after bladder decompression and this should be the first attempt at interventional therapy. We have also seen significant improvement in fetuses who have undergone serial bladder decompression. Since bladder aspiration is technically easier than shunt insertion and also not associated with the same long-term complications, serial sampling as both a diagnostic and therapeutic procedure should be considered in a fetus, especially at gestations less than 20 weeks. Another reason for initial conservative, i.e. observational, management is that megacystis sometimes resolves spontaneously. This appears to happen in fetuses with muscular, thick-walled bladders that may be able to generate the pressures required to overcome the urethral obstruction.

Fetuses with persistent megacystis who have ultrasound and biochemical evidence of adequate renal function represent the group most likely to benefit from shunting [28] and until the value of shunting procedures is established, treatment should be restricted to this group. Intervention in a fetus with significantly impaired renal function is unlikely to be beneficial and is not advisable [29]. Antenatal detection of lung hypoplasia remains difficult and it is not yet possible to accurately

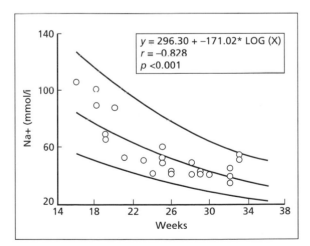

Fig. 11.2 Reference ranges for fetal urinary sodium used at University College Hospital, London. Mean and 95% confidence limits throughout gestation [26].

Table 11.4 Aims of vesico-amniotic shunting.

Reduce pressure in the urinary tract
Prevent further damage due to raised pressure
Promote normal growth and maturation of nephrons
Allow the formation of amniotic fluid
Improve the freedom of fetal movements and reduce compression
Promote pulmonary growth and maturation
Prevent gross distension of the urinary tract and abdominal wall (prune belly)

predict those fetuses at risk [3]. Oligohydramnios is associated with poor pulmonary function and should be regarded as a poor prognostic sign, unless serial ultrasound scans have proved that it had a short duration. The aims of vesico-amniotic shunting are summarized in Table 11.4 (p. 111). The last aim, prevention of gross distension, has been previously underestimated and is very significant. The atonic, dilated urinary tract may present more management difficulties postnatally than renal failure, for which dialysis and transplantation are available and successful. A number of patients with a poor fetal prognosis refuse termination of pregnancy and insist on shunting in order to give the fetus every possible chance. This requires careful consideration, but can occasionally result in a surprisingly favourable outcome.

Thoraco-amniotic shunting

Pleural effusions and cysts may be an isolated unilateral or bilateral finding or be associated with other abnormalities, such as generalized skin oedema and ascites, pericardial effusions and polyhydramnios (Fig. 11.3). In neonates, the commonest cause of an isolated pleural effusion is chylothorax, which is diagnosed by demonstrating chylomicrons in a milky-coloured pleural fluid after the first feed [30]. However, in the fetus the pleural fluid is a clear golden colour and it is not possible to distinguish between cases of congenital chylothorax and hydrothorax from other causes. Some authors have claimed to have made an antenatal diagnosis of congenital chylothorax by demonstrating high mononuclear cell counts in aspirated pleural fluid [11,31]. However, we have not been able to detect any difference in lymphocyte count and lipoprotein electrophoresis between fetuses confirmed neonatally to have chylothoraces and those with hydrothoraces from other causes (C. Aldrich & C. Rodeck, unpublished observations). Hydrops fetalis may occur in a wide variety of fetal and maternal disorders, including haematological, cardiovascular, pulmonary, gastrointestinal, metabolic and chromosomal abnormalities, congenital infections, neoplasms and malformations of the placenta and umbilical cord [32]. Even after a detailed assessment with ultrasound and fetal blood sampling, the cause frequently remains unknown. However, most cases of massive unilateral or bilateral pleural effusions are

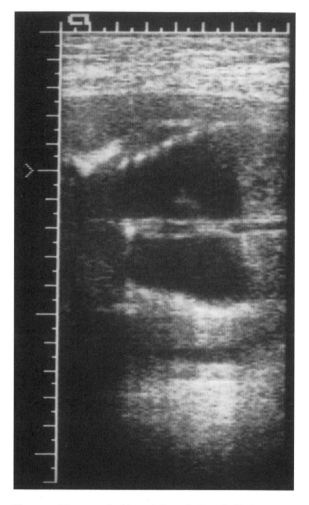

Fig. 11.3 Ultrasound of large bilateral pleural effusions. Gross hydrops and skin oedema was present.

chylothorax, and the presence of hydrops or ascites is a secondary effect.

Pulmonary cysts may be seen in cases of CAM (type 1), which is a rare malformation that may also result in pulmonary hypoplasia, hydrops and perinatal death. Other causes of pulmonary cysts, such as pulmonary sequestration, bronchogenic cysts and mediastinal cystic teratoma, may be rarely diagnosed antenatally [33]. These and associated effusions may also require treatment should they reach a significant size.

Serial ultrasound assessment of any intrathoracic fluid collection should be performed, as isolated pleural and pericardial effusions or pulmonary cysts may resolve spontaneously [34,35]. In some instances they have been managed conservatively and treated effectively during labour [36], or after birth [37], with no evidence of pulmonary hypoplasia.

In certain cases, when there is significant compression and mediastinal shift, simple percutaneous aspiration with a 22-gauge spinal needle may be required to allow the diagnosis of an underlying cardiac abnormality or other intrathoracic lesion to be made. Aspiration may also be useful in the prenatal diagnosis of pulmonary hypoplasia when the lung often fails to expand after decompression [12]. Spontaneous resolution has also been demonstrated after thoracocentesis [11], and short-term drainage by single or repeated aspiration should be considered, especially in cases of low gestational age when the chest may be too small for the shunt. In the majority of cases, however, the fluid reaccumulates within 24 hours and repeated procedures are required, which are likely to be more traumatic cumulatively than thoraco-amniotic shunting [12].

Shunt insertion should be considered, irrespective of the cause, in cases where the fluid reaccumulates and is large enough to produce significant pulmonary compression and/or mediastinal shift that has resulted in hydrops and polyhydramnios. Thoraco-amniotic shunting in these circumstances can allow the rapid expansion of the lungs and a simultaneous shift of the heart to its normal position, with resolution of fetal hydrops and polyhydramnios. The aims of thoraco-amniotic shunting are summarized in Table 11.5.

Table 11.5 Aims of thoraco-amniotic shunting (drainage of pleural effusions and pulmonary cysts).

Remove fluid and reduce intrathoracic pressure
Promote resolution of hydrops and polyhydramnios,
  reducing risk of preterm delivery and fetal death
Prevent development of hydrops and polyhydramnios
Promote pulmonary growth and development
Prevent pulmonary hypoplasia
Assist respiration and ventilation in the neonate

Ventriculomegaly

Shunting is not indicated for the reasons mentioned earlier and because a suitable shunt that will remain *in situ* without becoming blocked is not available.

Ascites

Peritoneo-amniotic shunts have been inserted in only a few cases with variable results. We have on occasion used it for urinary ascites after the amniotic end of a vesico-amniotic shunt has been pulled back into the peritoneal cavity, and there has been a high risk of pulmonary hypoplasia due to diaphragmatic compression. The main worry is the shunt coiling around and damaging gut or mesenteric vessels.

Techniques of shunt insertion

Shunting procedures should only be performed in centres with sufficient expertise and workload to maintain skills, i.e. a tertiary or quaternary referral centre. Before giving written consent, both parents must be counselled about the procedure and understand fully the risks and benefits, and be willing to attend for follow-up studies. Consultation with an appropriate paediatric specialist may be helpful, as is psychological support.

Fetal shunting may be performed as an outpatient procedure and only rarely is maternal and fetal sedation required. Diazemuls (5–10 mg i.v.) may be administered to the mother, and if fetal movements are vigorous fetal paralysis can be achieved with pancuronium (1–2 mg) injected into the umbilical vein. Some centres give prophylactic antibiotics and tocolytic agents but this has not been our practice. Whether the fetus should specifically be given some form of analgesia may also require consideration [38].

Types of shunts

We use the Rocket fetal catheter developed in 1982 [39] (Rocket of London Ltd, Watford, UK). It is a double-pigtail silastic catheter with external and internal diameters of 2.1 and 1.5 mm respectively, with radio-opaque stainless steel inserts at each end and lateral holes around the coils (Fig. 11.4). The amniotic

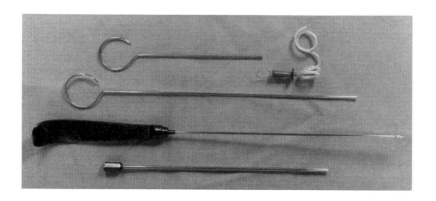

Fig. 11.4 Cannula, trochar, long and short obturators and double pigtail catheter used in shunting procedures. (De Elles Instruments, Coulsdon, Surrey, UK.)

coil is at right angles to the rest of the catheter and is therefore less likely to be removed by the fetus or become entangled with the umbilical cord. This shunt is available in one size and we have found it suitable for both thoraco-amniotic and vesico-amniotic shunting. It is introduced down a cannula, now made by D.C. Ellis Instruments (Coulsdon, Surrey, UK). The external diameter is 2.5 mm and it is 18 cm long. The trocar must have a very sharp tip in order to make introduction through the maternal and fetal abdominal walls easier and less painful.

Alternative shunts are available and include the following.

1 Harrison fetal bladder stent (Cook Urological, Spencer, Indiana, USA), a polyethylene catheter that is introduced over the outside of a needle. It has side holes at both ends, a flare at the amniotic cavity end and resumes a curled end once inserted [9]. It is available in different lengths and calibres, but there have been many technical problems with this catheter.

2 The Denver shunt was developed for the treatment of ventriculomegaly but has been found to be unsatisfactory. It is made of silicone rubber and has a rubber flange to maintain its position within the ventricle. Unlike other shunts it has a one-way valve to prevent reverse flow [13].

Procedure

High-resolution ultrasound scanning should be used to obtain the best transverse section of the fetal target. Curvilinear transducers are particularly convenient.

Holding the transducer in one hand, parallel to the intended course of the cannula, an entry site in the maternal abdomen is chosen. The placenta should not be transversed and the site should be away from the maternal uterine vessels, with the needle trajectory as short as possible.

The site is cleaned with antiseptic solution (chlorhexidene 0.5% in spirit) and the mother's lower abdomen draped with sterile towels. Local anaesthetic (1% lignocaine) is infiltrated into the maternal skin and subcutaneous tissue, down to the myometrium. If there is oligohydramnios a 20-gauge needle is first passed into the amniotic cavity and an amnio-infusion given with 150–200 ml of warmed normal saline. This may improve the image and allow the anomaly scan to be finished, but its main purpose is to facilitate the deposition of the intra-amniotic end of the catheter.

Under continuous ultrasound guidance the fetal target is fixed on one side of the ultrasound screen and the metal trocar and cannula are introduced into the amniotic cavity and then inserted through the chest or abdominal wall into the target fluid collection. After ensuring that the cannula is in the correct position, the trocar is removed and the drainage of fluid confirms the correct positioning of the cannula. Only minimal drainage should be allowed as decompression will reduce the size of the target and may result in the cannula becoming dislodged. To prevent this, the end of the catheter can be blocked temporarily with the operator's thumb. The fetal catheter is straightened out on its guide wire and inserted into the cannula. After the guide wire has been withdrawn, the shorter obturator pushes

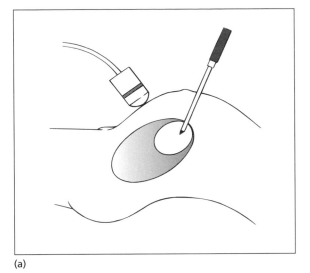

(a)

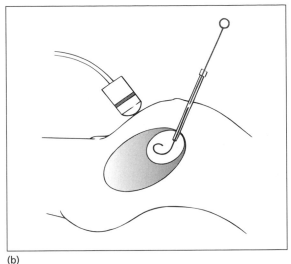

(b)

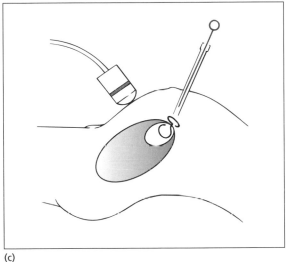

(c)

Fig. 11.5 Technique of shunt insertion. (a) The trochar and cannula have been inserted transamniotically into the fetal target. (b) The double pigtail catheter has been passed into the cannula and the short obturator used to deposit half the catheter within the fluid collection. (c) The cannula and long obturator have been withdrawn leaving the shunt *in situ*.

half of the catheter out and this coils up in the fetal fluid collection. The cannula is then slowly drawn back into the amniotic cavity, where the other half of the catheter is deposited by the longer obturator. This is the most difficult part of the procedure and requires the presence of fluid in the amniotic cavity. The technique of shunt insertion is illustrated in Fig. 11.5.

BLADDER SHUNTING

Oligohydramnios is a frequent finding in cases of obstructive uropathy; in severe cases, amnio-infusion as a first step greatly facilitates the procedure and avoids the outer end of the catheter being inadvertently left extra-amniotically. To avoid other anatomical structures the site of fetal insertion should ideally be suprapubic and away from the midline (Fig. 11.6). After the shunt has been inserted there should be a rapid decompression of the bladder, which subsequently cannot usually be identified; indeed only the presence of the inner tip of the shunt allows its localization. Intravesical pressure may be measured but its value is uncertain [40]. A

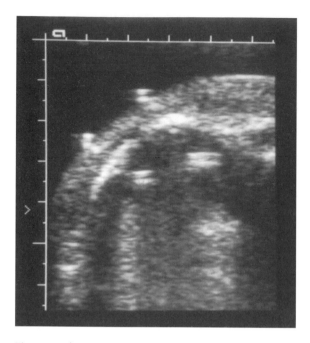

Fig. 11.6 Ultrasound of pleuro-amniotic shunt *in situ*.

sample of urine should be sent for biochemical analysis and possibly for karyotyping.

THORAX

In cases of polyhydramnios, amnio-drainage may

initially be performed to improve both visualization and access to the fetal target. The shunt should be inserted in the mid-thoracic region, extreme caution being taken to avoid the fetal heart, which ideally should be on the side furthest away from the cannula (Figs. 11.7 and 11.8). In cases of bilateral hydrothorax, if drainage of the contralateral lung is required the appropriate fetal position may be achieved by rotation of the fetal body using the tip of the cannula, avoiding a repeat puncture of the mother. A sample of pleural fluid should be sent for lymphocyte count and/or karyotyping.

ASCITES

A lateral approach to the fetal trunk is best, so as to

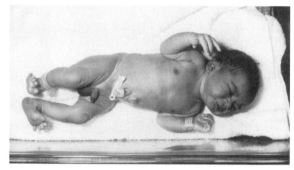

Fig. 11.7 Neonate with vesico-amniotic shunt *in situ*.

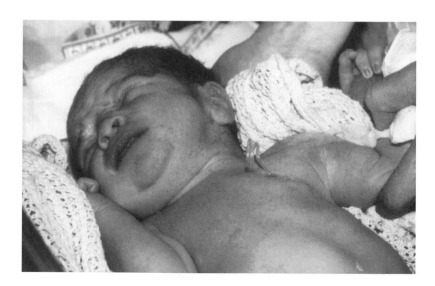

Fig. 11.8 Neonate with pleuro-amniotic shunt *in situ*.

avoid the umbilicus. The target should be just above the bladder where the depth of ascites is greatest, reducing the risk of trauma and of the intrafetal coil snaring bowel.

Complications

The procedure-related death rate of vesico-amniotic shunting has been reported by IFMSS to be in the order of 4.8% and that of ventriculo-amniotic shunting 10.25% [15]. No multicentre figures are available for thoraco-amniotic shunting but in our centre the procedure is associated with a 2% fetal loss rate, which is similar to that of vesico-amniotic shunting.

Elder *et al.* [41] reported a complication rate of 44% following shunting for obstructive uropathy. However, this report was a collection of several small series and case reports and reflects poor case selection and inexperience with the technique. The most common complications were inadequate shunt drainage or migration (19%), followed by preterm labour (12%), urinary ascites (7%) and chorioamnionitis (5%). These problems and fetal trauma are minimized by operator experience, careful site selection and continuous monitoring throughout the procedure. Poor drainage is a frequent complication and blockage of the shunt may occur due to vernix, blood or protein exudate. Fetal movement and growth may also result in shunt displacement. Our experience with the technical performance of the Rocket shunt has been very good and complications have been rare. Intrauterine infection is rare and may be reduced by ensuring a 'sterile' non-touch technique. Prophylactic antibiotics are unlikely to be helpful. Precautions against uterine stimulation and the ensuing premature labour may be taken by the administration of a tocolytic to the mother but is also unlikely to be useful unless there is considerable polyhydramnios.

Other specific complications have been described in the literature and include the formation of fetal urinary ascites, which can be managed by insertion of a peritoneo-amniotic shunt [1]. Uteroperitoneal amniotic fluid leakage following thoraco-amniotic shunting has been reported [42]. This can result in gross maternal ascites and acute fetal distress due to oligohydramnios and cord compression. Vesico-amniotic shunting has also been associated with a fetal paramedian abdominal wall defect and herniation of the small bowel has been described [43]. Shunts are occasionally drawn into the peritoneal or thoracic cavities and may have to be removed surgically postnatally.

Follow-up

Following shunt insertion close observation is essential. However, not all cases need to be seen at the treatment centre and frequently serial ultrasound scans can be performed at the referring hospital. These should be done at weekly intervals to determine whether the fluid collections have reaccumulated and also to monitor other features, such as improvement of fetal hydrops and normalization of amniotic fluid volume. When necessary, reassessment in the treatment centre is performed in order to evaluate progress. If there are signs of shunt malfunction (due to migration or blockage), such as reaccumulation of urine or fluid, a further shunt placement will have to be considered.

After vesico-amniotic shunting, fetal hydroureter and hydronephrosis frequently persist, whereas renal parenchymal hyperechogenicity tends to progressively reduce, although this echographic pattern does not necessarily indicate good renal function [3]. Reaccumulation of amniotic fluid also suggests that major renal impairment has not occurred, although this too is not a specific sign. Failure of amniotic fluid to collect indicates severe irreversible renal failure. Antenatal prediction of pulmonary hypoplasia remains difficult, but improvement of amniotic fluid volume after decompression is likely to be an important factor in fetal lung development and maturation [28].

Thoraco-amniotic shunting should result in a rapid resolution of pulmonary compression, mediastinal shift, polyhydramnios and fetal hydrops within 1–3 weeks. It may also help to differentiate between hydrops due to a primary pleural effusion, in which case the ascites and skin oedema may resolve after shunting, and other causes of hydrops, in which drainage does not necessarily prevent worsening hydrops. In cases of thoraco-amniotic shunting, a poor prognosis has been associated with the presence of associated malformations, bilateral effusions, hydrops and polyhydramnios that did not resolve within 1–3 weeks of shunt insertion [12]. Persistence of the effusion with failure of the lungs to expand and fill the chest indicates pulmonary hypoplasia and a poor prognosis, whereas the reverse suggests normal-sized lungs and a good prognosis [12,44].

Delivery and shunt removal

Providing no serious complications arise after shunt insertion, the pathology is corrected and the fetus continues to grow normally, delivery should be at term and ideally spontaneous and by the vaginal route. If paediatric surgery is required soon after birth, then an elective delivery may be more appropriate either by induction of labour or Caesarean section. An experienced neonatologist should always be present at the birth.

The neonate with urinary problems may need immediate ventilatory support, but the urinary tract and renal function can usually be investigated at leisure. The shunt may continue to function until definitive treatment has been achieved and can be left *in situ*. At delivery, there is only limited experience with chest drains and their management remains controversial. Immediate clamping and removal to avoid the development of pneumothoraces has been advocated [1]. In our hospital, the baby is electively intubated and transferred to the neonatal unit where an early chest X-ray is performed. Once the position of the shunt is confirmed, it is removed in a more controlled manner with local anaesthetic. We have found a very low incidence of pneumothoraces using this protocol. The shunt may be used to drain further collections of pleural fluid. A shunt that is not found at birth may be in the baby, in the mother or it may have been thrown away inadvertently. The mother and baby should undergo radiography as the steel tips of the shunt are radio-opaque.

Outcome

Obstructive uropathy is treated surgically by urinary bypass or diversion in postnatal life and it is illogical to assume that this should not be appropriate in prenatal life. Indeed, if it is believed that treatment is more successful at an early stage of a pathological process, then prenatal treatment is to be preferred to postnatal. The difficulty is in the selection of cases. There are some in whom surgical treatment is not required, and others in whom the pathology is so severe that treatment is hopeless. Many of the reports in the literature deal with such cases and this has led to a pessimistic view

of the value of shunting [41,45]. It is clearly futile to try to assess a treatment in cases that have no chance. Most centres have experience of some patients in whom shunting was unquestionably beneficial, but much evidence is anecdotal.

There are unfortunately no randomized trials and no detailed long-term follow-up studies, despite the efforts of IFMSS. Several facts emerged from the register that was kept for some years [15]: firstly, the correct diagnosis was often not made antenatally, particularly when urinary reflux was present as well; secondly, the neonatal survival rate was 76% in cases of PUV, which was better than expected; and lastly, many of the cases that were submitted were from centres that had experience of only one or two cases. Crombleholme *et al.* [46] looked at their experience with low urinary tract obstruction and found a higher survival rate in the groups (both good and poor prognosis) that had intervention compared with those that did not.

Unfortunately, the best human evidence that shunting can modify the natural history in a beneficial way still remains uncontrolled and anecdotal. A major worry is that if shunting does have a therapeutic effect on the urinary tract, could cases that would have died without treatment be converted into chronically ill survivors? This consequence probably happens and is in general undesirable. However, shunting has other beneficial effects on organ distension, amniotic fluid volume and lung growth as well. Some follow-up information is now becoming available through our collaboration with the Department of Paediatric Urology at Great Ormond Street Hospital, London. A number of fetuses with urinary tract dilatation but normal amniotic fluid volume have done worse than expected. This would argue for *in utero* shunting at an earlier stage of pregnancy and in fetuses less severely affected than before. However, if such a policy was adopted randomization into treated and untreated groups would be important.

In some respects, shunting for thoracic fluid and cysts is more straightforward. In all centres, reversal of hydrops and polyhydramnios has been observed and neonatal respiration is trouble-free in the majority of cases [12,44] with a better survival rate than expected from the literature. The contrary view is that if the lungs are already severely hypoplastic, shunting is unlikely to be able to reverse this. However, there are again no randomized studies and we do not know the long-term effects of treatment.

Conclusions

It is obvious that much more information is needed about the issues surrounding whether to treat, how and when. There has been much debate over whether to divert the urine percutaneously by shunting or by open surgery [47,48]. The latter has to some extent been encouraged by the problems that some centres have had with shunt patency and migration. As mentioned above, we have had excellent experience with our shunts and we do not regard obstructive uropathy, chest fluid or thoracic cysts as an indication for open fetal surgery.

New developments in endoscopic and laser technology may have an impact in the future. An Angiocath optic fibre bundle of 0.8 mm diameter can now be passed down an 18-gauge needle for investigation. A laser has been used to create a suprapubic cystotomy [49] and fetal suprapubic cystoscopy has been performed and enabled both fulguration of the valves and insertion of a stent into the posterior urethra [50]. We are also hopeful that proton nuclear magnetic resonance spectroscopy of urine will be useful in the assessment of renal function [51].

Improved selection of cases for treatment remains important and more information about developmental physiology is required. Finally, it can be speculated that studies in basic developmental biology may open up possibilities for treating damaged and dysplastic kidneys and lungs with embryonic precursor cells and growth factors.

References

1 Lynch L, Mehalek K, Berkowitz RL. Invasive fetal therapy. In: Rodeck CH (eds) *Fetal Medicine*, vol 1. Oxford: Blackwell Scientific Publications, 1989:118–153.

2 Fisk NM, Rodeck CH. Antenatal diagnosis and fetal medicine. In: Roberton NRC (ed) *Textbook of Neonatology*, 2nd edn. London: Churchill Livingstone, 1992:121–150.

3 Nicolini U, Rodeck CH. Fetal urinary diversion. In: Chervenak FA, Isaacson GC, Campbell S (eds) *Ultrasound in Obstetrics and Gynaecology*. Boston: Little Brown and Co., 1993:1277–1282.

4 Nicolaides KH, Azar GB. Thoracoamniotic shunting. In: Chervenak FA, Isaacson GC, Campbell S (eds) *Ultrasound in Obstetrics and Gynaecology*. Boston: Little Brown and Co., 1993:1289–1293.

5 Clewell WH. Hydrocephalus shunts. In: Chervenak FA, Isaacson GC, Campbell S (eds) *Ultrasound in Obstetrics and Gynaecology*. Boston: Little Brown and Co., 1993: 1283–1287.

6 Harrison MR, Nakayama DK, Noall RA, de Lorimier AA. Correction of congenital hydronephrosis *in utero* II. Decompression reverses the effects of obstruction on the fetal lung and urinary tract. *J Pediatr Surg* 1982;17: 965–974.

7 Glick PI, Harrison MR, Noall RA, Villa RL. Correction of congenital hydronephrosis *in utero* III. Early mid-trimester ureteral obstruction produces renal dysplasia *J Pediatr Surg* 1983;18:681–687.

8 Harrison MR, Ross NA, Noall RA, de Lorimier AA. Correction of congenital hydronephrosis *in utero* I. The model: fetal urethral obstruction produces hydronephrosis and pulmonary hypoplasia in fetal lambs. *J Pediatr Surg* 1983;18:247–256.

9 Glick PI, Harrison MR, Adzick NS, Noall RA, Villa RL. Correction of congenital hydronephrosis *in utero* IV. *In utero* decompression prevents renal dysplasia. *J Pediatr Surg* 1984;19:649–657.

10 Petres RE, Redwine FO, Cruickshank DP. Congenital bilateral chylothorax. Antepartum diagnosis and successful intrauterine surgical management. *JAMA* 1982;248:1360–1361.

11 Benacerraf BR, Frigoletto FD. Mid trimester fetal thoracocentesis. *J Clin Ultrasound* 1985;13:202–204.

12 Rodeck CH, Fisk NM, Fraser DI, Nicolini U. Long-term *in utero* drainage of fetal hydrothorax. *N Engl J Med* 1988;319:1135–1138.

13 Clewell WH, Johnson ML, Meier PR. A surgical approach to the treatment of fetal hydrocephalus. *N Engl J Med* 1982;306:1320–1325.

14 Vintzileos AM, Ingardia CJ, Nochimson DJ. Congenital hydrocephalus: a review and protocol for perinatal management. *Obstet Gynecol* 1983;62:539–549.

15 Manning FA, Harrison MR, Rodeck CH and members of the International Fetal Medicine and Surgery Society. Catheter shunts for fetal hydronephrosis and hydrocephalus. *N Engl J Med* 1986;315:336–340.

16 Potter EL, Craig JM. *Pathology of the Fetus and Infant*. Chicago: Year Book Medical Publishers, 1976: 434–475.

17 Gembruch U, Hansmann M. Artificial instillation of amniotic fluid as a new technique for the diagnostic evaluation of cases of oligohydramnios. *Prenat Diagn* 1988;8:33–45.

18 Nicolaides KH, Rodeck CH, Gosden CM. Rapid

karyotyping in non-lethal fetal malformations. *Lancet* 1986;i:283–287.

19 Lipitz S, Robson SC, Ryan G, Haeusler MCH, Rodeck CH. Management and outcome of obstructive uropathy in twin pregnancies. *Br J Obstet Gynaecol* 1993;100:879–880.

20 Lebowitz RL, Griscom NT. Neonatal hydronephrosis: 146 cases. *Radiol Clin North Am* 1977;15:49–59.

21 Stiller RJ. Early ultrasonic appearance of fetal bladder outlet obstruction. *Am J Obstet Gynecol* 1989;160:584–585.

22 Mahoney BS, Filly RA, Callen PW, Hricak H, Globus MS, Harrison MR. Fetal renal dysplasia: sonographic evaluation. *Radiology* 1984;152:143–146.

23 Glick PI, Harrison MR, Golbus MS *et al.* Management of the fetus congenital hydronephrosis II. Prognostic criteria and selection for treatment. *J Pediatr Surg* 1985;20:376–387.

24 Nicolini U, Rodeck CH, Fisk NM. Shunt treatment for fetal obstructive uropathy. *Lancet* 1987;ii:1338–1339.

25 Grannum PA, Ghidini A, Scioscia A, Copel JA, Romero R, Hobbins JC. Assessment of fetal reserve in low level obstructive uropathy. *Lancet* 1989;i:281–282.

26 Nicolini U, Fisk NM, Rodeck CH. Fetal urine biochemistry: an index of renal maturation and dysfunction. *Br J Obstet Gynaecol* 1992;99:46–50.

27 Muller F, Dommergues M, Mandelbrot L, Aubry MC, Nichoul-Fekete C, Dumez Y. Fetal urine biochemistry predicts postnatal renal function in children with bilateral obstructive uropathies. *Obstet Gynecol* 1993;82:813–820.

28 Evans MI, Sacks AJ, Johnson MP, Robichaux III AG, May M, Moghissi KS. Sequential invasive assessment of fetal renal function and intrauterine treatment of fetal obstructive uropathies. *Obstet Gynecol* 1991;77:54–55.

29 Harrison MR, Golbus MS, Filly RA *et al.* Management of the fetus with congenital hydronephrosis. *J Pediatr Surg* 1982;17:728–742.

30 Chernick V, Reed MH. Pneumothorax and chylothorax in the neonatal period. *J Pediatr* 1970;76:624–632.

31 Elser H, Borutto F, Schneider A, Schneider K. Chylothorax in a twin pregnancy of 34 weeks sonographically diagnosed. *Eur J Obstet Gynecol Reprod Biol* 1983;16:205–211.

32 Keeling JW, Gough DJ, Iliff PJ. The pathology of non-rhesus hydrops. *Diagn Histopathol* 1983;6:89–111.

33 Adzick NS, Harrison MD. Management of the fetus with a cystic adenomatoid malformation. *World J Surg* 1993;17:342–349.

34 Lien JM, Colmorgan GHC, Gehret JF, Evantash AB. Spontaneous resolution of fetal pleural effusion diagnosed during the second trimester. *J Clin Ultrasound* 1990;18:54–56.

35 Jaffe R, Di Segni E, Altaras M, Loebel R, Benaderat N. Ultrasonic real-time diagnosis of transitory fetal pleural and pericardial effusion. *Diagn Imag Clin Med* 1986;55:373–375.

36 Schmidt W, Harms E, Wolf D. Successful prenatal treatment of non-immune hydrops fetalis due to congenital chylothorax. *Br J Obstet Gynaecol* 1985;92:685–687.

37 Pijpers L, Reuss A, Stewart PA, Wladimiroff JW. Noninvasive management of isolated bilateral fetal hydrothorax. *Am J Obstet Gynecol* 1989;161:330–332.

38 Giannakoulopoulos X, Sepulreda W, Kourlis P, Glover V, Fisk NM. Fetal plasma cortisol and B endorphin response to intrauterine needling. *Lancet* 1994;344:77–81.

39 Rodeck CH, Nicolaides KH. Ultrasound guided invasive procedures in obstetrics. *Clinics Obstet Gynecol* 1983;10:515–540.

40 Nicolini U, Tannirandorn Y, Vaughan J, Fisk NM, Nicolaidis P, Rodeck CH. Further predictors of renal dysplasia in fetal obstructive uropathy: bladder pressure and biochemistry of fresh urine. *Prenat Diagn* 1991;11:159–166.

41 Elder JS, Duckett JW, Snyder HM. Intervention for fetal obstructive uropathy: has it been effective: *Lancet* 1987;i:1007–1010.

42 Ronderos-Dumit D, Nicolini U, Vaughan J, Fisk NM, Chamberlain PF, Rodeck CH. Uterine–peritoneal amniotic fluid leakage: an unusual complication of intrauterine shunting. *Obstet Gynecol* 1991;78:913–915.

43 Robichaux III AG, Mandell James, Greene MF, Benacerraf BR, Evans MI. Fetal abdominal wall defect. A new complication of vesicoamniotic shunting. *Fetal Diagn Ther* 1991;6:11–13.

44 Thompson PJ, Greenough A, Nicolaides KH. Respiratory function in infancy following pleuro-amniotic shunting. *Fetal Diagn Ther* 1993;8:79–83.

45 Reuss A, Wladimiroff JW, Stewart PA, Scholtmeijer RJ. Noninvasive management of fetal obstructive uropathy. *Lancet* 1988;ii:949–951.

46 Crombleholme TM, Harrison MR, Golbus MS *et al.* Fetal intervention in obstructive uropathy: prognostic indicators and efficiency of intervention. *Am J Obstet Gynecol* 1990;162:1239–1244.

47 Harrison MR, Adzick NS, Flake AW. Prenatal management of the fetus with a correctable defect. In: Callen PW (ed) *Ultrasonography in Obstetrics and Gynaecology,* 3rd edn. Philadelphia: WB Saunders, 1994:536–547.

48 Evans MI, Drugan A, Manning FA, Harrison MR. Fetal surgery in the 1990's. *Am J Dis Child* 1989;143:1431–1436.

49 MacMahon RA, Renou PM, Shekelton PA, Paterson PJ. *In utero* cystectomy. *Lancet* 1992;340:1234.

50 Quintus R, Hume R, Smith C *et al*. Percutaneous fetal cystoscopy and endoscopic fulguration of posterior urethral valves. *Am J Obstet Gynecol* 1995;172:206–209.

51 Foxall PJD, Bewley S, Robson SC, Rodeck CH, Neild GH, Nicholson JK. Analysis of fetal and neonatal urine using proton nuclear magnetic resonance spectroscopy. *Arch Dis Child (Fetal and Neonatal)* 1995;73:F153–F157.

Chapter 12/Fetal umbilical cord catheterization under ultrasound guidance

DIDIER LÉMERY, JOAQUIN SANTOLAYA-FORGAS,
LAIRD WILSON, ANDRE BIENIARZ,
PHILIPPE VANLIEFERINGHEN and BERNARD JACQUETIN

Percutaneous umbilical blood sampling (PUBS) is a diagnostic procedure used in most fetal medicine units and is described elsewhere in this book. PUBS allows direct access to the fetal circulation for diagnostic and therapeutic purposes, including fetal transfusions, exchange transfusions and intravascular infusions of drugs. The authors have described a technique of catheterization of the umbilical cord under ultrasound guidance for human intrauterine exchange transfusions [1,2]. Ultrasound-guided chronic catheterization of umbilical vessels and chronic intra-amniotic tolerance in animal studies have also been reported [3–5]. Recently, an artificial training model for endoscopically guided cord catheterization has been reported but is very difficult to perform (Yves Ville, personal communication). In this chapter the operative guidelines, technique for human exchange transfusions and description of an animal model for testing chronic fetal tolerance of the catheters are reviewed.

Indications for umbilical vein catheterization in humans

In humans, ultrasound-guided fetal cord catheterization has only been reported for blood transfusion purposes. Several fetal medicine units (M.H. Poissonnier & Y. Brossard unpublished data) have used fetal intravascular catheters for long-term infusion of albumin in cases of hydrops fetalis. The technique was developed to avoid cord and/or placental injuries due to dislodgement of the needle after fetal movements while performing intrauterine exchange transfusion [6]. Although fetal curarization can be used to inhibit fetal movements [7], it cannot control iatrogenic and operator-dependent dislodgements due to small needle movements during long procedures. Needle dislodgements may lead to fetal

exsanguination [8] or to the infusion of blood into Wharton's jelly leading to cord tamponade [9].

Operative guidelines for human umbilical cord catheterization (see ref. 6)

Fetal umbilical cord catheterization under ultrasound guidance has been performed only in cases of anterior insertion of the placenta. The technique may be possible in lateral or fundal insertion if there is a direct path to the root of the umbilical vein without any transamniotic passage. A posterior placental insertion precludes the use of this technique because it makes necessary a transamniotic passage of the catheter, which can then be removed from the cord by the fetus. If necessary, a direct path to the root of the umbilical vein can be made possible by moving the uterus after a laparotomy. However, due to the current limited experience we recommend using the technique in the less invasive manner.

Guidelines for chronic fetal catheterization are similar to those described for PUBS. However, umbilical cord catheterization must be performed in an operating room under complete sterile conditions. General anaesthesia is only required if a laparotomy or a more invasive procedure is anticipated.

Technique of cord catheterization

Prior to the procedure, a fetal non-stress test is performed, which will allow comparison with intraoperative and postoperative tests. Throughout the procedure a continuous heart rate recording is obtained by attaching the fetal heart rate transducer to the maternal abdominal wall with sterile adhesive tape. Syringes containing prediluted solutions (1 ml/500 g of fetal weight) of atropine, furosemide, adrenaline, isopropyl noradrenaline and vecuronium are prepared and ready to use [2].

The technique is best performed by a team of two operators experienced in diagnostic and interventional ultrasound, which allows one of them to have both hands free at certain points of the intervention. A key step in the procedure is to choose the correct site of entry of the catheterization device. It should be chosen in such a way that direct access to the vein is possible and the maternal bowel avoided. A local anaesthetic (lignocaine 1%) is administered at the chosen site. Two alternatives are then possible: (i) direct placement of the catheter through a needle or (ii) a modified ultrasound-guided Seldinger technique. PUBS is then undertaken, adjusting the tip of the needle through the placenta into the root of the umbilical vein and avoiding, as previously mentioned, any transamniotic passage. A fetal blood sample is obtained, the purity confirmed and appropriate testing performed according to indication.

If the direct technique is used, an epidural Tuohy needle (16 gauge) is required. A 1-mm epidural catheter (Périfix) is then introduced through the needle and the needle is removed when fetal blood has been aspirated, confirming the intravascular location of the catheter. Alternatively, a thin-walled 18-gauge spinal needle with a 1-mm lumen (Becton Dickinson) may be used. For the modified Seldinger technique, a 20-gauge regular spinal needle that has been previously sheathed with a short 16-gauge peripheral Teflon catheter is used. The sheathed needle is then introduced in the vessel root via a 1-mm skin incision. After blood sampling, a guide wire from a 1-mm diameter central venous catheter (Seldiflex 1 × 300 mm, Plastimed) is introduced into the vein. The echogenicity of the metal allows good control of its progress (Figs 12.1 & 12.2). Once this wire is correctly inserted, the needle is removed leaving the peripheral catheter in the abdominal wall and the wire in the cord. The central catheter is then pushed

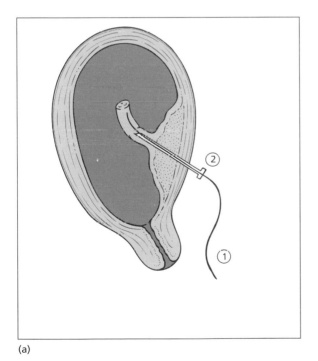

(a)

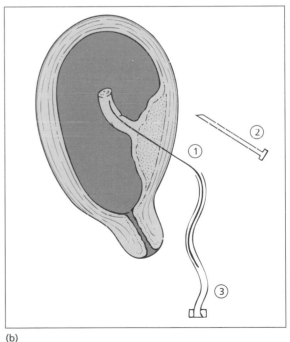

(b)

Fig. 12.1 (a) After regular PUBS the guide wire of the catheter (1) is introduced into the umbilical vein through a 20-gauge needle (2).

(b) The needle (2) has been removed. The guide wire remains in the umbilical vein (1). The catheter (3) is pushed into the vein and guided by the wire.

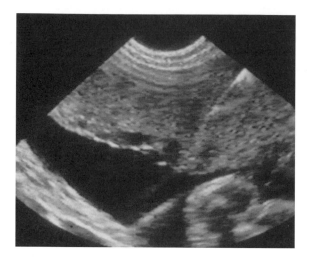

Fig. 12.2 Echogenic visualization of the guide wire during placement.

toward the vein guided by both wire and peripheral catheter. Finally, the wire is pulled out, while the short catheter will protect the intravascular line from bending and compression by the abdominal wall or uterine contraction. In both techniques, approximately 5 cm of catheter are threaded into the umbilical vein. After catheter insertion an infusion of saline will create some echogenic turbidity in the vein, allowing visualization of the catheter and confirmation of its correct location.

Non-human primate animal model

For research purposes, chronic open cannulation of fetal vessels is commonly performed. The majority of animal fetal catheterization models require a fetal part to be exteriorized through a hysterotomy: we have found only one report of ultrasound-guided cannulation of the umbilical vein [5]. Nevertheless, this method is clearly a less invasive approach to the study and evaluation of the fetus and therefore had to be considered. The authors chose the baboon (*Papion anubis*) model to test the feasibility of chronic umbilical vein catheterization because these primates have a haemochorial monodiscoid placenta similar to the human and different to that of the rhesus monkey, which normally has a bilobed placenta [10]. Baboons have a mean duration of pregnancy of 184 ± 2 days. In this study all animals were operated on between 134 and 161 days. Before

the operation, ultrasonographic evaluation of the fetus was performed to determine fetal viability, fetal size, amniotic fluid volume, placental location and umbilical cord insertion. All animals had an ultrasonographically proven anterior placenta. During the operation, anaesthesia was maintained with halothane. A midline laparotomy was then performed. A 5-MHz ultrasound probe within a sterile plastic sleeve was used to carefully locate the umbilical cord insertion. The umbilical vein was then cannulated with a 0.52×0.82 mm vinyl cannula via an 18-gauge thin-walled spinal needle (Becton-Dickinson). The needle was introduced transplacentally into the vein under continuous ultrasound guidance. Approximately 10 cm of cannula were threaded into the umbilical vein. Two additional cannulae were inserted, also under ultrasound guidance, into the amniotic cavity to allow for amnio-infusions (before cord catheterization to improve visualization of the cord) and to monitor uterine contractions after the procedure. The three intrauterine cannulae were then anchored to the uterine serosa with 3-0 silk suture and were exteriorized via a midlateral flank incision. The abdominal incision was then closed with Vycril suture. The maternal femoral vein and artery were then dissected in the groin area of the leg and cannulated. These cannulae were anchored and exited subcutaneously toward the midlateral flank incision with tunnelling needles. The five cannulae were then led subcutaneously to a midline dorsal incision at the level of the scapula with a tunnelling needle. The incisions for tunnelling were then closed. A nylon mesh jacket was placed on the animal and the cannulae led out through a 60-cm flexible stainless steel tether connecting the back of the jacket to a swivel on the side of the cage. The amniotic fluid cannulae were connected to a pressure transducer and pressure changes recorded on a four-channel polygraph. The cannulae in the umbilical vein, femoral vein and artery were attached to syringes on an infusion pump. Heparin was infused to keep the cannulae patent; Cephazolin 1 g daily was also infused. The postoperative follow-up of the mother consisted of evaluation for potential infection and bleeding. Fetal viability was determined ultrasonographically twice daily and fetal blood samples obtained daily. Uterine contractions were monitored 24 hours per day and throughout labour and delivery. Figure 12.3 shows maternal and fetal haematological values after chronic umbilical vein catheterization in a baboon.

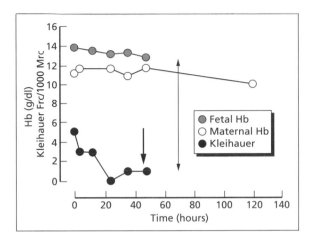

Fig. 12.3 Maternal and fetal haemoglobin (Hb) concentrations in baboon model of chronic umbilical cord catheterization. Parallel evolution of Kleihauer–Betke smears in mother also shown. Single arrow, fetal death; double arrow, delivery. Frc = fetal red cells; Mrc = maternal red cells.

Follow-up, tolerance and complications in humans

Umbilical vein catheterization for short periods of time is feasible and a safe procedure in humans. This technique has only been used to perform fetal blood exchange transfusions. The indication for the first attempt at this procedure was to transfuse a fetus haemorrhaging due to a cord root injury caused by fetal movements at the beginning of an intravascular transfusion procedure [2]. Eight other catheterizations in four fetuses between 27 and 34 weeks' gestation have since followed. Time to place the catheter has always been <5 min and catheters have remained within the umbilical vein for 30–210 min. The catheter to be used should be selected according to the indication. If epidural catheters instead of central venous catheters are used we have experienced difficulties infusing, and more so while aspirating, blood. Blood cultures performed before catheter removal were always negative. No thrombosis or haematomas within Wharton's jelly or the placenta nor histological findings of chorioamnionitis were detected after birth. Three fetuses were delivered by Caesarean section and one vaginally between 9 and 64 days after the first catheterization procedure [6].

Conclusions

Experimental fetal medicine using non-human primate animal models will be the final arbiter in determining if this technique can be safely used in humans. Animal experiments and research in fetomaternal physiology, endocrinology, haematology, immunology, nutrition, fetal surgery, etc. are needed before such a technique is attempted in humans. Umbilical cord catheterization, subcutaneous tunnelling of the catheter and connection to an infusion chamber, such as those used for chemotherapy, may be foreseen as an alternative treatment modality in the following circumstances.

1 Parenteral supplementation of growth-restricted fetuses. The use of nutrient supplementation as well as the restoration of normal oxygenation and metabolic status may improve fetal growth in cases of placental insufficiency.

2 Intraoperative and postoperative monitoring of fetal metabolic status and treatment of fetal pain and infection. Chronic fetal catheterization performed preoperatively may become indispensable for open fetal surgery as well as for endoscopic fetal surgery.

3 Gene therapy may also benefit from this technique, which could allow administration of several doses of stem or transfected cells. Monitoring the fetal reaction to these treatments may also be possible using only one interventional procedure.

References

1 Daffos F, Cappella-Pavlovsky M, Forestier F. A new procedure for fetal blood sampling *in utero*: preliminary results of 53 cases. *Am J Obstet Gynecol* 1983;**146**:985.

2 Lemery D, Urbain MF, Vanlieferinghen P, Micorek JC, Jaquetin B. Intra-uterine exchange transfusion under ultrasound guidance. *Eur J Obstet Gynecol Reprod Biol* 1989;33:161–168.

3 Rosen M. Anesthesia and monitoring for fetal intervention. In: Harrisson MR, Golbus MS, Filly RA (eds) *The Unborn Patient*. Philadelphia: WB Saunders, 1990.

4 Wilson L, Parson MT, Flouret G. Inhibition of spontaneous uterine contractions during the last trimester in pregnant baboons by an oxytocin antagonist. *Am J Obstet Gynecol* 1990;**163**:1875–1882.

5 Taylor PM, Silver M, Fowden AL. Intravenous catheterization of fetus and mare in late pregnancy: management and respiratory, circulatory and metabolic effects. *Equine Vet J* 1992:391:396.

6 Lemery D, Urbain MF, Micorek JC, Jacquetin B. Fetal umbilical cord catheterization under ultrasound guidance. *Fetal Ther* 1988;3:37.

7 Weiner C. Pancuronium protects against fetal bradycardia following umbilical cord puncture. 11th Society of Perinatal Obstetricians Annual Meeting, Meeting Abstrac. *Am J Obstet Gynecol* 1991;**164** part 2:335.

8 Rightmire DA, Ertmoed EE. Fetal exsanguination following umbilical cord sampling. 11th Society of Perinatal Obstetricians Annual Meeting, Meeting Abstrac. *Am J Obstet Gynecol* 1991;**164**: 339.

9 Moise KJ, Carpenter RJ, Huhta JC *et al*. Umbilical cord hematoma secondary to *in utero* intravascular transfusion for Rh isoimmunization. *Fetal Ther* 1987;2: 65–70.

10 Lemery D, Santolay-Forgas J, Wilson L *et al*. A non-human primate model for the *in utero* chronic catheterization of the umbilical vein. A preliminary report. *Fetal Diagn Ther* 1995;10:326–332.

Chapter 13 / Intrauterine pressure

ALEXANDRA BENACHI, DAVID TALBERT
and NICHOLAS M. FISK

Introduction

The study of human fetal physiology has, until recently, been limited by the relative inaccessibility of the intrauterine environment. Direct evaluation of the intrauterine and fetal environment began in the 1960s with the first invasive procedures [1] and expanded in the 1980s with the increase in indications for ultrasound-guided needling procedures [2,3].

Prior to this, studies of intra-amniotic pressure in the human concentrated almost entirely on its change with uterine activity and therefore on labouring women at term. They were achieved via a needle or catheter inserted transabdominally into the amniotic cavity [4–6] or transcervical catheters inserted either extra-amniotically or in patients with ruptured membranes [7–9]. It was not until the mid to late 1980s that oligohydramnios [10,11] and polyhydramnios [12,13] came to be recognized as specific indications for invasive procedures. The resultant studies paved the way for better understanding of the effects of normal and abnormal amniotic fluid volume and pressure on fetal well-being [14–16].

Early animal [17,18] and human [19] studies attempted to evaluate fetal pressures, but in many cases failed to account for alterations in surrounding intra-amniotic pressure, which varies with gestation, uterine activity and maternal and fetal movements [14].

Intrauterine manometric technique in human pregnancy

Definition

Pressure is defined as force per unit area with units in pascals (N/m^2). These are very small units and thus kilopascals (kPa) are more usually used in medicine. To get a feel for this unit consider the following: 1 ml of water weighs about 1 g. If four walls, 1 cm wide were glued to a surface to form a container and then filled with water to a height of 1 cm, the water would exert a pressure of $1 g/cm^2$ anywhere over the area of that surface contained within the walls. If the level were raised to 10 cm, 10 g of water would be pressing on the same area and the pressure would be $10 g/cm^2$, which is approximately 1 kPa [20]. Thus the pressure in a fairly tall mug of coffee varies from nothing at the surface to about 1 kPa at the bottom.

Although a variety of geometric shapes have been used to describe the uterine cavity [21], most authors accept that in order to apply Laplace's law the uterus may be considered as equivalent to a sphere [22–24], a mathematical simplification of the composite radii of little consequence for intrauterine pressure. Pressure within the sphere is a function of T/r, where T is the wall tension and r the radius. The initial application of this law to non-living matter held that pressure fell with increasing r, and this was the basis for an assumption that resting amniotic pressure (AP) falls in late gestation [25]. This simple hydrostatic model, however, is complicated within a musculo-elastic structure like the uterus by the effects of stretch (increasing r) or T. This in turn is modulated by wall thickness, myocyte length and the effects of pregnancy hormones. Furthermore, distension (implying an increase in pressure) is an important stimulus for uterine growth and thus further increase in r. Therefore the development of AP in pregnancy reflects the relative rate of change of T/r. On this basis it has alternatively been suggested that AP rises in late pregnancy with tension increasing at a greater rate than radius [21]. These theoretical conflicts highlighted the need for direct pressure studies.

Materials and methods

AMNIOTIC PRESSURE

Different studies have used different apparatus to measure AP. Older studies of basal intrauterine pressure were performed via transcervical catheters inserted in early labour either extra-amniotically or in patients with ruptured membranes, and therefore were not standardized [9,24]. New invasive techniques allow measurement of pressures in pregnant women undergoing clinically indicated invasive procedures in ongoing pregnancies or at termination of pregnancy. Two main types of transducers can be used: fluid-filled transducers with a fluid-filled line to transmit pressure from the measured part to the transducer, or pressure-tip transducers.

Our group used a 20-gauge needle inserted under ultrasound guidance into the amniotic cavity and attached to a saline-filled catheter. This was linked to a silicon strain-gauge transducer, although more modern disposable transducers have recently been used (Fig. 13.1) [14,15]. Initially, the output was observed on a chart recorder for 60–90 seconds to ensure stable readings free of artefact before reading actual pressures by meter. It was then found that AP reading instability could be adequately discerned from observation of the

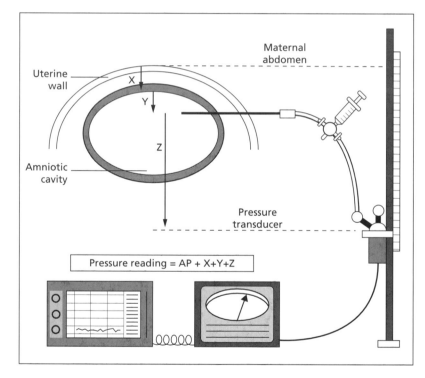

Fig. 13.1 Fluid-filled manometry system for measurement of amniotic pressure (AP) in human pregnancies undergoing invasive procedures. For ease of interpretation of the components of measured AP, this example shows the transducer positioned beneath the amniotic cavity: the pressure recorded at the level of the transducer equals, in addition to that due to uterine tone (AP), the sum of the height of the fluid column in the catheter below the needle (Z) and the height of the fluid column within the amniotic cavity above the needle (Y). X represents the distance between skin and amniotic cavity. Given that the density of overlying fat and muscle approximates that of water, fluid pressure at the transducer equals AP + X + Y + Z. When the transducer is elevated on the sliding attachment pole to be level with, and thus referenced to, the maternal skin, X + Y + Z = 0 and the recorded pressure will equal AP. Referencing the apparatus at the maternal skin surface thus eliminates the gravitational component. (From Fisk *et al.* [15], with permission).

meter, and subsequent readings were then taken directly from the meter when stability had been maintained. Fluid-filled manometer systems self-compensate for the position of the needle within the amniotic cavity, as discussed below.

AP is defined as the pressure within the amniotic cavity over and above that exerted gravitationally by the height of the amniotic fluid column. The pressure measured by a fluid-filled system will, in addition to the pressure due to uterine tone, reflect the sum of the gravitational pressure in the column of fluid above the needle plus the gravitational pressure in the tubing between the needle and transducer. If AP was zero this would be the same as if the open end of the needle was laid on top of the mother's abdomen. The system is in fact zeroed using this as a reference point. Any extra pressure registered when the needle is inserted must therefore be due to uterine wall tension.

Thus variation in position of the needle within the amniotic cavity will not alter the pressure recorded at the transducer. Referencing at the top of the amniotic cavity is impractical and potentially inaccurate; this point would need to be determined ultrasonically, and then somehow translated laterally to reference the transducer. However, as the maternal soft tissue overlying the top of the amniotic cavity comprises both muscle (more dense than water) and fat (less dense), their combination is considered to approximate the density of water. Accordingly the skin surface has been chosen as the reference point, and considered the highest point of a virtual amniotic cavity whose vertical dimension is larger by the overlying soft tissue thickness.

Other groups have used different techniques. Weiner *et al.* [26] used the fetal heart as the reference point. This technique depends on the position of the fetal heart, which may vary between pregnancies and within any single pregnancy with fetal movement. In another method [27,28], the needle's hub was attached directly to a pressure-tip transducer. Pressure was displayed digitally and the angle of the needle measured by a digital meter. Before any measurement was taken, the solid pressure transducer with attached needle was zeroed at an angle of 45° from the horizontal. Actual AP was then calculated after correcting for angle deviations from 45° because the angle determines the vertical distance between transducer and tip of the needle. This essentially measures pressure at the needle tip, whose position may obviously vary depending on its location.

Our group prefers the use of fluid-filled transducers because the simple referencing system reduces variability from the use of different measurement locations within the uterine cavity. Indeed for accurate measurement with the pressure-tip transducer one would need to insert the transducer into the amniotic cavity, via a thin probe for example, which is not very practicable with ultrasound-guided invasive procedures.

INTRAFETAL PRESSURES

Just as intravascular pressure recordings in adults and children are referenced to atmospheric pressure at the level of the heart, intravascular and intracavitary pressures in fetuses should be referenced to the surrounding AP [29]. Subtraction recordings of supra-amniotic pressure are thus necessary [14], not only as a means of reference but also to control for the considerable fluctuations in AP that occur with uterine contractions and maternal respiratory activity. The usual technique in human fetuses consists of two separate 20-gauge needles with fluid-filled lines connecting each to a pressure transducer. The first is located within the amniotic cavity to record AP on one channel of a multichannel recorder, and the second positioned within the fetus (umbilical vein, peritoneal cavity, bladder, etc.). The resultant absolute and relative pressures can then be displayed on a meter or chart recorder.

Another technique [26] uses a single catheter to measure both fetal and amniotic pressures. After insertion into the fetus, the first pressure is measured, then the needle is withdrawn from the fetus into the amniotic cavity where AP is also measured. The second pressure is then subtracted from the first. Although less invasive, this technique may be less accurate, being based on the assumption that AP remains stable throughout the invasive procedure.

When measuring vascular pressure, care must be taken to identify the vessel accurately and to be sure that the needle aperture is not up against the vessel wall otherwise the pressure measured will be higher.

Sources of error

Potential sources of error are plenty, and the lack

of standardization of technique as well as recording method accounts in no small part for the disparate findings reported.

One source of error is the reference point. The ideal system for measuring AP would involve subtraction of amniotic fluid pressure from surrounding maternal intraperitoneal pressure. Although suitable for animal studies, the additional insertion of a paracentesis needle [30] in women is now considered unethical. Caldeyro *et al.* [30] circumvented this problem by measuring intravesical pressure via a urethral catheter considering this to reflect maternal intra-abdominal pressure when intravesical volume was < 20 ml. Subtraction of intra-abdominal from intrauterine pressure was deemed important in these older studies of uterine activity during labour, in order to distinguish contractions from maternal straining and respiratory effort. In the non-labouring patient at rest, it seems unlikely that maternal intra-abdominal pressure comprises a significant component of measurement of stable AP. However, pressure recordings made through a single needle system require a reproducible reference point, such as the top of the maternal abdomen. The accuracy of readings zeroed at the level of anatomical landmarks in the fetus is likely to be impaired by variations in maternal and fetal position, and by changes in uterine and fetal size with gestation. Nevertheless, changes in maternal position may alter the height of the amniotic 'fluid column' necessitating re-zeroing of the system.

Fluid-filled transducers, in contrast to pressure-tip transducers, may produce damping if the tubing is of excessive length. However, this is only a problem with respect to pulse pressures and is not considered to affect stable pressures [29]. Another disadvantage of fluid-filled systems is the potential for inaccuracy in the presence of bubbles, which can be avoided by repeated flushing and visual inspection of both the transducer dome and pressure lines.

A further potential source of error is electrical drift, usually due to changes in transducer temperature and so is relatively slow. Re-zeroing the system before each reading and recalibrating before each patient can minimize this type of error.

Artefacts causing elevated pressures include contraction provoked by the introduction of any needle through the uterine wall, artefactually high readings in anxious women who tense their abdominal muscles, and pressure exerted if the operator inadvertently leans on the maternal abdomen while scanning.

There are thus two components to AP: firstly, that due to uterine tension, which according to Pascal's law is equal and uniform within the uterus; and secondly, a gravitational component that varies vertically. AP referenced to a variable point will thus vary with the position of that point within the cavity.

Amniotic pressure

Amniotic pressure in normal pregnancy

Although AP has been extensively investigated over the last four decades, the emphasis has been almost exclusively on its change with uterine activity. Numerous studies of intrauterine pressure have been performed in labouring women at term. AP has also been studied in the first and second trimester prior to or during termination of pregnancy. The rationale for these investigations was the characterization of pressure changes during spontaneous and pharmacologically induced contractions. Resting AP has only been studied as a baseline against which the effects of oxytocic drugs were assessed. Such reports present AP readings graphically, with typical scales of 0 to 100–250 mmHg, rendering accurate interpretation of resting AP impossible. Another problem has been the lack of uniform reference point as discussed above. Although some authors standardized readings at the maternal umbilicus [31] or against maternal intraperitoneal or intravesical pressure [5,32], most deemed no reference point necessary to calculate changes in AP with contractions.

Two groups [14,16,26] have recently reported AP measurements at ultrasound-guided needling to show that intra-amniotic pressure increases linearly over the last half of gestation, presumably due to an increase in uterine tone secondary to stretching of myometrial fibres (Fig. 13.2). The results from our group are consistent with data obtained at term of basal AP (8–12 mmHg) in early labour [32]. However they are only half as high as those of Weiner *et al.* [26] who recorded AP after fetal blood sampling and used a variable reference point (fetal heart). In contrast we measured AP before other procedures to avoid stimulating contractions and used a fixed reference point comparable between subjects [16].

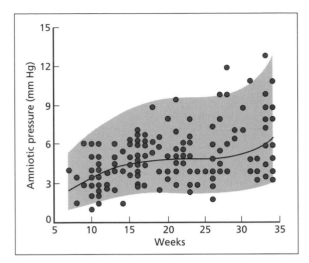

Fig. 13.2 Amniotic pressure in 171 singleton pregnancies with normal amniotic fluid volume. The line represents the estimated mean ($\log_e (y + 1) = 0.12 + 0.23x - 0.010x^2 + 0.00015x^3$, $R^2 = 0.19$, $P < 0.001$ where y is amniotic pressure in mmHg and x is gestation in weeks) and the shaded area the 95% reference range. (From Fisk *et al.* [16], with permission.)

In contrast to these results, Sideris and Nicolaides [27] found that the mean AP decreased exponentially with gestation, from 9 mmHg at 10 weeks to a plateau at 5 mmHg from 30 weeks. However, as discussed above, their methodology involved a pressure-tip transducer attached to the needle hub with measurements referenced to its tip; consequently, they measured pressure at the variable position of the needle tip, rather than gravity-independent pressure within the amniotic cavity attributable to uterine tone. Accordingly, it is understandable that they found a decline in pressure with gestation, given that with advancing gestation it is likely that an increasingly larger proportion of the needle would be introduced beneath the reference point used by others.

The reference range in Fig. 13.2 is independent of maternal age, parity and gravidity; allowing for limited numbers studied, it may also be applicable to twin pregnancies [16]. In that study, there was no correlation of AP with amniotic fluid index, which reflects amniotic fluid volume [33], suggesting that intrauterine volume is not a primary determinant of AP. Instead it seems

that gestational age is the main factor influencing AP. Furthermore, the relationship of AP to increasing gestation is different from that of amniotic volume, which increases to 22 weeks and does not change significantly thereafter [34]. This study demonstrated that AP rises in late pregnancy, whereas it had previously been assumed to fall, due to a stable uterine radius and thus volume. If development of AP with advancing gestation is assumed to reflect the relative change of T/r, the weakly sigmoid-shaped normal AP curve suggests that P, and thus T relative to r, increases more rapidly in the first and third trimesters than in mid-pregnancy. T could not be deduced, since uterine radius was not measured. However, a planimetric ultrasound study has suggested that uterine radii increase in a near-linear fashion throughout pregnancy [35]. AP thus appears mediated by gestation-specific anatomical and hormonal influences on gravid uterine musculature.

Amniotic pressure in abnormal fluid volume

POLYHYDRAMNIOS

Amniotic pressure and effect of fluid drainage

Polyhydramnios is associated with a high rate of maternal and fetal complications. Maternal ones include abdominal discomfort, respiratory embarrassment and uterine irritability. Preterm delivery occurs more frequently, with a rate of 22% corrected for congenital anomalies, as also does premature rupture of the membranes [36]. The incidence of pre-eclampsia is also increased [37]. Similarly there is an increased incidence of postpartum haemorrhage, attributed to uterine atony [36], and gross enlargement of the uterus may rarely result in ureteric obstruction [38]. The above maternal complications are similar to those encountered in high-order multiple pregnancies, and many authors have attributed them to uterine distension [39]. The incidence of Caesarean section is also increased in polyhydramnios [40], due largely to unstable fetal lie. A further risk is abruption, which has been associated with rapid decompression of the uterus as amniotomy [41,42].

Three main variables influence perinatal survival in polyhydramnios: presence of congenital anomalies, gestational age at delivery and severity of polyhydramnios

[43,44]. The most severe form of polyhydramnios occurs in mid-trimester fetofetal transfusion syndrome [45]. Untreated perinatal mortality rates are 80–100% [46], although these have fallen to around 33% in recent series employing aggressive management [46–49]. Approximately one-third of the losses are intrauterine deaths, and in this regard fetal hypoxaemia and acidaemia have been demonstrated at fetal blood sampling [15]. The remainder are due to prematurity and consequently much attention has recently focused on developing therapies against polyhydramnios.

Treatment of polyhydramnios, usually only considered in severe or acute cases in the mid or early third-trimester, has two aims: relief of maternal symptoms and prolongation of gestation. Polyhydramnios secondary to fetofetal transfusion syndrome is the most frequent indication.

The first description of therapeutic drainage of amniotic fluid [50] came from Queen Charlotte's Hospital in London in 1933. Numerous case reports and small series have since described relief of maternal symptoms and prolongation of gestation with this procedure in both singleton and twin pregnancies [51]. Although some authors have found that rapid reaccumulation of amniotic fluid rendered drainage of little benefit [52,53] without significant improvement in outcome [54], recent series of polyhydramnios secondary to fetofetal transfusion syndrome suggest that it may be beneficial in prolonging gestation [48,55,56]. The small number of such patients seen in any one centre renders it unlikely that the efficacy of this procedure, known as amnioreduction or therapeutic or decompression amniocentesis, can be evaluated without a multicentre randomized trial.

Initially, most authors removed only small quantities of fluid at amnioreduction [51], in view of concerns regarding precipitation of abruption or preterm labour [57]. However the good results of the Phoenix group [46,49,58] in draining volumes of 1–5 litres without significant complications led to widespread adoption of their practice of aggressive therapeutic amnioreduction, whereby all the excess fluid is removed to restore amniotic fluid volume to normal. Elliot *et al.* [58] reported only three complications in a series of 200 therapeutic amnioreductions (1.5%): one rupture of the membranes 24 hours after the procedure at 26 weeks, one chorioamnionitis at 31 weeks 18 hours

after the procedure and one abruptio placentae at 38 weeks in an anencephalic fetus after removal of 10.2 litres. The last case prompted them to restrict therapeutic amnioreduction to a maximal removal of 5 litres per procedure.

An alternative to drainage is medical amnioreduction with prostaglandin synthetase inhibitors [59]. Although the reduction in urine output is less with sulindac than indomethacin, in general the former is now preferred because of the lower incidence of side-effects, in particular premature closure of ductus [60,61].

Almost all authors attribute the complications of polyhydramnios to uterine distension. Implicit in the concept of distension of a sealed container is a rise in internal pressure. Csapo *et al.* [62] incrementally increased intrauterine volume in postpartum rabbits and although there was little initial change in resting pressure, an exponential increase accompanied further increase in volume. There have been reports evaluating intrauterine pressure in polyhydramnios [63,64]. Notwithstanding the difficulties discerning exact details from such observational reports characteristic of the older literature, it appears that some cases of polyhydramnios had normal pressure, while in others it was markedly raised to 25 mmHg. Recent studies on ultrasound-guided needling in ongoing pregnancies [14,16,26] have clearly shown that resting AP is raised in polyhydramnios. As shown in Fig. 13.3 AP in polyhydramnios lies above the reference mean and exceeds the upper limit of the reference range in just over half of cases; this may explain previous conflicting reports of AP in polyhydramnios. In contrast to Caldeyro-Barcia *et al.* [32], who contended that there were two separate types of polyhydramnios (normal and high pressure), our group has suggested that raised pressure simply reflects the degree of increased amniotic fluid volume. AP appears a linear function of severity, as assessed semi-quantitatively by both the deepest pool measurement and the amniotic fluid index (AFI) (Fig. 13.4). In those with mildly increased amniotic fluid volume (deepest pool < 12 cm or AFI < 40 cm) AP often lay within the reference range, while gross elevations in AP were found only where the deepest pool exceeded 15 cm and the AFI 50 cm. This is consistent with the known properties of skeletal and uterine muscle, in which resting tension increases initially only slightly with increasing length as the elastic and inelastic muscle

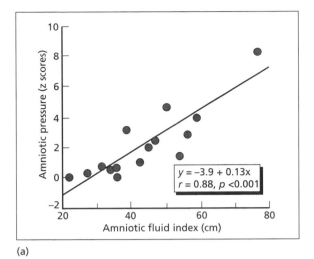

(a)

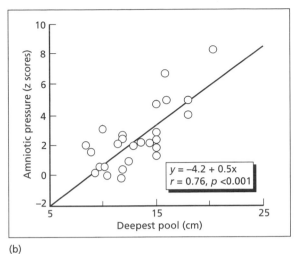

(b)

Fig. 13.3 (a) The relationship, in pregnancies with polyhydramnios, between amniotic pressure in z scores and semi-quantitative amniotic fluid volume expressed as the amniotic fluid index ($y = -3.9 + 0.13x$, where y is amniotic pressure z score and x is amniotic fluid index in cm, $r = 0.88$, $P < 0.001$). (b) The relationship, in pregnancies with polyhydramnios, between amniotic pressure in z scores and semi-quantitative amniotic fluid volume expressed as the deepest vertical pool measurement (y is amniotic pressure z score and x is deepest pool in cm). (From [65], with permission)

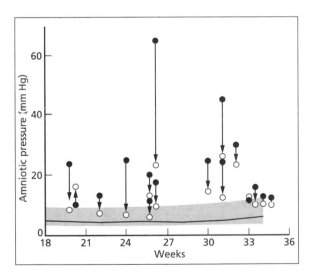

Fig. 13.4 The acute effect of drainage of 100–1100 ml of amniotic fluid on amniotic pressure ●, before drainage; ○, after drainage; shaded area, reference range). (From Fisk [65], with permission.)

fibres slide over each other, until the resting length is exceeded producing a large rise in tension due to stretching of inelastic fibres.

Elevated AP in gross polyhydramnios is consistent with the clinical features of this condition and can be normalized by drainage of excess fluid [15]. Indeed, it is possible that normalization of pressure rather than volume could be the more appropriate therapeutic aim, at least in the short term. AP in pregnancies with polyhydramnios with high basal AP (above the upper limit of reference range) can be restored towards normal by drainage of amniotic fluid (Fig. 13.5). In contrast, no significant change in AP occurs with drainage in those with normal AP (within the reference range) [65]. The volumes drained in the group with raised AP were relatively small (mean 679 ml), considering that amniotic fluid volumes (and their drainage) of up to 7–10 litres have been reported in association with gross polyhydramnios.

Impaired uteroplacental perfusion

Tabor and Maier [66] speculated that raised AP impairs uteroplacental perfusion in polyhydramnios, based on their observation of cardiotocographic changes in a case of transient iatrogenic polyhydramnios during intrapartum amnio-infusion. Indeed, in twin–twin transfusion syndrome it has recently been suggested that raised

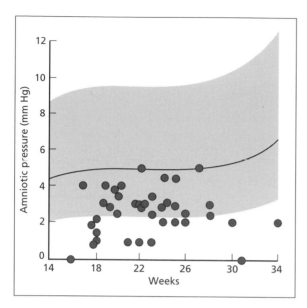

Fig. 13.5 Amniotic pressure in pregnancies complicated by oligohydramnios shown against the reference range for pregnancies with normal amniotic fluid volume. ●, severe oligohydramnios. (From Fisk [65], with permission.)

pressure in the recipient's sac secondary to polyhydramnios impairs placental perfusion in the donor twin, and that this results in further hypovolaemia and oliguria in the donor. This suggestion arose from an unexpected observation in recent series of fetofetal transfusion syndrome treated by serial amniocenteses, whereby removal of sufficient fluid to normalize volume in the recipient's sac was accompanied by normalization of amniotic fluid volume in the previously anhydramniotic donor's sac [46,48,49,55] and, in some cases, resolution of hydrops.

Our group [67] have suggested that raised AP might explain the high frequency of fetal hypoxaemia and acidaemia and therefore the 6–14% of antenatal death in normal (without congenital anomalies or preterm labour and rupture of membranes) singletons with polyhydramnios. Of 22 fetuses from pregnancies with polyhydramnios investigated by fetal blood sampling, eight (36%) had a pH value and 16 (73%) a Po_2 value below the reference range. Both fetal pH and Po_2 were significantly negatively linearly correlated with the degree of elevation in AP. Although some of these fetuses were hydropic, had congenital anomalies

or were from multiple pregnancies, univariate and multiple logistic regression analyses indicated that the above associations could not be accounted for by these potentially confounding variables. In order to determine the effect of raising AP on fetal blood gas status in the absence of confounding variables, 5–15 litres of saline were infused intra-amniotically in sheep, producing a rise in AP of 1.0 ± 0.013 (mean ± SE) mmHg/litre infused but no significant change in fetal acid–base status [68]. This failure to impair normal fetal blood gas status may have been due to the modest rise in AP achieved or instead might reflect species differences in placentation. Animals studies have indicated that uteroplacental perfusion needs to be reduced by 50% before any major effect on fetal blood gas status is demonstrated [69]. Increases in uterine pressure during contractions have been shown to produce alterations in uterine artery Doppler waveform [70]. Two groups [71,72] studied the effect of therapeutic amniocentesis on uterine artery velocimetry, using measurement of impedance index values from Doppler flow–velocity waveform, to demonstrate acute changes in amniotic fluid volume alter uteroplacental perfusion. They concluded that severe polyhydramnios can result in reduction in uterine blood flow, as fluid removal improves it.

Amnioreduction is currently performed in cases of polyhydramnios associated with maternal symptoms and as standard treatment for twin–twin transfusion syndrome. Measuring the AP in polyhydramnios has been useful in terms of understanding the complications of this phenomenon. It has been demonstrated that largest vertical pocket of amniotic fluid greater than 15 cm was always associated with elevated AP and most of the time with some maternal symptoms.

OLIGOHYDRAMNIOS

Amniotic pressure

Perinatal mortality is significantly increased in oligohydramnios, as a result of the underlying aetiology, such as congenital malformations and intrauterine growth retardation, of preterm delivery and of the sequelae of oligohydramnios, such as pulmonary hypoplasia (PH) [73,74]. The severity of oligohydramnios influences prognosis, with a mortality rate of 88% in severe compared with 11% in mild/moderate mid-trimester oligohydramnios [75].

Some of the fetal complications in oligohydramnios may be attributed to reduced amniotic fluid volume, such as PH and skeletal deformities, while others result from the underlying condition, such as intrauterine growth retardation or premature rupture of membranes.

Oligohydramnios is also associated with an increased risk of fetal distress and birth asphyxia [76]. Variable decelerations in oligohydramnios are attributed to umbilical cord compression as shown in rhesus monkeys, in which acute drainage of amniotic fluid resulted in variable decelerations that were eliminated by restoration of amniotic fluid volume [77].

The complications of oligohydramnios have been widely attributed to compression of the fetus and umbilical cord. Implicit in this concept is a rise in the surrounding AP. In contrast, several studies [14,15,26] have now demonstrated that AP is in fact low in oligohydramnios (Fig. 13.6). Indeed, descriptive data in labouring rabbits suggest that removal of 300–700 ml of amniotic fluid by amniocentesis results in a fall in basal AP [78]. This finding, that AP is decreased with reduced amniotic fluid volume, is broadly consistent with hydrostatic principles governing contents within inelastic confines. However, abnormal AP in oligohydramnios is confined to severe degrees of derangement in amniotic fluid volume, as it is in pregnancies complicated by polyhydramnios. This further supports the suggestion that the relationship between AP and intrauterine volume is non-linear, presumably reflecting the different physical principles determining pressure within a musculoelastic structure like the human uterus, as discussed earlier.

The finding of low AP in oligohydramnios is not surprising if the law of Laplace is considered [79]. A decrease in the quantity of amniotic fluid sufficient to cause persistent contact between fetal parts and the uterine wall isolates pockets of amniotic fluid. As the theoretical radius of these amniotic fluid pockets increases with decreasing amniotic fluid volume, AP should thus fall and approach infinity.

Low amniotic pressure and concept of fetal compression

Prolonged oligohydramnios is associated with a variety of fetal manifestations including PH, characteristically flattened facies and postural deformities such as contractures and talipes equinovarus. These phenomena were first considered, with bilateral renal agenesis, to be part of a specific syndrome [80]; however reports of their presence in association with reduced amniotic fluid volume from other causes, and their absence in fetuses with bilateral renal agenesis and normal amniotic fluid volume, led to their recognition as sequelae of oligohydramnios [81]. Accordingly many authors have attributed the sequelae of oligohydramnios to compression of the fetus by the uterine walls in the absence of amniotic fluid [82–84].

Clinical studies indicate that the likelihood of PH after oligohydramnios depends on three variables: gestation at onset, duration and severity of oligohydramnios [84–86]. Amniorrhexis is unlikely to result in PH when membrane rupture occurs after the second trimester [84,87]. Although a causal relationship between oligohydramnios and PH has been well established, the mechanism involved remains controversial [88,89]. Different hypotheses have been suggested.

Compression by intrathoracic space-occupying lesions, such as viscera in diaphragmatic hernia, pleural effusions

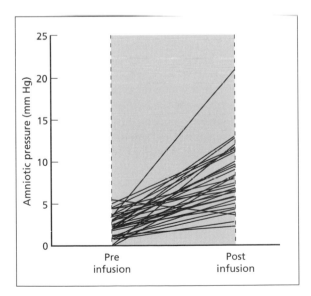

Fig. 13.6 The effect of infusion of normal saline on amniotic pressure (mmHg) in 60 pregnancies complicated by oligohydramnios; mean 4.3 mmHg. (From Fisk [65], with permission.)

and tumours, is known to impair fetal lung growth. The fetus is widely held to be compressed in prolonged oligohydramnios, and thus extrathoracic compression has been assumed as the mechanism for oligohydramnios-related PH [90]; however, it is now known that AP is decreased in that situation [15]. Furthermore, restoration of amniotic fluid volume is not accompanied by any change in fetal breathing movement or umbilical artery Doppler indices, biophysical variables considered affected by fetal compression in oligohydramnios [91,92]. The finding in oligohydramnios of low AP in the presence of soft-tissue manifestations considered indicative of compression (talipes, flattened facies, arthrogryposis, etc.) appears paradoxical. However, amniotic fluid no longer completely surrounds the fetus in severe oligohydramnios. Thus with decreasing amniotic fluid volume, the entire tension of the uterine wall becomes exerted over some fetal parts (head, extremities) that happen to be the internal 'pillars' of the uterus. Fetal compression by the surrounding uterine wall could thus still be mediated through these pillars, even though pressure in the amniotic fluid pockets is low. However, Harding *et al.* [93] have recently shown in sheep that pressures within fetal body cavities (i.e. pleural, peritoneal) do not change with removal and then restoration of amniotic fluid volume, which suggests that direct transmission of uterine tone to the fetal trunk via splinted extremities does not occur. Accordingly, fetal soft-tissue manifestations of oligohydramnios may instead be due to restriction of movement by the uterine wall. Indeed several authors have implicated immobility of fetal extremities in the aetiology of these sequelae [94].

Impairment of fetal breathing is now known not to be the mechanism for oligohydramnios-related PH [95–97], whereas loss of lung liquid from the airways into the amniotic cavity could be implicated in this condition. During gestation, lung liquid travels from the alveolae down the upper airways (the direction of net flow being always away from the lung) from where it is either swallowed or drains into the amniotic cavity [98]. Retention of this liquid within the future airways is required to maintain the lungs at an appropriate level of expansion in order to stimulate their growth [99]. This has been demonstrated by experimental tracheal ligation on fetal sheep, which leads to increases in lung weight and volume [100,101] and reverses PH

associated with oligohydramnios [102]. This phenomenon can be found in human fetuses with Fraser syndrome [103]. Normally, the upper airways produce resistance to the egress of lung liquid, creating a standing tracheal pressure of 1.5–3.0 mmHg above AP, and lung liquid acts as an internal stent around which the lung grows.

This last hypothesis is based on the fact that net outflow of lung liquid along the trachea must adhere to principles of fluid dynamics (tracheal pressure must exceed AP). Therefore, increased escape of lung liquid in oligohydramnios could be due to an increase in the tracheal pressure–AP gradient, secondary to a reduction in AP [79]. However, Fisk *et al.* [104] using an animal model have demonstrated that this might not be true because mimicking low AP in the upper airway by chronic fetal pharyngeal drainage does not impair lung development in fetal sheep.

Notwithstanding this, the pathogenesis of oligohydramnios-related PH is not fully understood. Indeed, Harding *et al.* [105] have reopened the debate by demonstrating that tracheal flow rates during non-labour uterine contractions were more than doubled in the presence of oligohydramnios due to increased fetal intrathoracic and intra-abdominal pressures, although these pressures do not change with oligohydramnios when the uterus is quiescent.

Effect of amnio-infusion

Amnio-infusion has both a diagnostic and therapeutic role in oligohydramnios. In cases of severe oligohydramnios, accurate sonographic visualization of fetal anatomy can be difficult and amnio-infusion is thus used for diagnostic purposes [11,106,107]. Fisk *et al.* [95] reported that diagnosis of the underlying aetiology was revised in 13% as a result of the procedure, unsuspected anomalies were revealed in 9–18% and ruptured membranes was demonstrated by liquor leakage and/ or membranous detachment. Concomitant fetal blood sampling can be done for fetal karyotyping.

Oligohydramnios is responsible for complications that theoretically should be obviated by amnio-infusion. Our group [15] showed that amnio-infusion in pregnancies with oligohydramnios significantly increased AP (Fig. 13.7). The rise in AP with infusion was greatest in those with severe oligohydramnios and those with a

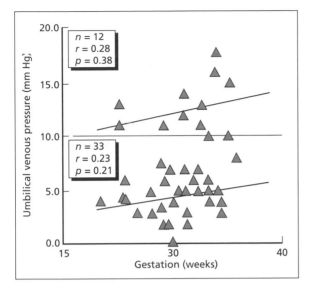

Fig. 13.7 Scattergram of 45 fetuses in which umbilical venous and amniotic fluid pressure were measured. Two distinct populations are seen: *n* = 12 refers to those fetuses with an umbilical venous pressure > 2SD above the norm (i.e. > 10mmHg); *n* = 33 are all normal. (From Weiner *et al.* [26], with permission.)

preinfusion AP beneath the reference range, consistent with preinfusion AP being the main variable determining this rise and the suggestion, made earlier with reference to polyhydramnios, that restoration of fluid volume restores AP towards normal.

Amnio-infusion, by restoring normal AFI, can prevent PH as established in animal models [108], in which restoration of amniotic fluid volume in fetuses with bladder outlet obstruction has significant beneficial effects on lung development. Our group [106] reported that serial amnio-infusion may be associated with a low incidence of sequelae of oligohydramnios. In this uncontrolled study 51 patients underwent a single amnio-infusion and nine patients serial infusions. Talipes occurred in 15% of pregnancies in the first group compared with none in the second group. There was also evidence of a degree of hypoplasia in 22% of pregnancies complicated by severe oligohydramnios diagnosed at or before 22 weeks compared with the 60% reported in severe oligohydramnios diagnosed at or before 28 weeks [109]. In a preliminary report of a cohort study, Vergani *et al.* [110] found that

prophylactic transabdominal amnio-infusion is associated with a significantly lower risk of PH than with expectant management. The prevalence of PH was significantly lower among the amnio-infusion cases compared with the controls (46% vs. 86%).

We previously recommended that because ruptured membranes have been noticed after amnio-infusion, AP should be measured intraprocedurally to avoid an excessive rise in AP. However our recent experience is that this is no longer necessary, providing one takes care to infuse only sufficient fluid to restore amniotic fluid volume to within the lower end of normal range.

Van den Wijngaard *et al.* [111] attributed normalization of a highly resistant umbilical artery waveform after amnio-infusion in a patient with severe oligohydramnios to relief of cord compression, documenting recurrence of the Doppler abnormality with return of oligohydramnios 5 days later. An alternative explanation to cord compression for these cardiovascular changes might be fetal head compression, which in fetal lambs is also followed by bradycardia [112]. In this light, the same group [111] have shown increased peripheral resistance in Doppler studies of the cerebral arteries in human fetuses with oligohydramnios. Although considered to be the result of fetal head compression in that study, these changes can also be induced by excessive transducer pressure [113], an unwitting possibility in any study requiring high ultrasonic resolution in the presence of severe oligohydramnios.

Oligohydramnios is also responsible for fetal distress during labour due to umbilical cord compression. Intrapartum restoration of amniotic fluid volume has been shown to reduce the frequency of fetal heart rate deceleration patterns [114–116] and to decrease morbidity from meconium aspiration [117]. The introduction of an intrauterine pressure catheter to allow intrauterine pressure readings, in addition to both AFI and fetal heart rate monitoring, has been advocated during intrapartum amnio-infusion in order to minimize complications such as uterine overdistension, elevated AP [118] and amniotic fluid embolism [119].

Fetal pressures

Vascular pressures

Access to human fetal compartments and evaluation of

different intrafetal pressures began only recently with the development of clinically indicated fetal invasive procedures. Animal experiments started earlier [17,18] and largely concentrated on physiology. Human studies of fetal pressures using subtraction manometry (see Introduction) allowed investigation of naturally occurring pathologies like hydrothorax [120] and urinary tract obstruction [121].

The development of ultrasound-guided fetal blood sampling has facilitated access to the circulation of the human fetus. The umbilical vein is the vessel most commonly punctured. Weiner *et al.* [26] found a mean umbilical venous pressure (UVP) of 5.3 ± 2.3 mmHg (range 2–11) in normal fetuses, and abnormal fetuses with a UVP > 10 mmHg had either heart failure or hepatomegaly. Nicolini *et al.* [14] reported similar values, (both studies reported UVP unrelated to gestational age) with a mean UVP of 4.5 mmHg. They also measured intrahepatic vein pressures, which ranged from 2 to 11 mmHg, and arterial pressure, which ranged from 14 to 22 mmHg. UVP should approximate to central venous pressure in the inferior vena cava. Because of the parallel fetal circulatory system and the preferential streaming of umbilical venous blood to the left atrium, UVP measurements may be even more sensitive to left ventricular dysfunction than the inferior vena cava [26]. UVP was higher than both intervillous space and fetal intraperitoneal pressure, which is consistent with continuous forward umbilical venous flow from the placenta to the fetus.

Most studies have failed to account for the effects of intra-amniotic pressure [122,123] and few used subtraction manometry. Castle and MacKenzie [124] in 1986 found lower values than the two previous studies, mean 2.2 mmHg, probably due to methodological and calibration differences.

Weiner [125] also applied the measurement of UVP, during diagnostic cordocentesis, to the evaluation of non-immune hydrops fetalis. Cardiac dysfunction, presumably inadequate cardiac output, resulted in an elevated UVP. The finding of a normal UVP essentially eliminates the heart as the cause of hydrops even if a cardiac malformation is present, although one must be aware, in a non-hydropic fetus with tetralogy of Fallot, that a cardiac malformation that permits transmission of arterial pressure to the venous system will also elevate the UVP in spite of adequate cardiac output.

Intrauterine transfusion

Early attempts at intrauterine therapy of anaemic fetuses were by intraperitoneal transfusion [126]. Mean intraperitoneal pressure (IPP) (2.5 mmHg) is normally lower than mean intraumbilical pressure (IUP), necessarily to enable flow along the umbilical vein from the placenta to the inferior vena cava. Animal studies indicate that embarrassment of umbilical venous return results from increased IPP (IPP > IUP) secondary to intraperitoneal transfusion, as the umbilical vein in its intra-abdominal portions traverses the peritoneal cavity [17]; Dunnihoo [123] measured IPP during intraperitoneal transfusion in monkey fetuses and found that bradycardia occurred only when IPP exceeded 10 cmH$_2$O. This explains the risk of complications in 20% of procedures associated with intraperitoneal transfusion compared with the 1–3% perinatal loss rate associated with intravascular transfusion [127]. Nicolini *et al.* [128] reported 11 cases of IPP measurements during transfusions. IPP before transfusion in fetuses without ascites was 2.5 mmHg and no correlation was observed with gestational age. Mean IPP increased to 8.3 mmHg after transfusion. In transfusion unassociated with complications or ascites, IPP rose by 1–9 mmHg (Fig. 13.8). In patients in whom fetal tachycardia or bradycardia occurred during transfusion, the rise in IPP was much greater (16–26 mmHg) than the maximum rise in IPP seen in uncomplicated procedures. Thus pressure monitoring may have a role in obviating undue pressure rises during intraperitoneal transfusion, although this information may be more simply inferred from fetal heart rate changes. The latter is our usual practice.

The intraperitoneal route was the only method of fetal transfusion until 1981, when Rodeck *et al.* [129] performed the first direct fetal intravascular transfusion under fetoscopic visualization. Then Daffos *et al.* [2] developed the ultrasound-guided technique of umbilical vein blood sampling. Two methods of fetal intravascular transfusion have been described: direct (with or without adjunctive peritoneal transfusion) [130] and exchange [131]. The direct technique is easier to perform and the procedure time shorter, but it may compromise the cardiovascular system of the fetus by rapidly increasing intravascular volume. Nicolini *et al.* [128] and Weiner *et al.* [132] showed that the direct or bolus technique increases umbilical pressure. Nicolini *et al.* [128]

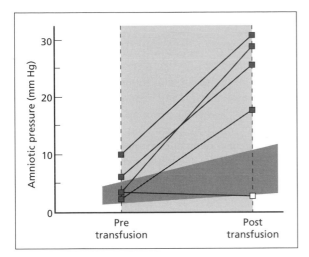

Fig. 13.8 Increase in intraperitoneal pressure with transfusion in uncomplicated procedures (Δ intraperitoneal pressure = 5.8 mmHg, P < 0.0005; stippled area, range). Changes in intraperitoneal pressure before and after transfusion are also shown for fetuses with fetal heart rate changes during transfusion (■) and one with pre-existing ascites (□). (From Nicolini *et al.* [128], with permission.)

reported a rise of mean UVP from 4.5 to 9.1 mmHg after transfusion. This rise in UVP correlated positively with the increase in haematocrit and negatively with gestational age. This elevation of UVP may have been caused by acute filling of a limited vascular capacitance with a large volume of blood or, alternatively, by generalized vasoconstriction possibly mediated by catecholamines in response to either hypoxia or triggering of baroreceptors. The greater increase at earlier gestational ages may be due to the maturational asynchrony of sympathetic and parasympathetic development or the reduction in catecholamine sensitivity that occurs with gestation. Moise *et al.* [133] showed that the mean UVP rise of 1.7 ± 2.8 mmHg during transfusion was associated with a decline in left and right ventricular outputs of 19 and 22%, respectively.

Nicolini *et al.* [134] and Moise *et al.* [135] reported that a combination of intravascular and then intraperitoneal transfusion allows a greater quantity of blood to be administered so that the interval between transfusions may be safely increased. The volume infused into the peritoneal cavity is considerably less than

that used for intraperitoneal transfusion alone, which reduces the related risk of this procedure alone. The direct intravascular route for fetal transfusion, with or without intraperitoneal transfusion, is now preferred to the intraperitoneal route alone.

Hallak *et al.* [136] evaluated whether abnormal elevations in UVP during intravascular transfusion predict adverse fetal outcome and whether this elevation could be used to direct therapy. They studied 14 fetuses with Rhesus incompatibility; after intravascular transfusion, five fetuses died within 24 hours after transfusion and nine survived. The only difference between the groups was the change in UVP during transfusion (5.0 mmHg for survivors, 18.1 mmHg for non-survivors). They concluded that an increase in UVP of 10 mmHg or more predicted fetal death with a sensitivity of 80% and specificity of 89%. Similar values were reported by Radunovic *et al.* [137]. Several groups advocate UVP measurement during transfusion. If the change in UVP approaches 10 mmHg, the procedure is discontinued; if the change exceeds 10 mmHg, blood is removed and replaced with an equal volume of saline. In general, however, most fetuses that begin intravascular transfusion with a normal UVP have a pressure < 10 mmHg at the end of the procedure [125,138].

Nicolini *et al.* [139] have demonstrated that fetal complications may be predicted by abnormal changes in acid–base parameters during intravascular transfusion but only in some cases not in all. This technique might not be reliable. On the contrary, pressure-guided intravascular transfusion is effective but fetal intolerance to a large and rapid intravascular volume load is generally manifested in fetal heart rate abnormalities [140].

We do not think that it is necessary to perform a pressure measurement when it would seem simpler instead to monitor fetal heart rate changes. Fetal distress can be detected by the monitoring of fetal heart rate by observation of the umbilical artery pulsations on colour flow Doppler or, using regular Doppler, by the loss of the end-diastolic flow during the procedure [141].

As all the above studies have shown a rise in venous pressure, it may be that in future this can be deduced from central venous waveforms, such as in the ductus venosus. Further studies are indicated.

Pressures within fetal body cavities

Pressures in different body cavities have been measured essentially to understand better the pathophysiology of disease states such as obstructive uropathies. Nicolini *et al.* [14] also recorded fetal urinary pressures in fetuses with low obstructive uropathies to be around 6–8 mmHg, similar to those seen in control subjects. Low bladder pressure was even found in fetuses with high urinary sodium, suggestive of major renal damage [121]. In another study, Nicolini *et al.* [142] concluded that there was no correlation between bladder pressure and the degree of impairment of renal function in fetuses with urinary obstruction, suggesting that intravesical pressure measurement was of no clinical value. In addition, to facilitate the sometimes difficult differential diagnosis by ultrasound of multicystic kidney from hydronephrosis Nicolini *et al.* [143] recorded intrarenal pressures. Readings within hydronephrotic kidneys were similar to those in the bladder, whereas the cystic spaces of a multicystic kidney had very low pressures. In general, urine biochemistry appears a more reliable guide to distinguishing the two conditions.

The aim of management of fetuses with primary fetal hydrothorax is to take the fetus to a safe gestational age to be delivered without hydrops. Vilos and Liggins [144] have shown that intrapleural pressure during apnoea is negative in fetal sheep. Nicolini *et al.* [14] described a technique for measuring pressure within the fetal pleural space using subtraction manometry and found the same data in a human fetus after complete aspiration of a bilateral hydrothorax. They reported raised baseline pressures of 2–10 mmHg with a decrease of those pressures with fluid drainage. The higher pressure was found on the side punctured first, as if decompression of the first side also decompressed the other side. Vaughan *et al.* [145] showed no relationship between the initial intrapleural pressure and gestational age in 11 fetuses with hydrothorax. They found raised intrapleural pressure before drainage of pleural fluid in all cases. In those that survived, the intrapleural pressures remained at or above zero after complete aspiration; in those that were subsequently diagnosed as having PH at autopsy, the postaspiration pressures were negative with respect to AP. These techniques contribute to our understanding of why some fetuses develop PH and why some develop hydrops.

Antenatal diagnosis of PH is still unreliable but some prognostic factors exist, such as age at diagnosis and at delivery, spontaneous resolution, hydrops and bilaterally. Shunting allows lung expansion and alleviates hydrops and polyhydramnios, but when the lungs do not expand after shunting, the fetus is likely to have PH [120,145]. There are too few data to suggest that intrapleural pressure monitoring could be of use in predicting the potential for lung re-expansion or the presence or absence of PH. We do not recommend clinical measurement of intrapleural pressure in cases of fetal hydrothorax but continue to use it for research purposes.

Conclusions

Human amniotic and intrafetal pressures have been studied over the last 10 years using simple fluid-filled transducer systems attached to ultrasound-guided needles. AP has been chiefly studied, and is known to increase with advancing gestation. AP is elevated in polyhydramnios in direct relation to its severity; this high AP is considered to mediate most of the complications of polyhydramnios. It appears that raised AP may impair uteroplacental perfusion, adding a further reason for restoring normal amniotic fluid volume as a therapeutic measure. AP measurements have also contributed to our understanding of the pathophysiology of the normal and abnormal fetus; for example, the time-honoured concept of fetal compression in oligohydramnios is not consistent with the finding of low AP, suggesting that other mechanisms such as increased lung liquid loss may be more relevant in generating sequelae of PH.

Intrafetal pressure studies have shown that the normal mean UVP is about 5 mmHg but rises with intravascular transfusion. IPP rises during intraperitoneal transfusion are associated with fetal heart rate changes; IPP exceeding fetal intra-abdominal pressure may explain the high loss rate associated with intraperitoneal transfusion. Pressure measurements within fetal body cavities have shown that obstructive uropathy is associated with low intravesical pressure, and that negative pleural pressure post aspiration of hydrothorax is suggestive of PH.

Although the above studies have been useful in understanding fetal pathophysiology and improving interventions such as manipulating amniotic fluid volume or intrauterine transfusion, manometry techniques, at this time, remain primarily a research tool.

References

1 Liley AW. Liquor amnii analysis in management of pregnancy complicated by rhesus sensitisation. *Am J Obstet Gynecol* 1961;**82**:1359–1370.

2 Daffos F, Capella-Pavlovsky M, Forestier F. Fetal blood sampling during pregnancy with use of a needle guided by ultrasound: a study of 606 consecutive cases. *Am J Obstet Gynecol* 1985;**153**:655–660.

3 Benacerraf BR, Frigoletto FD, Wilson M. Successful mid-trimester thoracocentesis with analysis of the lymphocyte subpopulation in the pleural effusion. *Am J Obstet Gynecol* 1986;**155**:398–399.

4 Wolf W. Aussere wehenmessung und wehenscmerz bemerkungen zu der arbeit von Dr S Lorand. *Zentralbl Gynakol* 1940;**64**:311–317.

5 Alvarez H, Caldeyro R. Contractility of the human uterus recorded by new methods. *Surg Gynecol Obstet* 1950;**91**:1–13.

6 Hendricks CH, Quilligan EJ, Tyler CW, Tucker GJ. Pressure relationships between the intervillous space and the amniotic fluid in human term pregnancy. *Am J Obstet Gynecol* 1959;**77**:1028–1037.

7 Williams EA, Stallworthy JA. A simple method of internal tocography. *Lancet* 1952;**i**:330–332.

8 Turnbull AC. Uterine contractions in normal and abnormal labour. *J Obstet Gynaecol Br Emp* 1957;**44**:321–323.

9 Steer PJ, Carter MC, Gordon AJ, Beard RW. The use of catheter-tip pressure transducers for the measurement of intrauterine pressure in labour. *Br J Obstet Gynaecol* 1978;**85**:561–566.

10 Hackett GA, Nicolaides KH, Campbell S. Doppler ultrasound assessment of fetal and uteroplacental circulations in severe second trimester oligohydramnios. *Br J Obstet Gynaecol* 1987;**94**:1074–1077.

11 Gembruch U, Hansmann M. Artificial instillation of amniotic fluid as a new technique for the diagnostic evaluation of cases of oligohydramnios. *Prenat Diagn* 1988;**8**:33–45.

12 Landy HJ, Isada NB, Larsen JW. Genetic implications of idiopathic hydramnios. *Am J Obstet Gynecol* 1987;**157**:114–117.

13 Carlson DE, Platt LD, Medearis AL, Horenstein J. Quantifiable polyhydramnios: diagnosis and management. *Obstet Gynecol* 1990;**75**:989–993.

14 Nicolini U, Fisk NM, Talbert DG *et al.* Intrauterine manometry: technique and application to fetal pathology. *Prenat Diagn* 1989;**9**:243–254.

15 Fisk NM, Tannirandorn Y, Nicolini U, Talbert DG, Rodeck CH. Amniotic pressure in disorders of amniotic fluid volume. *Obstet Gynecol* 1990;**76**:210–214.

16 Fisk NM, Ronderos-Dumit D, Tannirandorn Y, Nicolini U, Talbert DG, Rodeck CH. Normal amniotic pressure throughout gestation. *Br J Obstet Gynaecol* 1992;**99**:18–22.

17 Crosby WM, Brobmann GF, Chang ACK. Intrauterine transfusion and fetal death. Relationship of intraperitoneal pressure to umbilical vein blood flow. *Am J Obstet Gynecol* 1970;**108**:135–138.

18 Reynold SRM, Paul WM. Pressures in umbilical arteries and veins of the fetal lamb *in utero*. *Am J Physiol* 1958;**193**:257–259.

19 Holt EM, Boyd ID, Gillmer MA, Naylor CJ, Thomas G. Fetal intraperitoneal pressure changes during intrauterine transfusion. *Br J Obstet Gynaecol* 1972;**79**:255–259.

20 Sykes MK, McNicol MW, Campbell EJM (eds). The mechanics of respiration. In: *Respiratory Failure*, 2nd edn. Oxford: Blackwell Scientific Publications, 1976:16–17.

21 Anderson ABM, Turnbull AC, Murray AM. The relationship between amniotic fluid pressure and uterine wall tension in pregnancy. *Am J Obstet Gynecol* 1967;**97**:992–997.

22 Reynolds SRM. The relationship of hydrostatic conditions in the uterus to the size and shape of the conceptus during pregnancy: a concept of uterine accommodation. *Anat Rec* 1946;**95**:283–293.

23 Coren RL, Csapo AI. The intra-amniotic pressure. *Am J Obstet Gynecol* 1963;**85**:470–483.

24 Csapo A. The diagnostic significance of the intrauterine pressure. *Obstet Gynecol Surv* 1970;**25**:403–543.

25 Reynolds SRM (ed.). Growth of the distended uterus. In: *Physiology of the Uterus*, 2nd edn. New York: Hafner, 1965:203–210.

26 Weiner CP, Heilskov J, Pelzer G, Grant S, Wenstrom K, Williamson RA. Normal values for human umbilical venous and amniotic fluid pressures and their alteration by fetal disease. *Am J Obstet Gynecol* 1989;**161**:714–717.

27 Sideris I, Nicolaides KH. Amniotic fluid pressure during pregnancy. *Fetal Diagn Ther* 1990;**5**:104–108.

28 Ville Y, Sideris I, Nicolaides KH. Amniotic fluid pressure in twin–twin transfusion syndrome: an objective prognostic factor. *Fetal Diagn Ther* 1996;**11**:176–180.

29 Rudolph AM, Heymann MA. Methods for studying the circulation of the fetus *in utero*. In: Nathanielsz PW (ed.) *Animal Models in Fetal Medicine*, vol I. New York: Perinatology Press, 1985:2–58.

30 Caldeyro R, Alvarez H, Reynolds SRM. A better understanding of uterine contractility through simultaneous recording with an internal and a seven channel external method. *Surg Gynecol Obstet* 1950;**91**:641–650.

31 Hellman LM, Tricomi V, Gupta O. Pressures in the human amniotic fluid and intervillous space. *Am J Obstet Gynecol* 1957;74:1018–1021.

32 Caldeyro-Barcia R, Alvarez H. Abnormal uterine action in labour. *J Obstet Gynaecol Br Commonw* 1952;59:646–656.

33 Moore TR, Cayle JE. The amniotic fluid index in normal human pregnancy. *Am J Obstet Gynecol* 1990;162:1168–1173.

34 Brace RA, Wolf EJ. Normal amniotic fluid volume changes throughout pregnancy. *Am J Obstet Gynecol* 1989;161:382–388.

35 Gohari P, Berkowitz RL, Hobbins J. Prediction of intra-uterine growth retardation by determination of total intrauterine volume. *Am J Obstet Gynecol* 1977;127:255–260.

36 Cardwell MS. Polyhydramnios: a review. *Obstet Gynecol Surv* 1987;42:612–617.

37 Desmedt EJ, Henry OA, Beischer NA. Polyhydramnios and associated maternal and fetal complications in singleton pregnancies. *Br J Obstet Gynaecol* 1990;97:1115–1122.

38 Seeds JW, Cefalo RC, Herbert WN, Bowes WA. Hydramnios and maternal renal failure: relief with fetal therapy. *Obstet Gynecol* 1984;64:26S–29S.

39 Steinberg LH, Hurley VA, Desmedt E, Beischer NA. Acute polyhydramnios in twin pregnancies. *Aust NZ J Obstet Gynaecol* 1990;30:196–200.

40 Zamah NM, Gillieson MS, Walters JH, Hall PF. Sonographic detection of polyhydramnios: a five-year experience. *Am J Obstet Gynecol* 1982;143:523–527.

41 Pritchard JA, Mason R, Corley M, Pritchard S. Genesis of severe placental abruption. *Am J Obstet Gynecol* 1970;108:22–25.

42 Green-Thompson RW. Antepartum haemorrhage. *Clin Obstet Gynaecol* 1982;9:479–515.

43 Carlson DE, Platt LD, Medearis AL, Horenstein J. Quantifiable polyhydramnios: diagnosis and management. *Obstet Gynecol* 1990;75:989–993.

44 Desmedt E, Henry OA, Steinberg LH, Beischer NA. Acute and subacute polyhydramnios in singleton pregnancies. *Aust NZ J Obstet Gynaecol* 1990;30:191–195.

45 Bebbington MW, Wittman BK. Fetal transfusion syndrome: antenatal factors predicting outcome. *Am J Obstet Gynecol* 1989;160:913–915.

46 Urig MA, Clewell WH, Elliott JP. Twin–twin transfusion syndrome. *Am J Obstet Gynecol* 1990;163:1522–1526.

47 Schneider KTM, Vetter K, Huch R, Huch A. Acute polyhydramnios complicating twin pregnancies. *Acta Genet Med Gemellol* 1985;34:179–184.

48 Pinette MG, Pan Y, Pinette SG, Stubblefield PG. Treatment of twin–twin transfusion syndrome. *Obstet Gynecol* 1993;82:841–846.

49 Elliott JP, Urig MA, Clewell WH. Aggressive therapeutic amniocentesis for treatment of twin–twin transfusion syndrome. *Obstet Gynecol* 1991;77:537–540.

50 Rivett LC. Hydramnios. *J Obstet Gynaecol Br Emp* 1933;40:522–525.

51 Feingold M, Cetrulo CL, Newton ER, Weiss J, Shakr C, Shmoys S. Serial amniocenteses in the treatment of twin to twin transfusion complicated with acute poly-hydramnios. *Acta Genet Med Gemellol* 1986;35:107–113.

52 Weiner CP. Diagnosis and treatment of twin to twin transfusion in the mid-second trimester of pregnancy. *Fetal Ther* 1987;2:71–74.

53 Chescheir NC, Seeds JW. Polyhydramnios and oligohydramnios in twin gestations. *Obstet Gynecol* 1988;71:882–884.

54 Saunders NJ, Snijders RJ, Nicolaides KH. Therapeutic amniocentesis in twin–twin transfusion syndrome appearing in the second trimester of pregnancy. *Am J Obstet Gynecol* 1992;166:820–824.

55 Mahoney BS, Petty CN, Nyberg DA, Luthy DA, Hickok DE, Hirsch JH. The 'stuck twin' phenomenon: ultrasonographic findings, pregnancy outcome, and management with serial amniocenteses. *Am J Obstet Gynecol* 1990;163:1513–1522.

56 Elliot JP, Urig MA, Clewell WH. Aggressive therapeutic amniocentesis for treatment of twin–twin transfusion syndrome. *Obstet Gynecol* 1991;77:537–540.

57 Cabrera-Ramirez L, Harris RE. Controlled removal of amniotic fluid in hydramnios. *South Med J* 1976;69:239–240.

58 Elliot JP, Sawyer AT, Radin TG, Strong RE. Large volume therapeutic amniocentesis in the treatment of hydramnios. *Obstet Gynecol* 1994;84:1025–1027.

59 Kirshon B, Mari G, Moise K. Indomethacin therapy in the treatment of symptomatic polyhydramnios. *Obstet Gynecol* 1990;75:202–205.

60 Carlan SJ, O'Brien WF, Jones MH, O'Leary TD, Roth L. Outpatient oral sulindac to prevent recurrence of preterm labor. *Obstet Gynecol* 1995;85:769–774.

61 Rasanen J, Jouppila P. Fetal cardiac function and ductus arteriosus during indomethacin and sulindac therapy for threatened preterm labor: a randomized study. *Am J Obstet Gynecol* 1995;173:20–25.

62 Csapo A, Takeda H, Wood C. Volume and activity of the parturient rabbit uterus. *Am J Obstet Gynecol* 1963;85:813–818.

63 Caldeyro-Barcia R, Pose SV, Alvarez H. Uterine contractility in polyhydramnios and the effects of withdrawal of the excess of amniotic fluid. *Am J Obstet Gynecol* 1957;73:1238–1254.

64 Wieloch J. Uber messungen des druckes im normal graviden und hydramniotischen uterus. *Zentralbl Gynakol* 1927;3:129–136.

65 Fisk NM. *Amniotic pressure in disorders of amniotic fluid volume*. PhD thesis, University of London, 1992.

66 Tabor BL, Maier JA. Polyhydramnios and elevated intrauterine pressure during amnioinfusion. *Am J Obstet Gynecol* 1987;156:130–131.

67 Fisk NM, Vaughan J, Talbert D. Impaired fetal blood gas status in polyhydramnios and its relation to raised amniotic pressure. *Fetal Diagn Ther* 1994;9:7–13.

68 Fisk NM, Giussani DA, Parkes MJ, Moore PJ, Hansoon MA. Amnioinfusion increases amniotic pressure in pregnant sheep but does not alter fetal acid–base status. *Am J Obstet Gynecol* 1991;165:1459–1463.

69 Skillman CA, Plessinger MA, Woods JR, Clark KE. Effect of graded reductions in uteroplacental blood flow on the fetal lamb. *Am J Physiol* 1985;249:H1098–H1105.

70 Bower SJ, Campbell S, Vyas S, McGirr C. Braxton Hicks contractions can alter uteroplacental perfusion. *Ultrasound Obstet Gynecol* 1991;1:46–49.

71 Bower SJ, Flack NJ, Sepulveda W, Talbert DG, Fisk NM. Uterine artery blood flow response to correction of amniotic fluid volume. *Am J Obstet Gynecol* 1995;173:502–507.

72 Guzman ER, Vintzileos A, Benito C, Houlihan C, Waldron R, Egan S. Effects of therapeutic amniocentesis on uterine and umbilical artery velocimetry in cases of severe symptomatic polyhydramnios. *J Mat Fetal Med* 1996;5:299–304.

73 Manning FA, Hill LM, Platt LD. Qualitative amniotic fluid volume determination by ultrasound: antepartum detection of intrauterine growth retardation. *Am J Obstet Gynecol* 1981;139:254–258.

74 Chamberlain PF, Manning FA, Morrison I, Harman CR, Lange IR. Ultrasound evaluation of amniotic fluid volume I. The relationship of marginal and decreased amniotic fluid volumes to perinatal outcome. *Am J Obstet Gynecol* 1984;150:245–249.

75 Moore TR, Longo J, Leopold GR, Casola G, Gosink BB. The reliability and predictive value of an amniotic fluid scoring system in severe second trimester oligohydramnios. *Obstet Gynecol* 1989;73:739–742.

76 Manning FA, Hill LM, Platt LD. Qualitative amniotic fluid volume determination by ultrasound: Antepartum detection of intrauterine growth retardation. *Am J Obstet Gynecol* 1981;139:254–258.

77 Gabbe SG, Ettinger BB, Freeman RK, Martin CB. Umbilical cord compression associated with amniotomy: laboratory observations. *Am J Obstet Gynecol* 1976;126:353–355.

78 Csapo A, Takeda H, Wood C. Volume and activity of the parturient rabbit uterus. *Am J Obstet Gynecol* 1963;85:813–818.

79 Nicolini U, Fisk NM, Rodeck CH, Talbert DG, Wigglesworth JS. Low amniotic pressure in oligohydramnios: is this the cause of pulmonary hypoplasia? *Am J Obstet Gynecol* 1989;161:1098–1101.

80 Potter EL. Bilateral renal agenesis. *J Pediatr* 1946;29:68–76.

81 Perlman M, Williams J, Hirsch M. Neonatal pulmonary hypoplasia after prolonged leakage of amniotic fluid. *Arch Dis Child* 1976;51:349–353.

82 Wigglesworth JS, Winston RML, Bartlett K. Influence of the central nervous system on fetal lung development. *Arch Dis Child* 1977;52:965–967.

83 Thibeault DW, Beatty EC, Hall RT, Bowen SK, O'Neill DH. Neonatal pulmonary hypoplasia with premature rupture of fetal membranes and oligohydramnios. *J Pediatr* 1985;107:273–277.

84 Rotschild A, Ling EW, Puterman ML, Farquharson D. Neonatal outcome after prolonged preterm rupture of the membranes. *Am J Obstet Gynecol* 1990;162:46–52.

85 Kilbride HW, Yeast J, Thibeault DW. Defining limits of survival: lethal pulmonary hypoplasia after midtrimester premature rupture of membranes. *Am J Obstet Gynecol* 1996;175: 675–681.

86 Moore TR, Longo J, Leopold GR, Casola G, Gosink BB. The reliability and predictive value of an amniotic fluid scoring system in severe second trimester oligohydramnios. *Obstet Gynecol* 1989;73:739–742.

87 Nimrod C, Varela-Gittings F, Machin G, Campbell D, Wesenberg R. The effect of very prolonged membrane rupture on fetal development. *Am J Obstet Gynecol* 1984;148:540–543.

88 Wigglesworth JS, Desai R. Effects on lung growth of cervical cord section in the rabbit fetus. *Early Hum Dev* 1979;3:51–65.

89 Dornan JC, Ritchie JWK, Meban C. Fetal breathing movements and lung maturation in the congenitally abnormal human fetus. *J Dev Physiol* 1984;6:367–375.

90 King JC, Mitzner W, Butterfield AB, Queenan JT. Effect of induced oligohydramnios on fetal lung development. *Am J Obstet Gynecol* 1986;154:823–830.

91 Fisk NM, Talbert DG, Nicolini U, Vaughan J, Rodeck CH. Fetal breathing movements in oligohydramnios are not altered by amnioinfusion. *Br J Obstet Gynaecol* 1992;99:464–468.

92 Fisk NM, Welch R, Ronderos-Dumit D, Tannirandorn Y, Nicolini U, Rodeck CH. Relief of presumed compression in oligohydramnios: amnioinfusion does not affect umbilical Doppler waveforms. *Fetal Diagn Ther* 1992;7:180–185.

93 Harding R, Hooper SB, Dickson KA. A mechanism

leading to reduced lung expansion and lung hypoplasia in fetal sheep during oligohydramnios. *Am J Obstet Gynecol* 1990;**163**:1904–1913.

94 Pringle KC. Human fetal lung development and related animal models. *Clin Obstet Gynecol* 1986;**29**:502–513.

95 Fisk NM, Ronderos-Dumit D, Soliani A, Nicolini U, Vaughan J, Rodeck CH. Diagnostic and therapeutic transabdominal amnioinfusion in oligohydramnios. *Obstet Gynecol* 1991;**78**:270–278.

96 Kilbride HW, Thibeault DW, Yeast J, Maulik D, Grundy HO. Fetal breathing is not a predictor of pulmonary hypoplasia in pregnancies complicated by oligohydramnios. *Lancet* 1988;**i**:305–306.

97 Dickson KA, Harding R. Fetal breathing and pressures in trachea and amniotic sac during oligohydramnios in sheep. *J Appl Physiol* 1991;**70**:293–299.

98 Strang LB. Fetal lung liquid: secretion and reabsorption. *Physiol Rev* 1991;**71**:991–1016.

99 Hooper SB, Harding R. Fetal lung liquid: a major determinant of the growth and functional development of the fetal lung. *Clin Exp Pharmacol Physiol* 1995;**22**:235–247.

100 Moessinger AC, Fewell JE, Stark RI *et al.* Lung hypoplasia and breathing movements following oligohydramnios in fetal lambs. In: Jones CT, Nathanielsz PW (eds) *The Physiological Development of the Fetus and Newborn.* London: Academic Press, 1985:273–278.

101 Alcorn D, Adamson TM, Lambert TF, Maloney JE, Ritchie BC, Robinson PM. Morphological effects of chronic tracheal ligation and drainage in the fetal lamb lung. *J Anat* 1977;**123**:649–660.

102 Adzick NS, Harrison MR, Glick PL, Villa RL, Finkbeiner W. Experimental pulmonary hypoplasia and olygohydramnios: relative contributions of lung fluid and fetal breathing movements. *J Pediatr Surg* 1984;**19**:658–665.

103 Wigglesworth JS, Desai R, Hilopp AA. Fetal lung growth in congenital laryngeal atresia. *Pediatr Pathol* 1987;**7**:515–525.

104 Fisk NM, Parkes MJ, Moore PJ, Hanson MA, Wigglesworth J, Rodeck CH. Mimicking low amniotic pressure by chronic pharyngeal drainage does not impair lung development in fetal sheep. *Am J Obstet Gynecol* 1992;**166**:991–996.

105 Harding R, Hooper SB, Dickinson KA. A mechanism leading to reduced lung expansion and lung hypoplasia in fetal sheep during oligohydramnios. *Am J Obstet Gynecol* 1990;**163**:1904–1913.

106 Fisk NM, Ronderos-Dumit D, Soliani A, Nicolini U, Vaughan J, Rodeck CH. Diagnostic and therapeutic transabdominal amnioinfusion in oligohydramnios. *Obstet Gynecol* 1991;**78**:270–278.

107 Owen J, Henson BV, Hauth JC. A prospective randomized study of saline solution amnioinfusion. *Am J Obstet Gynecol* 1990;**162**:1146–1149.

108 Nakayama DK, Glick PH, Harrisson MR, Villa RL, Noall R. Experimental pulmonary hypoplasia due to oligohydramnios and its reversal by relieving thoracic compression. *J Pediatr Surg* 1983;**18**:347–353.

109 Moore TR, Longo J, Leopold GR, Casola G, Gosink BB. The reliability and predictive value of an amniotic fluid scoring system in severe second trimester oligohydramnios. *Obstet Gynecol* 1989;**73**:739–742.

110 Vergani P, Locatelli A, Strobelt N, Mariani S, Cavallone M, Ghidini A. Amnioinfusion for prevention of pulmonary hypoplasia in second trimester rupture of membranes (abstract). *Am J Obstet Gynecol* 1997;Suppl **86**:280.

111 Van den Wijngaard JAGW, Wladimiroff JW, Reuss A, Stewart PA. Oligohydramnios and fetal cerebral blood flow. *Br J Obstet Gynaecol* 1988;**95**:1309–1311.

112 O'Brien WF, Davis SE, Grissom MP, Eng RR, Golden SM. Effect of cephalic pressure on fetal cerebral blood flow. *Am J Perinatol* 1984;**1**:223–226.

113 Vyas S, Campbell S, Bower S, Nicolaides KH. Maternal abdominal pressure alters fetal cerebral blood flow. *Br J Obstet Gynaecol* 1990;**97**:740–747.

114 Miyazaki FS, Nevarez F. Saline amnioinfusion for relief of repetitive variable decelerations: a prospective randomised study. *Am J Obstet Gynecol* 1985;**153**:301–306.

115 Nageotte MP, Freeman RK, Garite TJ, Dorchester W. Prophylactic intrapartum amnioinfusion in patients with preterm premature rupture of membranes. *Am J Obstet Gynecol* 1985;**153**:557–562.

116 Strong TH, Hetzler G, Sarno AP, Paul RH. Prophylactic intrapartum amnioinfusion: a randomised clinical trial. *Am J Obstet Gynecol* 1990;**162**:1370–1375.

117 Hofmeyer GJ. Amnioinfusion for meconium-stained liquour in labour. In: Keirse MJNC, Renfrew MJ, Nrilson JP, Crowther C (eds) *Pregnancy and Childbirth Module.* London: Cochrane Database of Systematic Reviews, BMJ Publishing Group, 1993.

118 Posner MD, Ballagh SA, Paul RH. The effect of amnioinfusion on uterine pressure and activity: a preliminary report. *Am J Obstet Gynecol* 1990;**163**:813–818.

119 Maher JE, Wenstrom KD, Hauth JC, Meis PJ. Amniotic fluid embolism after saline amnioinfusion: two cases and review of the literature. *Obstet Gynecol* 1994;**83**:851–854.

120 Rodeck CH, Fisk NM, Fraser DI, Nicolini U. Long-term *in utero* drainage of fetal hydrothorax. *N Engl J Med* 1988;**319**:1135–1138.

121 Glick PL, Harrison MR, Golbus MS *et al.* Management of the fetus with congenital hydronephrosis II. Prognostic criteria and selection for treatment. *J Pediatr Surg* 1985;**20**:376–387.

122 Holt EM, Boy ID, Gillmer MA, Naylor CJ, Thomas G. Fetal intraperitoneal pressure changes during intrauterine transfusion. *J Obstet Gynaecol Br Commonw* 1972;79: 255–259.

123 Dunnihoo DR. Intrauterine fetal transfusion: monitoring intraperitoneal pressures. *Am J Obstet Gynecol* 1982;142: 241–242.

124 Castle BM, Mackenzie IZ. *In vivo* observations on intravascular blood pressure in the fetus during mid-pregnancy. In: Rolfe P (ed.) *Fetal Physiological Measurements*. London: Butterworth, 1986:65–69.

125 Weiner CP. Umbilical pressure measurement in the evaluation of nonimmune hydrops fetalis. *Am J Obstet Gynecol* 1993;168:817–823.

126 Liley AW. Intrauterine transfusion of fetus in haemolytic disease. *Br Med J* 1963;2:1107–1109.

127 Moise KJ. Intrauterine transfusion with red cells and platelets. *West J Med* 1993;159:318–324.

128 Nicolini U, Talbert DG, Fisk NM, Rodeck CH. Pathophysiology of pressure changes during intrauterine transfusion. *Am J Obstet Gynecol* 1989;160:1139–1145.

129 Rodeck CH, Kemp JR, Holman CA, Whitemore DN, Karnicki J, Austin MA. Direct intravascular fetal blood transfusion by fetoscopy in severe rhesus isoimmunisation. *Lancet* 1981;i:625–627.

130 Berkowitz RL, Chitkara U, Goldberg JD, Wilkins I, Chervenak FA, Lynch L. Intrauterine intravascular transfusions for severe red blood cell isoimmunization: ultrasound-guided percutaneous approach. *Am J Obstet Gynecol* 1986;155:574–581.

131 Grannum PA, Copel JA, Plaxe SC, Scioscia AL, Hobbins JC. *In utero* exchange transfusion by direct intravascular injection in severe erythroblastosis fetalis. *N Engl J Med* 1986;314:1431–1434.

132 Weiner CP, Pelzer GD, Heilskov J, Wenstrom KD, Williamson RA. The effect of intravascular transfusion on umbilical venous pressure in anemic fetuses with and without hydrops. *Am J Obstet Gynecol* 1989;161:1498–1501.

133 Moise KJ Jr, Mari G, Fisher DJ, Huhta JC, Cano LE, Carpenter RJ Jr. Acute fetal hemodynamic alterations after intrauterine transfusion for treatment of severe red blood cell alloimmunization. *Am J Obstet Gynecol* 1990;163:776–784.

134 Nicolini U, Kochenour NK, Greco P, Letsky E, Rodeck CH. When to perform the next intrauterine transfusion in patients with Rh alloimmunization: combined intravascular and peritoneal transfusion allows longer intervals. *Fetal Ther* 1989;4:14–20.

135 Moise KJ Jr, Carpenter RJ Jr, Kirshon B, Deter RL, Sala JD, Cano LE. Comparison of four types of intrauterine transfusion: effect on fetal hematocrit. *Fetal Ther* 1989;4:126–137.

136 Hallak M, Moise KJ, Hesketh DE, Cano LE, Carpenter RJ. Intravascular transfusion of fetuses with rhesus incompatibility: prediction of fetal outcome by changes in umbilical venous pressure. *Obstet Gynecol* 1992;80:286–290.

137 Radunovic N, Lockwood CJ, Alvarez M, Plecas D, Chitkara U, Berkowitz RL. The severely anemic and hydropic isoimmune fetus: changes in fetal hematocrit associated with intrauterine death. *Obstet Gynecol* 1992;79:390–393.

138 Moise JK Jr, Schumacher B. Anaemia. In: Fisk NM, Moise KJ (eds) *Fetal Therapy. Invasive and Transplacental*. Cambridge: Cambridge University Press, 1997:141–164.

139 Nicolini U, Santolaya J, Fisk NM *et al.* Changes in fetal acid/base status during intravascular transfusion. *Arch Dis Child* 1988;63:710–714.

140 Skupski DW, Wolf CFW, Bussel JB. Fetal transfusion therapy. *Obstet Gynecol Surv* 1996;51:181–192.

141 Schumarer B, Moise KJ Jr. Fetal transfusion for red blood cell alloimmunization in pregnancy. *Obstet Gynecol* 1996;88:137–150.

142 Nicolini U, Tannirandorn Y, Vaughan J, Fisk NM, Nicolaidis P, Rodeck CH. Further predictors of renal dysplasia in fetal obstructive uropathy: bladder pressure and biochemistry of fresh urine. *Prenat Diagn* 1991;11: 159–166.

143 Nicolini U, Vaughan JI, Fisk NM, Dhilon HK, Rodeck CH. Cystic lesions of the fetal kidney: diagnostic and prediction of postnatal function by fetal urine biochemistry. *J Pediatr Surg* 1992;27:1451–1454.

144 Vilos GA, Liggins GC. Intrathoracic pressures in fetal sheep. *J Dev Physiol* 1982;4:247–256.

145 Vaughan JI, Fisk N, Rodeck CH. Fetal Pleural Effusions. In: Harman C (eds) *Invasive Fetal Testing and Treatment*. Boston: Blackwell Science, 1995:218–239.

Chapter 14/Prenatal diagnosis and therapeutic techniques in twin pregnancies

YVES VILLE and KYPROS H.NICOLAIDES

Before 1974 a twin pregnancy was considered a contraindication for amniocentesis. Since then, a strong case has been made for obtaining fluid from both sacs based on the evidence that the risk of fetal anomaly in a twin pregnancy, meaning in at least one twin, is higher than that of a singleton [1].

Diagnosis of chorionicity

Before 8 weeks, monozygotic twins will appear within the same gestational sac and the intertwin membrane might be difficult to visualize. From 9 to 12 weeks' gestation, dichorionic twins will be separated by a thick membrane whose insertion on the placenta or the uterine wall will have a characteristic Y shape, whereas monochorionic twins will be separated by a thin hairy membrane inserting sharply on the placenta [2]. After 15 weeks, differentiating between monochorionic and dichorionic twins will be less accurate: different fetal genders will confirm dizygosity, whereas separate placental masses and thickness of the membranes will not be sufficient criteria. In these situations or situations in which the determination of chorionicity is needed in early prenatal diagnosis before gender is apparent, DNA techniques or invasively collected fetal tissue may be of use [3]. These indicate zygosity and thus are only of value in denoting dichorial placentation in the presence of dizygous results.

Amniocentesis

Traditionally, amniocentesis in a twin pregnancy has involved puncture of the first sac, withdrawal of amniotic fluid, injection of a dye and then a new needle insertion to puncture the second sac [4]. The dye allowed the operator to check that fluid aspirated after the second puncture was dye-free. The disadvantage of this method is that two skin and uterine entries are required, increasing the potential for complications. The rate of fetal loss is related to the number of insertions required to obtain amniotic fluid; in addition, with the injection of dyes, a foreign substance is introduced into the amniotic cavity of one of the fetuses, and neonatal bowel occlusions have been reported after intra-amniotic injection of methylene blue.

In order to avoid a second puncture, which could enhance uterine activity and increase the risk of intra-amniotic infection, we recommend the single-needle insertion technique. The site of needle insertion is determined mainly by the position of the membrane separating the two sacs. After entry into the first sac and aspiration of amniotic fluid, the needle is advanced through the dividing membrane into the second sac. To avoid contamination of the second sample with any amniotic fluid from the first sac still in the needle, the first 1 ml of fluid from the second sample is discarded. This method is simple and potentially less traumatic than the traditional procedure.

Despite a large number of small uncontrolled studies, the safety of amniocentesis in twin gestations is still debated. In early studies, the reported rate of fetal loss following amniocentesis in twins ranged from 5 to 17%. However, some of these studies did not use ultrasonographic guidance during the procedure and may have overestimated the risk of the procedure. Furthermore, it is uncertain whether fetal loss rate after invasive testing is due to the procedure itself or to the twin gestation. One retrospective study [5] matched twin pregnancies undergoing amniocentesis for genetic purposes and others undergoing ultrasonographic examination at the same gestational age that were conducted over a limited period of 5 years, when amniocenteses were performed with a consistent protocol entailing ultrasonographic guidance and separate needle insertions. Given a background fetal loss rate of 3.2% in their control population and that 20 times as many cases would be required for statistical analysis, this study suggested that procedure-related fetal loss rate is probably of the same magnitude as that in singletons.

Chorionic villous sampling

A combination of ultrasound, fetal sex determination and genetic studies using polymorphic markers may be required to differentiate the two samples; however, a single sample should be performed when the twins are obviously monochorionic with a single placental mass and a thin intertwin membrane with a sharp attachment to the placenta. When performed at 9–12 weeks, Pergament *et al.* [6] reported successful sampling in 99.2% of 128 procedures. There is no evidence for an increased fetal loss rate when compared with chorionic villous sampling (CVS) performed on singleton pregnancies.

CVS has several advantages and potential pitfalls. Chorionicity is theoretically easily determined at this stage of pregnancy (< 14 weeks). However, even when the two placental masses are clearly separated, the procedure can be technically difficult for one of the two biopsies. When chorionicity is uncertain, sampling at the insertion site of the umbilical cord can be helpful, although it could theoretically increase the risk of fetal loss.

At the time of the procedure, a detailed transabdominal ultrasound evaluation to determine chorionicity and amnionicity is most important for the indication and accuracy of prenatal diagnosis in twins. Crown–rump length of each fetus, location of each placenta and its margins relative to any other gestational sac, location and thickness of the dividing membrane and the sampling method (one or two needle insertions) can then be determined. Pregnancies with two distinct placental sites of implantation separated by a thick membrane will have each chorion sampled individually. A single sample will be performed in pregnancies with only one placental site and in which the dividing membrane is either thin or not seen.

Fetal blood sampling

Fetal blood sampling is facilitated by precise cord localization and therefore facilitates identification of a malformed or chromosomally abnormal fetus. Blood subgroup determination in each sample can be a useful adjunct to the rapid diagnosis of zygosity.

Twin to twin transfusion syndrome

Ultrasound examination demonstrates monochorionic diamniotic twin pregnancies with fetuses that are discordant in size. The larger twin (presumed recipient) has a distended bladder and is surrounded by polyhydramnios, whereas in the smaller twin (presumed donor) the bladder is always empty and the fetus appears to be fixed to the placenta or the uterine wall because of anhydramnios. The fetal biparietal diameter, head and abdominal circumferences and femur length are measured and the estimated fetal weight and intertwin difference in weight, expressed as a percentage of the weight of the recipient, are calculated. The degree of polyhydramnios is assessed by measurement of the deepest vertical pool of amniotic fluid.

Amniodrainage

For amniodrainage an 18-gauge needle is introduced into the uterus under ultrasound guidance. The amniotic fluid is allowed to drain freely into a sterile bag through a plastic tube attached to the hub of the needle over a period of 40–120 min until there is subjective normalization of amniotic fluid volume on ultrasonographic examination. Patients are assessed every week and further amniodrainage is performed if there is recurrence of polyhydramnios [7].

Laser coagulation of placental anastomoses

For laser coagulation, a detailed ultrasound examination including colour flow mapping is first performed to localize the placenta, the intertwin amniotic membrane, the placental insertion of the umbilical cords and the communicating blood vessels on the chorionic plate [8]. The appropriate site of entry on the maternal abdomen is chosen to avoid injury to the placenta or fetuses and to allow access to the suspected area of vascular communications. Under continuous ultrasound visualization, a rigid 2-mm diameter fetoscope (field of vision

75°) housed in a 2.7-mm diameter canula (KeyMed, Southend, UK or Storz, Tuttlingen, Germany) is introduced transabdominally into the amniotic cavity of the recipient twin. A 400-µm diameter Nd:YAG laser fibre (MBB, Munich, Germany) is passed down the side-arm of the cannula to 1 cm beyond the tip of the fetoscope.

A combination of ultrasonographic and direct vision is used to examine systematically the chorionic plate along the whole length of the intertwin membrane and identify the crossing vessels, which are coagulated by the administration of a total of 1000–4500 J delivered by 3-s shots using an output of 30–50 W at a distance of 1 cm [8]. Subsequently, amniotic fluid is drained through the fetoscope cannula over a period of 10–20 min to obtain subjective normalization of the amniotic fluid volume on ultrasonographic examination. The total procedure takes 30–90 min to complete.

Acardiac twins: selective feticide in monochorionic pregnancies

Acardiac twins is the most extreme manifestation of twin to twin transfusion syndrome and is found in approximately 1% of monozygotic twin pregnancies. This twin disorder has been named the twin-reversed arterial perfusion (TRAP) sequence because the underlying mechanism is thought to be disruption of normal vascular perfusion and development of the recipient twin due to an umbilical artery-to-artery anastomosis with the donor or pump twin. At least 50% of donor twins die due to congestive heart failure or severe preterm delivery as a consequence of polyhydramnios. All perfused twins die because of the associated multiple malformations.

Moore *et al.* [9] reported that the outcome of the donor twin depends on the weight of the acardiac fetus; when the percentage weight compared with the donor was >70, 50–70 and <50% the risk for congestive heart failure in the donor was 100, 70 and 8% respectively. However, the value of these data in the antenatal management of affected pregnancies is limited by our current inability to estimate accurately the weight of acardiac–anencephalic fetuses with varying degrees of hydrops.

Prenatal treatment has been attempted by serial amniodrainages or the administration of indomethacin to the mother [10,11]. Although such therapy can potentially prevent polyhydramnios-related preterm delivery, it does not reduce the risk of congestive heart failure and consequent intrauterine or neonatal death of the donor twin. More recently, attempts at therapy have concentrated on surgical removal of the acardiac twin or occlusion of its umbilical cord.

Selective removal of the acardiac fetus by hysterotomy was performed in seven cases at 19–26 (mean 22) weeks' gestation [12–14]. The patients remained in hospital for 5–34 days and received rigorous tocolytic therapy. In one case there was placental abruption and fetal death within 2 hours of the procedure and in the other six the healthy donor twins were delivered by Caesarean section at 27–37 (mean 33) weeks' gestation and survived. Emergency delivery was undertaken because of placental abruption in five cases, premature labour in two and preterm prelabour amniorrhexis in one.

The first attempts to arrest blood flow in the umbilical cord vessels of the acardiac twin were by ultrasound-guided injection of thrombogenic coils or fibrin. In one case there was immediate cessation of blood flow in the recipient cord and after an uneventful pregnancy the normal twin was delivered at term [15]. In two other cases, however, the donor twin also died [16].

Another technique for arresting flow in the umbilical cord vessels of the acardiac twin is endoscopic laser coagulation [17]. In four cases of TRAP sequence, presenting at 17, 20, 26 and 28 weeks' gestation respectively, an endoscope was introduced into the uterus under local anaesthesia and a Nd:YAG laser was used to coagulate the umbilical cord vessels. Laser coagulation was successful in the cases treated at 17 and 20 weeks and healthy infants were delivered after spontaneous labour at 29 weeks. The main limitation of the technique seems to be the size and water content of Wharton's jelly, which prevents laser coagulation after 20 weeks. Since in TRAP sequence perinatal mortality for the donor twin is at least 50% and the condition can be diagnosed easily by routine ultrasound examination in early pregnancy, it could be argued that in all cases prophylactic treatment should be considered at early or mid gestation. In patients presenting at later gestation with polyhydramnios and evidence of heart failure in the donor twin, early delivery or alternative techniques should be considered to interrupt the blood flow within the cord vessels. Embolization of both the arterial and the venous system can be achieved by ultrasound-guided cordocentesis using different approaches (primary right heart embolization versus direct cord tamponade) and different materials (thrombogenic coils or histoacryl glue); these rely on cordocentesis-related techniques [15,16]. The hazard to the healthy twin is the main risk with this technique, with a reported mortality rate in the healthy twin of approximately 50%. This is probably at least partly due to the learning curve of the procedure and of the embolization material.

The technique of endoscopic cord ligation involves the use of two ports introduced in the uterus under general analgesia, one for the endoscope and one for introduction of the suture. The suture must be passed around the cord and both ends brought outside for an extracorporeal knot to be tied and pushed on to the cord; the knot will be cut by scissors passed down one of the cannulae. In the first case, both fetuses died within 24 hours of the procedure, but in the second case the operation was successful and a healthy baby was delivered at 36 weeks' gestation [18,19]. Another four cases have recently been reported by Deprest *et al.* [20] with a 50% neonatal death rate, mainly due to prematurity as a consequence of preterm prelabour rupture of the membranes (PPROM) that complicated about 30% of the cases reported so far; the authors speculate that the use of two or more access ports is a risk factor for PPROM. In one case, cord ligation was achieved through a single port under ultrasound guidance only; this report showed the feasibility of the technique through a long-lasting procedure (45–60 min) [21]. This should be borne in mind when such a procedure is required and emphasis should be on early diagnosis and management with less invasive techniques.

References

1 Little J, Bryan E. Congenital anomalies in twins. *Semin Perinatol* 1986;10:50–64.

2 Kurtz AB, Wapner RJ, Mata J *et al.* Twin pregnancies, accuracy of first trimester abdominal ultrasound in predicting chorionicity and amnionicity. *Radiology* 1992; 185:759–762.

3 Brambati B, Tului L, Lanzani A *et al.* First trimester genetic diagnosis in multiple pregnancy: principles and potential pitfalls. *Prenat Diagn* 1991;11:767–774.

4 Filkins K, Russo J. Genetic amniocentesis in multiple gestations. *Prenat Diagn* 1984;4:223–230.

5 Ghidini A, Lynch L, Hicks C, Alvarez M, Lockwood C. The risk of second-trimester amniocentesis in twin gestations: a case–control study. *Am J Obstet Gynecol* 1993;169:1013–1016.

6 Pergament E, Schulman JD, Copeland K. The risk and efficacy of chorionic villus sampling in multiple gestations. *Prenat Diagn* 1992;12:377–384.

7 Saunders NJ, Snijders RJM, Nicolaides KH. Therapeutic amniocentesis in twin–twin transfusion syndrome appearing in the second trimester of pregnancy. *Am J Obstet Gynecol* 1992;166:820–824.

8 Ville Y, Hyett J, Hecher K, Nicolaides K. Preliminary experience with endoscopic laser surgery for severe twin to twin transfusion syndrome. *N Engl J Med* 1995;332: 224–227.

9 Moore TR, Galoe S, Bernishke A. Perinatal outcome of forty-nine pregnancies complicated by acardiac twining. *Am J Obstet Gynecol* 1990;163:907–912.

10 Platt LD, Devore GR, Bieniarz A, Benner P, Rao R. Antenatal diagnosis of acephalus acardia: a proposed management scheme. *Am J Obstet Gynecol* 1983;146:857–859.

11 Ash K, Harman CR, Gritter H. TRAP sequence, successful outcome with indomethacin treatment. *Obstet Gynecol* 1990;76:960–962.

12 Robie GF, Payne GG, Morgan MA. Selective delivery of an acardiac twin. *N Engl J Med* 1989;320:512–513.

13 Fries MH, Goldberg JD, Golbus MS. Treatment of acardiac–acephalus twin gestation by hysterotomy and selective delivery. *Obstet Gynecol* 1992;79:601–604.

14 Ginsberg NA, Applebaum M, Rabin SA *et al.* Term birth after mid-trimester hysterotomy and selective delivery of an acardiac twin. *Am J Obstet Gynecol* 1992;167:33–37.

15 Porreco RP, Barton SM, Haverkamp AD. Occlusion of umbilical artery in acardiac, acephalic twin. *Lancet* 1991;337:326–327.

16 Dommergues M, Mandelbrot L, Delezoide AL, Dumez Y. Twin-to-twin transfusion syndrome: selective feticide by embolisation of the hydropic fetus. *Fetal Diagn Ther* 1995;10:26–31.

17 Ville Y, Hyett J, Vandenbussche F, Nicolaides KH. Endoscopic laser coagulation of umbilical cord vessels in TRAP sequence. *Ultrasound Obstet Gynecol* 1994;4: 1–3.

18 McCurdy CM, Childers JM, Seeds JW. Ligation of the umbilical cord of an acardiac acephalus twin with an endoscopic intrauterine technique. *Obstet Gynecol* 1993;82:708–711.

19 Quintero RA, Reich H, Puder KS *et al.* Umbilical cord ligation of an acardiac twin by fetoscopy at 19 weeks of gestation. *N Engl J Med* 1994;300:469–471.

20 Deprest JA, Evrard VA, Van Schoubroeck D, Vandenberghe

K. Endoscopic cord ligation in selective feticide. *Lancet* 1996;348:890–891.

21 Lemery DJ, Vanlieferinghen P, Gasq M, Finkeltin F, Beaufrere AM, Beytout M. Fetal umbilical cord ligation under ultrasound guidance. *Ultrasound Obstet Gynecol* 1994;4:399–401.

Chapter 15/Pregnancy reduction in multifetal pregnancies

MARC DOMMERGUES, YVES DUMEZ and MARK I.EVANS

Introduction

Multiple pregnancies of high order almost always result from infertility therapies, including ovulation induction by parenteral gonadotrophins [1,2] with or without assisted reproductive technologies such as gamete intrafallopian transfer and *in vitro* fertilization but also by less powerful agents such as clomiphene citrate [3,4]. Perinatal mortality and morbidity are positively correlated to the number of fetuses [5], mainly due to a high rate of premature deliveries. The aim of multifetal pregnancy reduction (MFPR) is to improve perinatal outcome of multiple pregnancies of high order by reducing the risk of premature delivery. MFPR can be achieved by several techniques, including transcervical aspiration and intrathoracic KCl injection either transabdominally or transvaginally. All MFPR techniques are ultrasound guided and can be performed under local anaesthesia on an outpatient basis.

Although there is no definitive consensus regarding the optimal gestational age for MFPR, our opinion is that it is optimally done at 10–11 weeks. At this gestational age, the odds for spontaneous *in utero* death of one of the embryos are small and some gross birth defects can be identified or suspected, which may contribute to the choice of which embryos should be terminated.

Ultrasound guidance

The aim of preoperative sonography is to assess the number of live embryos and their growth, to map their respective locations and to check for interovular membranes (monochorial vs. multichorial type). The embryos not to be terminated should be precisely identified to avoid any trauma of their ovular cavities throughout the procedure. Careful mapping of the embryos to be reduced is also crucial, since survival after a failed attempt of feticide can potentially result in survival with sequelae. Therefore any attempt should be thoroughly completed. If there are no fetal abnormalities, the choice of the embryos to be terminated is mainly based on topographic criteria, and the easiest to reach should be chosen. If a set of monochorial embryos is recognized within a multiple pregnancy, both monochorial fetuses should be terminated together.

Transcervical aspiration

This technique was first published by Martene-Duplan *et al.* [6] in the early 1980s and we have been using it routinely since 1987 [7].

The patient is placed in the lithotomy position and ultrasound control is obtained using an abdominal probe. The uterine cervix is exposed by a single valve speculum, cleansed and gently grasped using a Pozzi tenaculum. Progressive cervical dilatation is achieved using Hegar dilators. A Karman cannula, connected to a 20-ml syringe, is then inserted transcervically and brought in contact with the embryo located next to the internal cervical os. The embryo is aspirated by a brisk depression operated manually. The corresponding placenta is not aspirated. The operation can be repeated if more than one embryo is to be terminated [3,6–8].

This technical approach has many disadvantages. Cervical dilatation is often required. Significant preoperative bleeding may occasionally occur. The procedure is easier with smaller embryos, i.e. at 9 weeks or earlier, a gestational age at which screening for fetal anomaly is not possible. In our hands, the miscarriage rate of the whole pregnancy following transcervical MFPR was twice that via the transabdominal route [3]. However, some authors have reported good results following transcervical MFPR [8].

Transabdominal needling

Under sonographic guidance by an abdominal probe, a 20-gauge needle is inserted through the mother's abdomen into the thorax of the embryo. In the earliest attempts, fetal demise was achieved by mechanical trauma or the injection of air or saline. However, mechanical trauma and saline injections were not always effective and air injection altered sonographic images. Therefore, transabdominal MFPR is now achieved by KCl injection [9–12], at a concentration of 1.3–2 mEq/ml. Fundal embryos are usually easier to needle than lower-lying ones. After the needle has been inserted into the embryo, a 2-ml syringe is attached to the needle. It is possible to check that the tip of the needle is located in the embryo and is not displaced into the amniotic cavity by operating a mild depression with the syringe. Then, 1–2 ml of KCl are injected gently, to prevent the embryo from being pushed away from the needle tip by the pressure of the fluid injected. Occasionally the fluid injected into the embryo can be seen as a trans-sonic image in the fetal mediastinum and pleura. When the needle is correctly inserted, the fetal heart stops within a few seconds following the injection. After the needle has been removed, the terminated embryo often seems to 'sink' passively in its amniotic cavity. The success of the procedure should be rechecked by ultrasound a few hours later or the following day, to avoid the risk of misdiagnosing a failed attempt.

Transvaginal needling

This approach is similar to the latter technique, but the needle is inserted through a transvaginal needle guide attached to a vaginal ultrasound probe and advanced through the vaginal and uterine wall into the gestational sac.

Although transvaginal needling can be done at earlier gestational ages, it is usually performed at 9.5–10 weeks. Originally a 17 to 19-gauge needle was inserted manually through the vagina and the myometrium into the embryo, and KCl was then injected into the fetal thorax. More recently, a thinner 21-gauge needle has been used, and insertion by an automated spring-loaded device has been described [13].

Earlier in gestation, at 7–8 weeks, MFPR can be achieved by mechanical trauma using the same trans-vaginal route. The tip of a 25-cm long needle with an external diameter of 1.6 mm connected by a catheter to a 20-ml syringe is placed in contact with the embryo. A brisk suction is applied, resulting in cessation of fetal heart activity [14]. This technique has the potential disadvantage of being performed at a gestational age at which sonographic evaluation of the structure of the embryo is not yet possible. However, performing MFPR earlier may be psychologically more acceptable to some patients. In addition, preliminary reports have suggested that the fetal loss rate is lower in early transvaginal procedures [15].

Postoperative follow-up

Spotting is usually noticed following transcervical aspiration, but not after transvaginal or transabdominal MFPR. The usefulness of prophylactic antibiotics, tocolytic agents or cervical suture has not been demonstrated. The major goal of subsequent obstetrical follow-up is to achieve prevention of prematurity. Since the risks of premature delivery are decreased but not completely eliminated by MFPR, this concern should be clearly explained to the patient. In addition, centres performing MFPR should obtain extensive perinatal follow-up of all their cases in order to provide continuous self-evaluation.

Preoperative counselling

The need for careful counselling prior to MFPR should not be underestimated. It is important to provide information both on the natural history of multiple pregnancies and on the expected obstetrical and perinatal results of MFPR, including the risk of premature delivery associated with multiple pregnancies of high order. Obstetrical benefits of MFPR should be weighed against potential drawbacks of the procedure, including fetal loss and maternal stress. The motivation of the couple should also be evaluated, and medical history should also be taken into account. For example, the subjective experience of a triplet pregnancy is likely to be extremely different in a young fertile multipara following a cavalier ovulation induction as opposed to a couple with a long history of infertility.

Following MFPR, spontaneous *in utero* death of one of the surviving embryos is infrequent. In contrast, miscarriage of the whole pregnancy before 24 weeks occurs in a significant number of cases (9–15%) [11], and these miscarriages often take place 4–8 weeks after the procedure. However, this relatively high pregnancy loss rate must be compared with the incidence of miscarriages in multiple pregnancies of high order. For example, in our institution, pregnancy loss before 24 weeks occurs in up to 10% of triplet pregnancies without MFPR.

The risk of miscarriage following MFPR has been shown to increase with the initial number of embryos, but also with the number of fetuses reduced [11]. It should also be stressed that there is a learning curve and that the miscarriage rate decreases with the experience of the operator [16].

While maternal complications are not infrequent in multiple pregnancies of high order, no significant maternal morbidity is associated with MFPR, apart from miscarriages. The use of local anaesthesia is recommended to avoid the potential side-effects of general anaesthesia, which is not used by the majority of centres.

Since in multiple pregnancies prematurity is the major factor of paediatric morbidity, gestational age at birth should be the prominent criterion to evaluate the efficacy of MFPR. MFPR has not been found to be associated with an increase in the incidence of intrauterine growth retardation or malformations in surviving fetuses. In the absence of MFPR, prematurity, as well as neonatal mortality and morbidity associated with multiple pregnancies, are correlated with the number of fetuses [5]. Nearly all quadruplets are delivered before 37 weeks; 30–40% of them are born before 32 weeks [17]. In our institution, 78% of potentially viable triplets deliver before 37 weeks, and 21% before 32 weeks. Similar results have been found by others [1].

The obstetrical follow-up of over 1000 MFPRs performed since 1981 [11,16] has shown that among potentially viable deliveries (≥24 weeks), mean gestational age at birth was 36 menstrual weeks. However, nearly half of the patients delivered after 37 completed weeks and more than 85% delivered later than 33 weeks.

The major factor correlated with gestational age at birth is the number of embryos left following MFPR [3,11]. Following a reduction to three embryos, 89% of patients delivered before 37 weeks and 33% before 32 weeks. With a reduction to two embryos, 52% of patients delivered before 37 weeks and 13% before 32 weeks. In contrast, with a reduction to one embryo, 30% of patients delivered before 37 weeks and 10% before 32 weeks.

These data and the results presented above suggest that MFPR clearly produces a major decrease in the risk of premature delivery in quadruplets or more. Benefits can also be expected from MFPR in triplets but this is more debatable than in pregnancies of higher order. Therefore, we feel that MFPR should be offered to patients with quadruplet pregnancies. In the case of triplets, parental autonomy should be given a high priority in the decision process after thorough counselling on the potential risks and benefits of MFPR. We do not perform MFPR in twins except in very exceptional circumstances.

The final number of embryos to be left following MFPR has also been debated. While leaving a single embryo is the most effective way of preventing prematurity, this approach is associated with a higher risk of miscarriage. Moreover, most couples with a long history of infertility wish to keep twins despite an increased risk of premature delivery.

The psychological distress of couples considering MFPR should never be underestimated. These pregnancies are extremely desired by parents who often undergo stressful and expensive infertility therapies, sometimes over many years. However, the birth of triplets or quadruplets is also perceived negatively. Many couples originally consider MFPR mainly for 'social' reasons and do not realize that maternal and paediatric outcomes may be significantly compromised in multiple pregnancies of high order. The tremendous guilt experienced by these parents is at least partly ameliorated when they receive accurate information.

Conclusions

The choice of a particular technique cannot be based on objective criteria only. While we and others have had better results with transabdominal MFPR than with transcervical aspiration [3,9], this has not been universally confirmed [8]. Whatever technique is used, the experience of the operator is an important factor in the safety of the procedure and we believe MFPR should be performed by experienced physicians. However, despite the relatively good results of MFPR, it must be stressed that this technique reduces but does not completely eliminate the increased risk of prematurity associated with multiple pregnancies of high order. Therefore, our major goal remains prevention of iatrogenic multiple pregnancies. During *in vitro* fertilization, this can be easily achieved by limiting the number of embryos transferred. However, despite careful monitoring, induction of ovulation can result in the recruitment of multiple follicles. In such cases, follicle aspiration is a potential alternative. It is clear that to obviate the need for MFPR, infertility specialists must continue to be vigilant in the use of fertility drugs.

References

1 Holcberg G, Biale Y, Lewenthal H, Insler V. Outcome of pregnancy in 31 triplet gestations. *Obstet Gynecol* 1982;59:472–479.

2 Schenker JG, Yarkoni S, Granat M. Multiple pregnancies following induction of ovulation. *Fertil Steril* 1981;35: 105–123.

3 Dommergues M, Nisand I, Mandelbrot L, Isfer E, Radunovic N, Dumez Y. Embryo reduction in the management of multifetal pregnancies following infertility therapy: obstetrical risks and perinatal benefits are related to the operative strategy. *Fertil Steril* 1991;55:801–811.

4 Evans MI, Fletcher JC, Zador IE. Selective first trimester termination in octuplet and quadruplet pregnancies: clinical and ethical issues. *Obstet Gynecol* 1988;71:289–296.

5 Botting BH, McDonald Davies I, McFarlane AJ. Recent trends in the incidence of multiple births and associated mortality. *Arch Dis Child* 1987;62:941–950.

6 Martene-Duplan J, Aknin AJ, Alamowitch R. Aspiration embryonnaire partielle au cours de grossesses multiples. *Contracept Fertil Sex* 1983;11:745–748.

7 Dumez Y, Oury JF. Method for first trimester selective abortion in multiple pregnancy. *Contr Gynecol Obstet* 1986;15:50–53.

8 Salat-Baroux J, Aknin J, Antoine JM, Alamowitch R. The management of multiple pregnancies after induction for superovulation. *Hum Reprod* 1988;3:399–401.

9 Berkowitz R, Lynch L, Chitkara U. Selective reduction of multifetal pregnancies in the first trimester. *N Engl J Med* 1988;318:1043–1047.

10 Bessis R, Milanese C, Frydman R. Partial termination of pregnancy. Presented at the 2nd Congress on the Fetus as a Patient, Jérusalem, Mai 1985.

11 Evans MI, Dommergues M, Wapner RJ *et al.* Efficacy of transabdominal multifetal pregnancy reduction: collaborative experience among the world's largest centers. *Obstet Gynecol* 1993;82:61–66.

12 Jeny R, Leroy B. Réduction sélective en cas de grossesses multiples. *Ann Radiol* 1983;26:446.

13 Timor-Tritsch IE, Peisner DB, Monteagudo A, Lerner JP, Sharma S. Multifetal pregnancy reduction by transvaginal puncture: evaluation of the technique used in 134 cases. *Am J Obstet Gynecol* 1993;168:799–804.

14 Itskovitz J, Boldes R, Thaler I, Bronstein M, Erlik Y, Brandes J. Transvaginal ultrasonography guided aspiration of gestational sacs for selective abortion in multiple pregnancy. *Am J Obstet Gynecol* 1989;160:215–217.

15 Itskovitzeldor J, Drugan A, Levron J, Thaler I, Brandes JM. Transvaginal embryo aspiration: a safe method for selective reduction in multiple pregnancies. *Fertil Steril* 1992;58.

16 Evans M, Dommergues M, Timor-Tritsch I *et al.* Transabdominal versus transcervical/vaginal multifetal pregnancy reduction: international collaborative study of more than 1000 cases. *Am J Obstet Gynecol* 1994;170: 902–909.

17 Pons JC, Le Moal S, Dephot N, Papernik E. La grossesse quadruple en France. In: Papiernik E (ed) *Les Grossesses Multiples*. Paris: Doin, 1991:319–328.

Section 2
Gynaecology

Chapter 16/Interventional ultrasound in daily obstetrical–gynaecological practice

RICHARD JAFFE, JOAQUIN SANTOLAYA-FORGAS
and DIDIER LÉMERY

Introduction

The bimanual examination is still the mainstay of the gynaecological examination. Gynaecologists use their experience and knowledge of anatomy to subjectively assess the status of the patient. They obtain information from the size and consistency of the pelvic structures and from any pain initiated by slight movement of the uterus and ovaries. Even with experienced hands, the bimanual examination can only furnish a limited assessment of the pelvic structures. Ultrasonography has improved the gynaecological examination by adding an objective component. While bimanual examination describes ovarian cysts in very limited terms, the ultrasonographic examination adds precise information on their size, internal structures and appearance. Under the bimanual examination the uterus can only be felt from the outside, whereas ultrasonography can add information regarding the myometrium and uterine cavity [1,2]. Furthermore, often bimanual examinations cannot be performed in patients with vaginal bleeding and chronic medical conditions (Fig. 16.1), or in children and young girls who have not experienced intercourse. For example, it is not uncommon to see girls with foreign bodies in the vagina causing pain, discharge and bleeding. Prompt diagnosis is important to prevent severe complications and ultrasound and vaginoscopy are easy to perform, well tolerated and may complement each other in the detection of foreign vaginal bodies. In these situations, ultrasonography has become an invaluable diagnostic aid.

In this chapter we discuss the different applications of office ultrasonography as related to invasive procedures performed by the gynaecologist.

The uterine cavity

Intrauterine device (IUD)

The most common uses of ultrasonography in association with an intrauterine device (IUD) are to confirm proper insertion of an IUD, to localize an IUD in the case of 'lost strings' and to evaluate the cause of pain and bleeding in patients using this type of contraception [3]. Ultrasonography may be employed to locate IUDs both within the uterus and outside the uterus in the case of perforation. Although transvaginal ultrasonography is superior in the accurate location of an IUD involved in a perforation, abdominal ultrasonography has a significant advantage over the transvaginal route in guiding the removal of an IUD with lost threads [4]. With the help of ultrasonography, the exact location and type of IUD can be determined. The device is frequently imaged as a hyperechoic density with shadowing and ring-down (Fig. 16.2). Myometrial invasion is diagnosed when any part of the IUD extends beyond the endometrium into the myometrium. Studies have demonstrated that the IUD is considered correctly positioned if the fundal distance measured on the longitudinal scan is no more than one-third greater than the thickness of the anterior or posterior uterine wall [4]. A common problem with IUDs is difficulty in extraction due to it being embedded in the endometrium. In these cases, the tip of the IUD often breaks and ultrasonography can be used to ensure the complete removal of the device (Fig. 16.3).

Minor uterine surgery

With the improved resolution offered by transvaginal ultrasonography, the uterine cavity and its contents can be easily recognized. This has been demonstrated to be

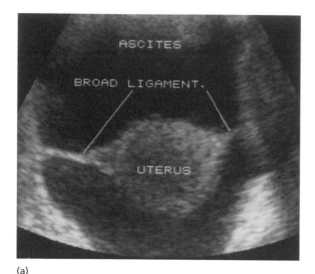

(a)

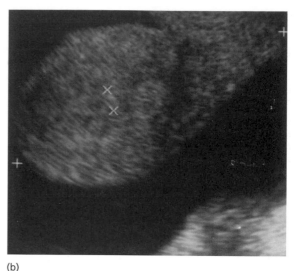

(b)

Fig. 16.1 (a) Visualization of the uterus and endometrial cavity in a patient with chronic renal failure referred for vaginal bleeding. (b) The nature of any free fluid within the peritoneal cavity can be safely determined under ultrasound guidance.

important in assisting in the performance of intrauterine surgical procedures, such as curettage, excision of polyps or intracavitary fibroids, and in the accurate location of instruments in the case of uncertainty of their position within the uterus (Fig. 16.4). Ultrasonography is also important in the evaluation of the uterine cavity during and following diagnostic curettage or pregnancy termination. In these patients this technique will assist in determining completion of the procedure, i.e. an empty uterine cavity.

Postpartum evaluation of the uterine cavity

Ultrasonography is frequently used to visualize the uterine cavity in cases of excessive postpartum bleeding or during the puerperium. This technique allows better indications for curettage and frequently eliminates the need for this invasive procedure, which is associated with a risk of infection and perforation. However, when retained parts of the placenta are detected, ultrasonographic guidance of the curette will reduce the risk of uterine perforation (Fig. 16.4).

Hysterosonography

A new approach to the anatomical evaluation of the uterine cavity is fluid-enhanced transvaginal ultrasonography or ultrasonohysterography (Fig. 16.5). With this technique the gynaecologist can distinguish between minimal intracavitary tissue and significant polyps or fibroids in women complaining of prolonged uterine bleeding [5].

Ultrasound-guided prenatal diagnostic procedures

Chorionic villous sampling, amniocentesis and fetal blood sampling can establish the presence or the aetiology and pathophysiology of fetal diseases and the reader is referred to previous chapters.

The fallopian tube

Ultrasonographically guided transcervical tubal catheterization can be performed in an ambulatory setting. This procedure has reduced the risk and morbidity of some surgical procedures on the fallopian tubes. Tubal catheterization has captured a permanent place in the treatment of tubal occlusion by replacing more invasive procedures, such as abdominal and laparoscopic surgery, and by enhancing *in vitro* fertilization procedures in patients with tubal obstruction. Visualization during the procedure can be performed with endoscopy, fluoroscopy

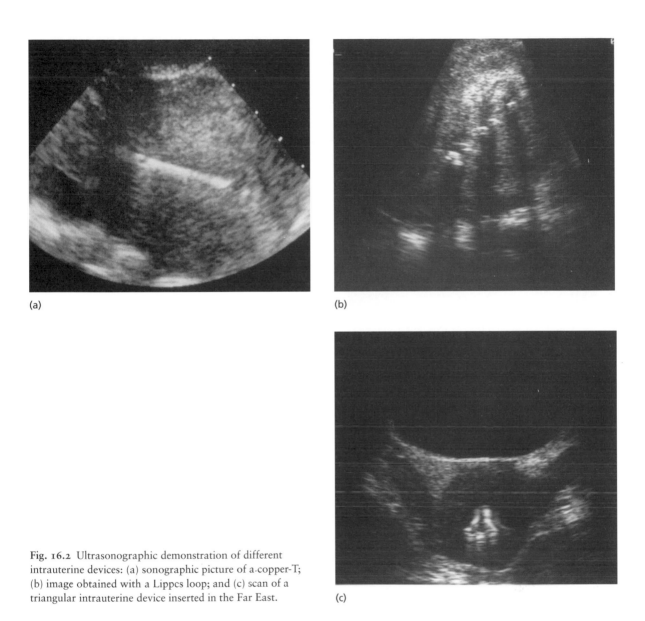

(a)

(b)

Fig. 16.2 Ultrasonographic demonstration of different intrauterine devices: (a) sonographic picture of a copper-T; (b) image obtained with a Lippcs loop; and (c) scan of a triangular intrauterine device inserted in the Far East.

(c)

or ultrasonography. Tubal catheterization performed under fluoroscopic visualization must be very carefully monitored so that the radiation dose to the ovaries does not exceed the acceptable limit. Ultrasonographic monitoring is inferior in resolution to that of fluoroscopy but, because of the elimination of radiation, this technique is quickly gaining popularity [6]. The use of ultrasonographic contrast media and Doppler imaging have improved the accuracy of this modality in the diagnosis of tubal disease during fertility work-up [7]. In addition to diagnosis of tubal disease, transcervical tubal catheterization has also been employed in the treatment of tubal occlusion. This procedure, called transcervical balloon tuboplasty, has been performed with both fluoroscopy and ultrasonography (Fig. 16.6). Fallopian tube catheterization has been successful in 80–90% of cases and pregnancy rates range from 20 to 40% [8,9]. Ectopic pregnancy has been reported to

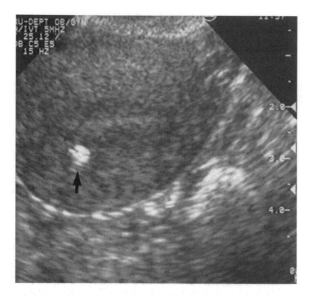

Fig. 16.3 Transvaginal ultrasonographic image of the tip (arrow) of an intrauterine device broken off at time of removal.

Fig. 16.4 During a dilatation and curettage procedure, ultrasound can safely guide the curette. (a) The curette is clearly seen within the uterine cavity, which is not empty of fetal tissue. (b) The curette is now emptying the uterine cavity.

occur in 5–15%. The main complications associated with the procedure are those related to anaesthesia and infectious processes. If pregnancy is established, close monitoring by hormonal levels as well as high-resolution transvaginal ultrasonography is advocated to demonstrate location of the developing sac (Fig. 16.7). With the early detection of tubal gestations, conservative treatment can be instituted to save the tube from irreversible damage.

Permanent contraception

Transcervical tubal catheterization has also been successfully employed for sterilization [10]. This can be performed in a similar way to balloon tuboplasty and different methods have been used for occlusion of the tubes. The reported methods include cryocoagulation, electrocoagulation, silicone plugs and chemical injection. These methods all suffer from high failure rates and do not yet compete successfully with surgical sterilization [11].

Assisted reproduction

Ultrasonographically guided tubal catheterization can also be performed for tubal placement of embryos and gametes. The main advantage of this procedure is the elimination of radiation and a relatively simple procedure.

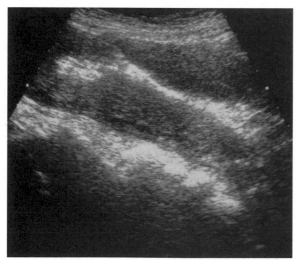

(a)

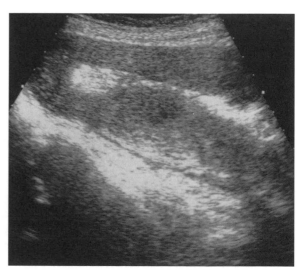

(b)

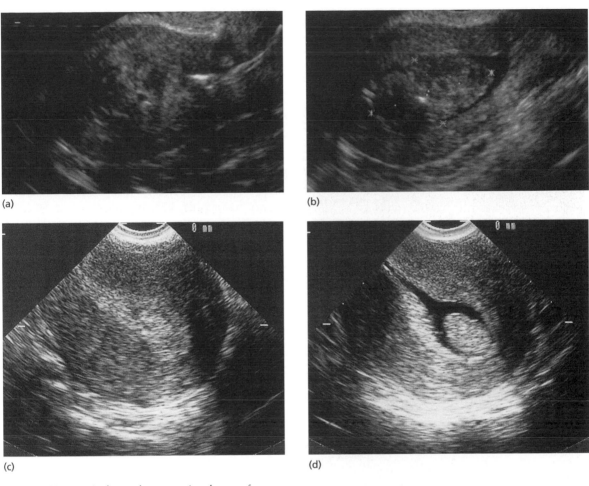

(a)

(b)

(c)

(d)

Fig. 16.5 Transvaginal scan demonstrating the use of ultrasonohysterography in evaluation of intrauterine masses. (a) The catheter has been inserted through the cervix. (b) After instillation of normal saline a pedunculated fibroid was delineated. (c) Irregular endometrium seen on transvaginal scan. (d) After saline infusion, a polyp can clearly be seen.

Ectopic pregnancies

As mentioned in Chapter 19, conservative treatment of tubal gestations is increasing in popularity due to the possibility of conserving the tube for future fertility [12]. In ectopic pregnancies detected early by transvaginal ultrasonography, local deposition of cytodestructive agents may reduce the amount of medication delivered

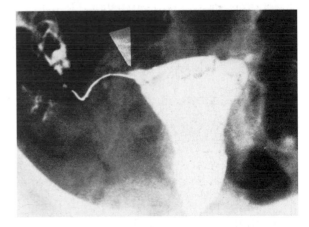

Fig. 16.6 Following dilatation of a proximal tubal occlusion (arrow) the balloon catheter is guided through the ostium and patency is confirmed.

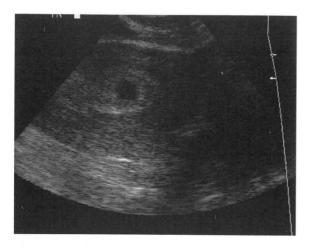

Fig. 16.7 Transvaginal scan detecting early intrauterine gestational sac.

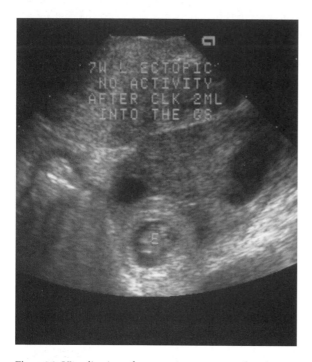

Fig. 16.8 Visualization of an ectopic pregnancy after the interruption of fetal heart activity following the transvaginal injection of 2 ml of potassium chloride.

and avoid serious side-effects (Fig. 16.8). The success of this technique depends on early detection of the pregnancy.

The cervix

Cervical incompetence is the inability of the uterus to maintain a pregnancy until term due to a cervical defect. The incidence is estimated to be 1–1.5% of all pregnancies and is generally based on a prior history of late abortions or preterm deliveries. The main aetiological factors are congenital anomalies of the cervix, cervical trauma due to instrumental cervical dilatation for pregnancy termination or dilatation and curettage, cone biopsy and cervical tumours [13–17]. In asymptomatic pregnant women with significant obstetrical history transvaginal ultrasonography is an objective method for assessment of cervical length and dilation and the presence or absence of fetal membranes within the cervix (Fig. 16.9). Cervical dilation of 2–2.5 cm or more and shortening of the cervix by over 50% indicates cervical incompetence [18]. However, several studies have demonstrated that in multiparous women and in the final weeks of pregnancy there may be an increase in cervical dilation without an increase in preterm delivery and these findings are therefore considered normal in these women [19]. It must be emphasized that vaginal examination is not a sensitive method for evaluating the cervix. Only part of the cervix can be palpated and the internal os is not assessed if the dilation does not involve the whole cervical length. The evidence from transabdominal ultrasound studies indicates that an internal os diameter of 2 cm or more is indicative of cervical incompetence [18]. However, the degree of bladder filling can alter the ultrasonographically measured internal os diameter and cervical length; therefore measurements should be made with both a filled and partially filled bladder [20]. Cervical length in pregnancy has been determined to be as high as 6 cm [21]. Shortening of the cervix occurs during the second half of pregnancy and more important than the actual length are the dynamic changes on serial examinations. Transperineal ultrasonography is performed with an empty bladder and has been shown to be more accurate than the transabdominal route [22]. In a study using the transperineal approach the mean cervical length in primiparous women was 4.7 cm. There was no increase in preterm deliveries when the cervical length was more than 2.5 cm [23]. Transvaginal ultrasonography is superior to both previous methods. With the close proximity of the probe to the scanned organs, a more

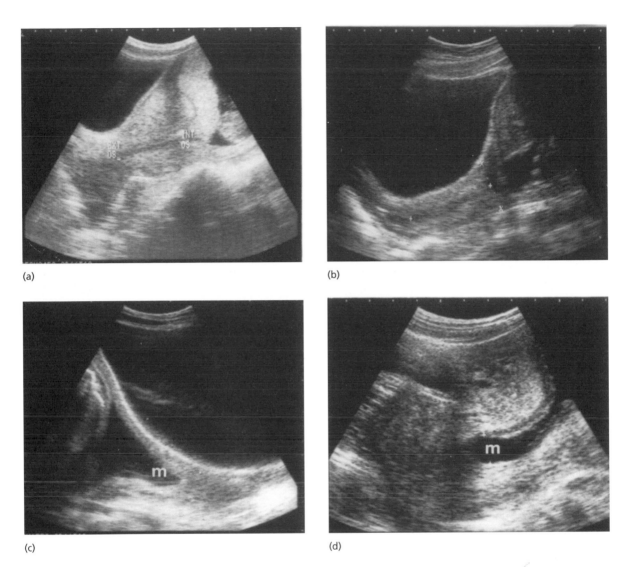

(a)

(b)

(c)

(d)

Fig. 16.9 (a,b) Assessment of cervical length in normal gestations. (c,d) Prolapse of fetal membranes (m) into a dilated cervical canal in cervical incompetence.

detailed anatomical evaluation can be performed and more accurate measurements obtained. The transvaginal route eliminates sound absorption by the symphysis and provides optimal delineation of the entire cervical length. This route also eliminates the need for a full bladder, which can hamper the evaluation. Using this technique, it has been established that the most important predictor of preterm birth before 30 weeks' gestation was an internal os dilation of 5 mm or more [24] and cervical

length of less than 2 cm. Cervical effacement begins at the level of the internal os and the effacement changes precede clinical manifestations by several weeks. With the help of ultrasonography, these early changes can be detected and patients treated with bedrest and tocolytics before the membranes protrude through the cervix and into the vagina. In cases of ruptured or collapsed membranes, abdominal ultrasonography is probably safer and reduces the risk of infection. Cervical cerclage has been the mainstay of treatment for cervical incompetence since Shirodkar first described its use in 1955 [25]. The procedure is performed at 13–14 weeks' gestation, except for rare cases where an emergency cerclage is placed in the second trimester due to bulging membranes. Ultrasonography has been employed to guide the placement of the suture and determine if the internal os is closed and good cervical length achieved. The use of ultrasonography is advantageous in providing the exact location of the internal os, the location of the membranes, decreased risk for puncturing of the amniotic sac and visualization of the actual closure of the cervix after placement of the suture [26]. The transabdominal approach is the most frequently employed method of directing the placement of the suture but a transrectal technique has also been reported [27]. These authors discussed that due to the close proximity of the probe to the cervix, the suture could be placed higher with this method than with the traditional transabdominal approach. Ultrasonographic follow-up after cervical cerclage has also been employed to detect early failure of the cerclage [28].

Conclusions

Ultrasonography has brought about an unprecedented change in the clinical practice of obstetrics and gynaecology. This imaging modality has become an integral part of patient care and is used daily in the evaluation of both obstetrical and gynaecological patients. Ultrasonography is used in general diagnoses, the evaluation of pelvic pain, bleeding disorders, infertility work-up, follow-up of treatments, screening for malignancies and as an aid in many surgical interventions. The employment of ultrasonographic guidance for common obstetrical and gynaecological procedures has also reduced their complication rate some common obstetrical and gynaecological procedures, resulting in greatly improved patient care.

References

1 Santolaya J. Physiology of the menstrual cycle by ultrasonography. *J Ultrasound Med* 1992;**11**:139–142.

2 Santolaya J, Ramakrishnan V, Scommegna A. The menstrual cycle: relations of biophysical and hormonal determinations in normal women of reproductive age. *Fertil Steril* 1992;**58**:1230–1233.

3 Aleem HA, Kamel HS, Abdoul-Oyoun ESM. Role of ultrasonography in managing IUD related complaints. *Contraception* 1992;**46**:211–220.

4 Bernaschek G, Deutinger J, Kratochwil A. *Endosonography in Obstetrics and Gynecology*. New York: Springer-Verlag, 1990:92–96.

5 Goldstein SR. Use of ultrasonohysterography for triage of perimenopausal patients with unexplained uterine bleeding. *Am J Obstet Gynecol* 1994;**170**:565–570.

6 Brosens I, Boeckx W, Delattin PH, Puttemans P, Vasquez G. Salpingoscopy: a new preoperative diagnostic tool in tubal infertility. *Br J Obstet Gynaecol* 1987;**94**:768–773.

7 Deichert U, Schlief R, van de Sandt M, Juhnke I. Transvaginal hysterosalpingo-contrast-sonography (HyCoSy) compared with conventional tubal diagnostics. *Hum Reprod* 1989;**4**:418–424.

8 Confino E, Friberg J, Gleicher N. Preliminary experience with transcervical balloon tuboplasty (TBT). *Am J Obstet Gynecol* 1988;**159**:370–375.

9 Thurmond A. Selective salpingography and fallopian tube recanalization. *AJR* 1991;**156**:33.

10 Cooper JM. Hysteroscopic sterilization. *Clin Obstet Gynecol* 1991;**35**:282.

11 Confino E. Transcervical tubal catheterization in the management of obstructions, gamete transfer, and treatment of ectopic gestations. In: Jaffe R, Pierson RA, Abramowicz JSA (eds) *Imaging in Infertility and Reproductive Endocrinology*. Philadelphia: JB Lippincott, 1995.

12 Stovall TC, Ling FW, Gray LA. Single-dose methotrexate for treatment of ectopic pregnancy. *Obstet Gynecol* 1991;**77**:754–757.

13 Golan A, Barnan R, Wexler S, Langer R, Bukovsky I, David MP. Incompetence of the uterine cervix. *Obstet Gynecol Surv* 1989;**44**:96–107.

14 McDonald IA. Cervical incompetence as a cause of spontaneous abortion. In: Bennet MJ, Edmonds DK (eds) *Spontaneous and Recurrent Abortion*. Oxford: Blackwell Scientific Publications, 1987:168–192.

15 Johnstone FD, Beard RJ, Boyde IE, McCarthy TG. Cervical diameter after suction termination of pregnancy. *Br Med J* 1976;**1**:68–70.

16 Ranney B. Congenital cervical incompetence in primigravidas. *Am J Obstet Gynecol* 1963;**86**:52–56.

17 Bennet MJ. Congenital abnormalities of the fundus. In: Bennet MJ, Edmonds DK (eds) *Spontaneous and Recurrent Abortion*. Oxford: Blackwell Scientific Publications, 1987:109.

18 Bernaschek G, Deutinger J, Kratochwil A. *Endosonography in Obstetrics and Gynecology*. New York: Springer Verlag, 1990;66–69.

19 Floyd WS. Cervical dilation in the mid-trimester of pregnancy. *Obstet Gynecol* 1961;**18**:380–381.

20 Confino E, Mayden KL, Giglia RV, Vermesh M, Gleicher N. Pitfalls in sonographic imaging of the incompetent uterine cervix. *Acta Obstet Gynecol Scand* 1986;**65**: 593–597.

21 Zemlyn S. The length of the uterine cervix and its significance. *J Clin Ultrasound* 1981;9:267–269.

22 Hertzberg BS, Bowies JD, Weber TM, Carroll BA, Kliewer MA, Jordan SG. Sonography of the cervix during the third trimester of pregnancy: value of the transperineal approach. *Am J Reprod* 1991;157:73–78.

23 Lumbroso P, Livache C, Lewin D. Le col de promipare. Une servie de 320 echographies perineales de principe. *J Gynecol Obstet Biol Reprod* 1983;12:489–494.

24 Okitsu O, Mimura T, Nakayama T, Aono T. Early prediction of preterm delivery by transvaginal ultrasonography. *Ultrasound Obstet Gynecol* 1992;2:402–409.

25 Shirodkar VN. A method of operative treatment for habitual abortion in the second trimester of pregnancy. *Antiseptic* 1955;52:299–300.

26 Wheelock JB, Johnson TRB, Graham D, Saucer GJ, Teal CL, Sanders RC. Ultrasound-assisted cervical cerclage. *J Clin Ultrasound* 1984;12:307–311.

27 Fleischer AC, Lombardi S, Kepole DM. Guidance for cerclage using transrectal sonography. *J Ultrasound Med* 1989;8:589–590.

28 Rana J, Davis SE, Harrigan JT. Improving the outcome of cervical cerclage by sonographic follow-up. *J Ultrasound Med* 1990;9:275–278.

Chapter 17/Ultrasound or endoscopy in the treatment of adnexal cystic masses

MICHEL CANIS, JEAN-ALAIN BOURNAZEAU, FRANÇOIS N.MASSON, REVAY BOTCHORISHVILI, ARMAND WATTIEZ, JEAN-LUC POULY, GERARD MAGE and MAURICE A.BRUHAT

Over the last few years several alternatives to the classical management by laparotomy of adnexal diseases such as adnexal cystic masses and ectopic pregnancies have been developed [1–8]. These changes are due to the development of endoscopic surgery and new ultrasound technologies including endovaginal probes. Together with these new techniques, the concept of minimal or even non-invasive surgery has been reported and advertised in the media, so that the classical treatment by laparotomy would nowadays appear unacceptable to many patients and even to many physicians.

Obviously these advances are very attractive for patients who wish to avoid surgery. However the problems associated with adnexal diseases have not changed: an ectopic pregnancy may still be a life-threatening condition. Therefore when using these new approaches we should not forget that treatment should be simple, reliable and safe.

Ultrasound-guided puncture of adnexal cystic masses

Puncture of malignant tumours

When proposing ultrasound-guided treatment of adnexal cystic masses, the controversies encountered in the development of laparoscopic surgery should not be obscured. Indeed the risk of spillage is probably the same whatever the technique used. Several conclusions can be drawn about the consequences of surgical puncture and/or rupture of malignant adnexal masses. The prognostic consequences are related to the delay between the puncture and the surgical treatment of the tumour. When the tumour is removed immediately, all the studies of the treatment of low malignant potential ovarian tumours have failed to demonstrate any incidence of intraoperative puncture or rupture of the tumour [9–14]. Despite the controversial results of univariate analysis [15–22], five studies [23–27] have reported that when an invasive tumour is removed immediately the risks of surgical puncture are more theoretical than real. This conclusion appears reasonable when studying the sensitivity of ovarian cytology in the diagnosis of malignancy: if many malignant cells were to be disseminated by the puncture, the cytological diagnosis would probably be much easier and more reliable [28–33]. However this conclusion should be regarded with caution as all the results available nowadays come from studies on drainage performed at laparotomy, not at laparoscopy or under ultrasound guidance. Moreover definitive conclusions about spillage are difficult, since the importance of a puncture is probably different for epithelial and germ-cell tumours, for small tumours of 3 cm and for large masses of 20 cm in diameter, for well or poorly differentiated tumours, etc. Obviously the prognosis of a malignant tumour will never be improved by a puncture, which should be avoided whenever possible.

Unfortunately several case reports and several national surveys have recently demonstrated that if the tumour is not removed immediately the prognosis of a malignant ovarian tumour is worsened by laparoscopic puncture or biopsy [34–41]. The two national surveys have also shown the following.

1 Many cases of unexpected malignant tumours have been adequately managed by an immediate vertical midline laparotomy.

2 Many patients were managed laparoscopically by surgeons not trained in oncological surgery, although the diagnosis of cancer was obvious.

3 Perfect preoperative selection appears very difficult since malignancy can be encountered among ultrasonographically benign masses [34].

Inadequate management is explained by the lack of expertise of the surgeon not by the technological approach used. Indeed inadequate surgical procedures were also performed by laparotomy as in a report from Helawa *et al.* [42] which included 40% of cancer not diagnosed at laparotomy and three cases treated inadequately by puncture, biopsy and cystectomy. However, the complications encountered when endoscopic surgery was being developed should be avoided during ultrasonographic management and therefore careful preoperative selection is essential. The rule proposed by Maiman *et al.* [34] should be followed: 'the ability to treat immediately and effectively an ovarian cancer is a prerequisite to the surgical management of adnexal cystic masses'. It should be emphasized that when using cytological examination and ultrasound puncture to diagnose a malignant ovarian tumour, the ovary is not removed immediately so that the risk of dissemination may be real. Secondary abdominal wall implants have also been reported after laparoscopic biopsy of borderline tumours [40]. Interestingly, Bonilla-Musoles *et al.* [43] reported that in seven cases they found no dissemination at laparotomies performed 2 days after an ultrasound puncture, whose site could even not be identified in six of the seven cases. They suggested that ultrasonographic puncture is safer since the needle is much smaller than that used at laparoscopy. Some authors are convinced that puncture and cytology will become a major tool in the diagnosis of ovarian cancer, as it is in the diagnosis of breast, kidney or liver cancer [43,44]. However there are differences between these tumours and ovarian cancer, which develops in the peritoneal cavity, where it spreads easily and early. Also, the cytological diagnosis of ovarian cancer is not reliable even in expert hands [28,33].

Puncture of benign masses

From laparoscopy we also learned that puncture of benign ovarian neoplasms is not a satisfactory treatment [45]. Indeed recurrence rates of 30–40% were reported as early as 1983. Moreover several recent papers have argued in favour of surgical treatment of benign ovarian neoplasms, the authors suggesting that benign neoplasms may be the precursors of ovarian cancer [46,47]. In the same way, Bourne *et al.* [48] recently reported that benign ovarian neoplasms are more

common in women with a familial history of ovarian cancer. Finally we observed three malignant recurrences after laparoscopic cystectomy performed to treat benign serous cysts in postmenopausal patients [49]. As these three malignant recurrences occurred more than 5 years after the initial laparoscopic treatment in a small group of 15 patients, we suggest that these patients may be at risk for ovarian cancer and that their ovaries should be removed. Ultrasound puncture appears unacceptable in such cases.

From the results of laparoscopic surgery, it should be emphasized that the classical complications attributed to the puncture have all been encountered. Granulomatous peritonitis after the puncture of teratomas occurs in about 1% of cases [1]. We observed only two cases of abdominal wall endometrioma after the treatment of 200 ovarian endometriomas, [50]; one was located on a previous suprapubic trocar site and can be attributed unequivocally to the laparoscopic procedure. This complication is rare and may be the consequence of an inadequate extraction of the cyst wall rather than that of the puncture. Finally we observed no case of pseudomyxoma peritonei following laparoscopic puncture and treatment of a benign mucinous cystadenoma, confirming that peritoneal dissemination of mucinous tumours occurs only in malignant masses and is almost never induced by a surgical puncture [51–56]. However, we recently treated by laparotomy one case of pseudomyxoma peritonei; we found 500 ml of a mucinous peritoneal fluid associated with a 15-cm benign mucinous cyst that had been punctured, diagnosed but not removed 18 months earlier in another department.

All these data emphasize that puncture and aspiration of benign masses is not a satisfactory treatment and cannot be proposed as an alternative to the classical or laparoscopic surgical treatment. In contrast, all the surgical series of adnexal cystic masses included 10–20% of functional cysts [57,58]. Although some functional cysts will always be encountered at laparoscopy performed for other indications, most of these lesions could have been treated with a non-surgical approach. Therefore there are indications for ultrasonographic management of adnexal masses.

Indications

Indications for ultrasound-guided puncture of adnexal

cystic masses can be summarized by answering three questions:

1 Is it necessary?
2 If necessary, is it possible and/or acceptable?
3 Is it enough?

IS ANY SURGICAL APPROACH NECESSARY?

Obviously, any surgical approach including ultrasound-guided puncture should be delayed to the next menstruation. In the same way, it is not necessary to puncture an uncomplicated, entirely cystic adnexal mass diagnosed in a pregnant patient, particularly if she has undergone ovarian hyperstimulation. Most cysts are functional and will disappear spontaneously without any surgical procedure.

In contrast, ultrasound puncture can be proposed as an alternative to expectant management or the 3-month treatment with the birth control pill often administered to patients diagnosed with entirely cystic masses. Several arguments can be advanced against expectant management.

1 The classical delay of 3 months will appear much too long in patients whose adnexal mass was in fact early ovarian cancer.
2 Follow-up may be difficult to obtain in young patients.
3 It may be simpler for a patient to have her cyst punctured than to comply with the rules of an adequate follow-up, which should include a monthly clinical and ultrasonographic examination.

Wolf *et al.* [59] recently demonstrated that using vaginal ultrasonography cystic adnexal masses were found in 14.8% of menopausal patients; however 16 of the 22 cysts found were less than 2 cm in diameter. It seems that such small lesions should not be punctured or operated. However prospective studies are required to demonstrate that this management, which sounds clinically reasonable, is valuable and safe.

Similarly, several authors have proposed expectant management for entirely cystic masses of less than 5 cm diagnosed in postmenopausal patients [3,60]. Although very attractive, this management should be used carefully. Indeed our results reported above demonstrated that the consequences of conservative treatment of ovarian masses in postmenopausal patients should be evaluated only with long-term results. At the moment,

only one group has reported long-term follow-up after expectant management [3]. Their results are promising, as all the entirely cystic masses operated on immediately were benign and only one of the 32 cysts followed increased in diameter and required surgical treatment.

IS IT POSSIBLE AND/OR ACCEPTABLE?

Preoperative selection is essential to make ultrasound-guided puncture safe and acceptable.

Clinical criteria

Clinical data, and particularly the previous medical history, can be very useful in understanding the aetiology of an adnexal mass discovered at ultrasound. A history of pelvic inflammatory disease suggests that a recently discovered cystic mass may be a hydrosalpinx rather than an ovarian tumour. In the same way, a history of endometriosis may be helpful in identifying an adnexal mass with echogenic contents. Clinical data are also essential to diagnose a functional cyst. In order to decide whether to perform a puncture the ultrasonographic appearance should be interpreted according to data such as age, date of the last menstrual period, previous surgical history, and diameter and bilaterality of the cyst.

An ultrasound-guided puncture should not be proposed in:

1 patients more than 5 years after the menopause except if bilateral oophorectomy has been performed under satisfactory conditions and a peritoneal cyst is suspected; or
2 patients whose ovarian activity is stopped by a medical treatment, except those who began a gonadotrophin-releasing hormone analogue treatment less than 2 months previously.

In contrast, ultrasound-guided puncture can be proposed in:

1 patients whose ovarian activity is not inhibited by any treatment;
2 pregnant patients before 14 weeks of gestation;
3 patients diagnosed previously with extensive pelvic adhesions and/or peritoneal cysts;
4 postmenopausal patients whose adnexal cyst was diagnosed after clinical signs similar to those observed by the patient when she was menstruating regularly.

Ultrasound-guided puncture has also been proposed

in very old patients in poor general condition [33,44]. This last indication is more controversial, since expectant management is also valuable in patients who would not be operated on even if the cyst was suspicious.

Ultrasound criteria

As ultrasound-guided puncture is generally proposed only in entirely cystic masses, ultrasonographic examination is the key step in managing adnexal cystic masses. The ultrasonographic appearance is clearly related to the pathological diagnosis, although most large series included some false-negative and a larger number of false-positive diagnoses of malignancy [61–63]. The results of ultrasonographic diagnosis have been improved by the development of the vaginal approach. However, in our recent experience, the incidence of malignant tumour among entirely cystic masses diagnosed with vaginal ultrasound was 1.9% (4 of 319 patients). Three of these tumours were of low malignant potential and one was a well-differentiated serous cystadenocarcinoma. All cases were diagnosed at laparoscopy. In two cases small intracystic vegetations (less than 1 mm in diameter) not visible at ultrasonography were found at laparoscopic inspection of the internal cyst wall. In one case the lesion was suspicious because of a thickened area on the cyst wall. In the fourth patient an unusually vascularized small cyst of 1 cm diameter was found beside a typical functional cyst of 3 cm diameter. The smaller lesion was a low malignant potential serous cystadenocarcinoma that was not seen at the preoperative ultrasonographic examination.

These data obtained from patients treated surgically suggest the following.

1 The incidence of malignant tumour is low among entirely cystic adnexal masses; indeed it is probably much lower than that reported here, as many anechogenic lesions are managed without surgery. In this study the incidence of functional cysts was only 13.2%, much lower than the incidence reported among entirely cystic masses [64].

2 Whatever the improvement of ultrasonographic transducers, some false-negatives will always be encountered in large studies.

3 The surgical diagnosis is still essential today.

4 An ultrasound-guided puncture should be considered as a surgical procedure and should be performed in an operating room.

Conflicting attitudes have been reported in the ultrasonographic management of septated masses. Although in our experience the incidence of malignant tumours among septated masses is not different from that found among entirely cystic masses, we think that septated masses should be managed cautiously as suggested by others [60,65,66]. A puncture is acceptable when the diagnosis of a functional cyst is very likely, in patients with previous ovarian hyperstimulation or in patients whose previous surgical history suggests that severe pelvic adhesions may explain the mass. However, many authors have included masses with thin septae in their ultrasonographic management [2,30,43,44,67,68].

Ultrasonographic puncture is contraindicated in masses with thick septae or with more complex appearances. Puncture of more complex masses has been used by Dordoni *et al.* [44] to confirm the diagnosis of malignancy in high-risk patients but this management should be further evaluated.

In the future the development of colour Doppler assessment and ultrasound scoring systems will improve

Table 17.1 Incidence of malignancy when combining an ultrasound scoring system and colour Doppler.

Reference	Incidence	High score low resistance	High score high resistance	Low score low resistance	Low score low resistance
Weiner *et al.* [71]	17/53 (32)	15/16 (94)	1/11 (9)	1/2 (50)	0/24 (0)
Schneider *et al.* [70]	16/55 (29)	13/16 (81)	1/4 (25)	2/16 (12)	0/19 (0)
Timor-Tritsch *et al.* [69]	16/94 (17)	14/14 (100)	1/11 (9)	1/2 (50)	0/67 (0)
Kawai *et al.* [72]	40/109 (37)	27/32 (84)	9/28 (32)	1/5 (20)	3/44 (7)
Total	89/311 (29)	69/78 (88)	12/54 (22)	5/25 (20)	3/154 (2)

Numbers in parentheses are percentages.

the preoperative selection process [69,70]. Colour Doppler has already been used by Bonilla-Musoles *et al.* [43] to select patients before ultrasound-guided puncture. Moreover one can see from Table 17.1 that combining preoperative colour Doppler and an ultrasound scoring system can improve the preoperative selection [69–72].

Can we improve the selection process using serum CA 125?

Selection before surgery may be improved using serum CA 125 [73]. However several reviews have confirmed that abnormal CA 125 is very common in premenopausal patients with benign disease and that about 50% of patients with stage I ovarian cancer have a normal serum CA 125 [74]. CA 125 is more useful in postmenopausal patients, in whom a threshold of 65 Ul/ml was proposed by Malkasian *et al.* [75]. An abnormal CA 125 should be considered as a contraindication to non-surgical managements in postmenopausal patients.

The value of intracystic tumour markers is more questionable, as these results are not available until a few days after the puncture, too late to minimize the consequences of the puncture. Cyst fluid CA 125 level cannot be used to distinguish benign and malignant tumors [76]. In contrast Dargent *et al.* [77] published very promising results on the correlation between the pathological diagnosis and the results of a panel of intracystic and serum levels of tumour markers. Unfortunately these results were not confirmed [78].

IS IT ENOUGH?

We know from laparoscopic and ultrasonographic studies

that the recurrence rate after puncture of benign ovarian neoplasms is very high, between 41 and 61% [44]. The recurrence rate is related to the diameter of the cyst and to the success of aspiration, recurrence being significantly more common after incomplete aspiration.

These results argue strongly for immediate surgical treatment of cysts diagnosed as ovarian neoplasms from the fluid appearance. The appearance of the cyst fluid is a valuable diagnostic tool. As shown in Table 17.2, the cyst fluid of a functional cyst is generally yellow or haemorrhagic. The colour of functional cyst fluid is described as 'saffron' yellow, whereas that of serous cyst is citrous, i.e. more whitish. Consequently, most patients can be treated in only one surgical procedure. When the cyst is yellow or haemorrhagic, the cyst may be functional and laparoscopy is not necessary. The diagnosis should be confirmed as soon as possible, using cytological examination and cyst fluid oestradiol (E2) and progesterone levels. Several years ago Abeille *et al.* [79] showed that high cyst fluid E2 levels were found in functional cysts. These results were confirmed by a recent study from Andolf *et al.* [80] who showed that an E2 level above 500 pg/ml was the single best predictor of no recurrence. Cytological examination is useful to distinguish functional and organic ovarian masses [81]. Unfortunately, ovarian cytology does not appear to be a reliable tool in the diagnosis of malignancy, as the sensitivity ranges from 27 to 93% [29–33]. All the results required to decide the management of the cyst should be available in less than 8 days. If the diagnosis of functional cyst is confirmed, an ultrasonographic examination is planned 3 months later. No further ultrasound follow-up is required, except in patients with recurrent clinical signs. As shown in Table 17.2, when the cyst fluid is clear, chocolate, dermoid or

Table 17.2 Correlation between the appearance of cyst fluid and the final pathological diagnosis in benign adnexal masses.

	Yellow	Clear	Haemorrhagic	Chocolate	Mucinous	Dermoid	Turbid
Pathology (*n*)	207	178	90	210	65	138	10
Functional (%)	46.4	4.5	55.6	3.8	1.5	0.0	0.0
Serous (%)	35.7	48.3	8.9	1.4	7.7	0.7	60.0
Mucinous (%)	9.2	11.8	1.1	0.5	72.3	0.7	40.0
Paraovarian (%)	6.8	31.5	2.2	0.0	0.0	0.0	0.0
Endometrioma (%)	1.4	1.7	31.1	94.3	3.1	0.7	0.0
Teratoma (%)	0.5	2.2	1.1	0.0	15.4	97.8	0.0

turbid, a functional cyst can be excluded in most cases and immediate laparoscopic treatment is necessary. Similarly when an organic cyst is diagnosed from the results of fluid analysis, ultrasonography is performed to confirm recurrence and surgical treatment is planned as soon as possible.

Interestingly, none of the fluid encountered in the four patients with entirely cystic masses reported above could be confused with the saffron-yellow fluid encountered in functional cysts [1]. Two were turbid, as often found in malignant tumours, and two were clear, as usual in serous cysts. Therefore if these masses had been punctured vaginally, three of them would have been diagnosed as non-functional from the appearance of the fluid. In contrast, diagnosis of the fourth patient would probably have been missed, since this small tumour was found beside a 3-cm diameter functional cyst that would probably have been the only lesion punctured. This small malignant mass could even have been missed at laparoscopy, since the laparoscopic appearance was unusual because of the presence of vessels rather than because it was highly suspicious.

Ultrasound-guided puncture has also been proposed as the first step in the treatment of ovarian endometrioma, the second step being medical treatment and the third a laparoscopic procedure that would be easier because of the preoperative drainage and medical treatment. The following comments can be made about this management.

1 From our experience in *in vitro* fertilization, it seems that endometriomas may be difficult to empty.

2 Puncture without postoperative medical treatment is useless [82].

3 Most patients with ovarian endometriomas can be treated laparoscopically in one step with satisfactory postoperative results.

4 In a recent report about 209 patients Zanetta *et al.* [83] concluded that drainage alone is ineffective as a therapeutic procedure, thus confirming previous reports [42,82].

5 The advantages of the three-step procedure have never been demonstrated by laparoscopy, so this management should be further evaluated.

Concluding, we suggest that ultrasound-guided puncture is one of the tools available in the management of adnexal cystic masses. However, it should be used following strict guidelines to avoid the spillage of unexpected malignant masses; benign ovarian neoplasms should be removed surgically.

Ultrasound-guided puncture is unnecessary prior to the next menses and in masses of less than 2 cm in diameter (even in postmenopausal patients).

Ultrasound-guided puncture is possible if the cyst is functional (hyperstimulation, less than 5 years after menopause); if the patient has undergone multiple previous surgical procedures and has extensive pelvic adhesions; if the mass is entirely cystic or has a thin septa; if CA 125 is below 35 ml, the mass entirely cystic and the patient postmenopausal; or if a thin septa is found and a functional cyst is very likely or pelvic adhesions are suspected.

Ultrasound-guided puncture is impossible if the cyst is not functional and the patient has no previous adhesions; if the mass is solid, mixed or septated; or if the CA 125 level is above 35 ml and the patient postmenopausal.

Ultrasound-guided puncture is sufficient if the cyst fluid is saffron yellow, the cyst fluid E2 level very high and the diagnosis of functional cyst is confirmed by cytological examination.

Ultrasound-guided puncture is not sufficient if the fluid is clear, dermoid, mucinous or chocolate; if the E2 level and cytological examination exclude the diagnosis of functional cyst; or if a recurrence is found.

In our clinic, ultrasound-guided puncture is used to treat: (i) functional cysts in patients who wish to avoid 3 months of treatment with the birth control pill and/ or of follow-up; (ii) patients with extensive adhesions who have either a functional cyst or peritoneal cysts already diagnosed and treated surgically. In this last indication, ethanol injection was recently proposed by Lipitz *et al.* [84] to prevent the recurrence of the cyst. The procedure is always performed in the operating room. Patients are always informed before the procedure about a possible laparoscopy and laparotomy.

Ultrasound-guided puncture of ectopic pregnancy

While the incidence of ectopic pregnancy has increased over the last 20 years [85], vaginal ultrasonography and improved immunological human chorionic gonadotrophin (hCG) and serum progesterone assays allow early diagnosis and conservative treatment in most cases [86–89]. Consequently the treatment of ectopic pregnancy has changed from laparotomy to laparoscopic surgery [90,91] and more recently to non-surgical treatments [4,6,8,92–95], such as expectant management or medical treatment with methotrexate (MTX) administered intramuscularly or in the tube. An early diagnosis of the ectopic is essential to avoid tubal rupture, which may be a life-threatening condition, to allow conservative and non-surgical treatments, and to avoid irreversible tubal damage thus decreasing the recurrence rate after conservative treatment [96].

Fertility results recently published strongly suggest that medical and ultrasonographic treatments are valuable alternatives to laparoscopic treatment [8,94,97]. Pregnancy rates after intramuscular and intrasaccular injection were 69.3% and 58.6% respectively [8,95]. In these studies, tubal patency on the side of the ectopic pregnancy was found in 82% and 90% of cases [8,95].

Our comments about other non-surgical approaches will be brief. Expectant management requires very careful preoperative selection and strict follow-up, not always very convenient for the patients. Moreover, failure rates of 27% have been reported in the best series [95]. It may be used only in very specific patients with a very low β-hCG level. Prostaglandins should no longer be used because of the complications reported [98]. RU 486 does not appear to be an effective treatment [99].

Laparoscopic treatment

Laparoscopic management has become the gold standard. Most patients who require surgical treatment can be treated endoscopically. Conservative laparoscopic treatment has been described before [5,90,91]. After aspiration of the haemoperitoneum, a linear salpingotomy is performed on the proximal third of the antimesenterial border of the haematosalpinx. A large aspiration lavage cannula is inserted in the tube. The ectopic pregnancy is separated from the tubal wall using an intratubal lavage and is then aspirated. Thereafter the tube is inspected, looking for persistent trophoblastic tissue; the contralateral tube is checked to evaluate the prognosis for future fertility. This last step is impossible in non-surgical treatments. Postoperative prognosis may be evaluated using hysterosalpingography. Postoperative follow-up of the decrease in hCG is necessary for early diagnosis of persistent ectopic trophoblastic tissue, which

Table 17.3 Fertility after salpingectomy for ectopic pregnancy.

	No.	Intrauterine pregnancy	Extrauterine pregnancy
Dubuisson *et al.* [103]	125	30 (24.0)	16 (12.8)
Pouly *et al.* [5]	39	18 (46.1)	0
Total	164	48 (29.3)	16 (9.7)

Numbers in parentheses are percentages.

occurs in about 6% of cases [100,101]. Postoperative management according to the level of β-hCG on postoperative day 2 has been reported previously [100]. Postoperative fertility is above 60% with a recurrence rate of 14% and the prognosis for fertility is related to the patient's medical history rather than to the diameter or location of the ectopic pregnancy [8].

Laparoscopic salpingectomy for ectopic pregnancy was reported by Dubuisson [102,103]. This procedure is easy and allows laparoscopic treatment of a ruptured ectopic if a powerful aspiration–lavage system that allows the quick identification and treatment of the bleeding is available. Postoperative fertility and recurrence rates are 29.3% and 9.7% respectively (Table 17.3).

Transvaginal intratubal injection of methotrexate under sonographic control

First reported by Feichtinger and Kemeter [4] in 1987 this technique is achieved under local anaesthesia by most authors. The ectopic sac must be visible at ultrasound, which should also be used to look for signs of normal or abnormal intrauterine pregnancy and for signs of haemoperitoneum. The ectopic sac is aspirated using 16- or 18-gauge needle and injected with MTX using either a standard dose of 50 mg or a dose of 1 mg/kg. The use of folinic acid is not necessary [8]. Close postoperative follow-up, including serial hCG titres and clinical and ultrasonographic examination, is required [6,8]. On postoperative day 2, a transient elevation of β-hCG is observed in about 30% of cases. In the same way, abdominal or pelvic pain is frequently observed within 24 hours of the injection and should be distinguished from tubal rupture using both clinical and

Table 17.4 Results of intratubal injection of methotrexate for the treatment of ectopic pregnancy.

	No.	Success	Patency	Intrauterine pregnancy	Extrauterine pregnancy
Feichtinger & Kemeter [4]	8	8	—	—	—
Ménard *et al.* [6]	8	6	—	—	—
Mottla *et al.* [106]	7	4	—	—	—
Fernandez *et al.* [8]	100	83 (83.0)	72/80 (90.0)	31/58 (53.4)	3/58 (5.2)
Darai *et al.* [97]	100	78 (78.0)	13/26 (56.5)	15/75 (20.0)	6/75 (8.0)
Total	223	179 (80.2)	85/106 (80.2)	46/133 (34.6)	9/133 (6.8)

Numbers in parentheses are percentages.

ultrasonographic examination. If the hCG titres increase steadily or if the clinical data suggest a tubal rupture, a laparoscopy should be performed.

From a review of some studies published recently this technique seems promising but slightly less effective than laparoscopy. Among selected patients, the success, fertility and recurrence rates were 80.2%, 41.3% and 16.3% respectively (Table 17.4). It should be emphasized that Fernandez *et al.* [8] and Stovall and Ling [94] were able to treat about 40% of their patients using this ultrasonographic approach. However several injections of MTX may be necessary; a decrease of less than 15% of the initial β-hCG titre 7 days after the first injection is used to decide on a second or third injection. Fernandez *et al.* [8] reported 11 failures among 55 patients 20% treated with one injection and 6 among 28 patients treated with two or three injections (21.8%).

Is an intratubal injection necessary?

Selection criteria for intramuscular and intratubal injection of MTX are similar [8,94]. As the success and postoperative fertility rates are similar, these two approaches should be carefully compared in prospective randomized trials.

A local injection decreases the systemic toxicity of MTX and Fernandez *et al.* [8] reported no stomatitis or neutropenia in a group of 100 patients. However, with a single injection, the systemic toxicity is also very low when the intramuscular route is used. Single-dose MTX treatment was reported to be successful in 94% of cases [94]. If similar results are reported by other authors, then systemic treatment will appear valuable.

Severe tubal damage has been reported after intratubal treatment of an ectopic pregnancy that had a β-hCG level of 15 000 IU/litre [104]. In contrast, Pansky *et al.* [105] have reported an interesting patency rate after laparoscopic MTX intratubal injection. Finally, although non-surgical treatment appears to be a very attractive alternative, poor results reported by others should be noted. Indeed, because of the very poor results obtained in the MTX group, Mottla *et al.* [106] discontinued a prospective randomized study designed to compare laparoscopic salpingotomy and laparoscopic injection.

Indications

Non-surgical management is becoming the standard for the treatment of interstitial and cervical pregnancies [107,108], as in such cases surgical treatment is often difficult and a conservative approach not always possible. An interstitial pregnancy should be injected using a vaginal approach. The ectopic gestational sac should be punctured through the myometrium whenever possible, thus minimizing the risk of bleeding induced by the puncture [108].

We choose between the non-surgical and the laparoscopic treatment of tubal ectopic pregnancies. The first rule is to confirm the diagnosis of ectopic pregnancy. Despite improvements in ultrasound, it may still be difficult to distinguish an early intrauterine pregnancy and an ectopic pregnancy. This question is even more important when deciding on non-surgical management, since MTX is an effective treatment of normal early intrauterine pregnancy! Non-surgical treatments are particularly useful in patients who are obese or have been previously operated many times. For instance, ectopic pregnancies after *in vitro* fertilization and embryo transfer are often diagnosed very early and are a very good indication of medical treatment in patients already operated on several times. In contrast, one may consider that in such cases it is essential to prevent recurrence and to perform laparoscopic salpingectomy.

The following criteria are required to propose ultrasound-guided treatment:
1 the ectopic gestational sac should be visible;
2 its diameter should be less than 3 cm;
3 the haemoperitoneum should be less than 100 ml;
4 the patient should be haemodynamically stable;
5 MTX treatment should be possible (normal platelet count, normal renal and liver function, normal coagulation tests);
6 β-hCG level should be less than 5000 mIU/ml;
7 there should be no cardiac activity in the ectopic sac. These last two criteria may be discussed, as some authors have reported successful treatment of very active ectopic pregnancies and recommend an intratubal injection only when ectopic cardiac activity can be identified [108]. However, from the results of Fernandez *et al.* [8] it appears that failure rates are much higher in patients with a β-hCG level > 5000 mIU/ml and in patients with ectopic cardiac activity (36% and 47% respectively). Therefore these criteria are probably reasonable contra-indications to ultrasound-guided treatment.

A pretherapeutic score has been proposed and used prospectively by Fernandez *et al.* [109] (Table 17.5). The success rate is 87% when the score is ≤ 12 and only 60% when it is > 12. A 60% success rate is satisfactory but not high enough for patients. Although this score may be difficult to use, as the progesterone assay is not available in all departments, the other clinical and biological criteria used in this scoring system should be considered before managing a patient.

Surgical treatment is used in the remaining cases. In experienced hands more than 98% of these patients are successfully treated by laparoscopy. The main question is to decide between salpingotomy and salpingectomy in order to preserve postoperative fertility and to prevent recurrences. In our department, a radical treatment was introduced several years after the conservative treatment so that we have been able to evaluate the limits and consequences of conservative treatment. The following conclusions can be proposed.

Table 17.5 Pretherapeutic score. (From Fernandez *et al.* [109], with permission.)

Score	1	2	3
Gestational age (weeks)	> 8	7–8	≤ 6
β-hCG level (mIU/ml)	< 1000	1000–5000	> 5000
Progesterone (ng/ml)	< 5	5–10	> 10
Pelvic pain	None	Induced	Spontaneous
Haematosalpinx (cm)	< 1	1–3	> 3
Haemoperitoneum (ml)	0	1–100	> 100

1 Except in the case of massive haemoperitoneum, most ectopic pregnancies can be treated conservatively whatever the diameter or the β-hCG level.
2 Fertility prognosis is not related to the diameter or location of the ectopic pregnancy, the volume of the haemoperitoneum or rupture of the tubal wall.
3 The indication for radical or conservative treatment should be decided according to the previous medical history and to the adhesions found at laparoscopy using a therapeutic score reported by Pouly *et al.* [5].
(a) score ≤ 4 perform salpingotomy;
(b) score = 5 perform salpingectomy;
(c) score ≥ 6 perform salpingectomy with a contralateral sterilization. Obviously this management may be used only if *in vitro* fertilization and embryo transfer is available.

References

1 Canis M, Mage G, Pouly JL, Wattiez A, Manhes H, Bruhat MA. Laparoscopic diagnosis of adnexal cystic masses: a 12 year experience with long term follow up. *Obstet Gynecol* 1994;**83**:707–712.
2 De Crespigny LC, Robinson HP, Davoren RAM, Fortune D. The 'simple' cyst: aspirate or operate. *Br J Obstet Gynaecol* 1989;**96**:1035–1039.
3 Kroon E, Andolf E. Diagnosis and follow up of simple ovarian cysts detected by ultrasound in postmenopausal women. *Obstet Gynecol* 1995;**85**:211–214.
4 Feichtinger W, Kemeter P. Conservative treatment of ectopic pregnancy by transvaginal aspiration under sonographic control and methotrexate injection. *Lancet* 1987;**i**:381.
5 Pouly JL, Chapron C, Mage G *et al.* Multifactorial analysis of fertility following conservative laparoscopic treatment of ectopic pregnancy in a series of 223 patients. *Fertil Steril* 1991;**56**:453–460.

6 Ménard A, Créquat J, Mandelbrot L, Hauuy J-P, Madelenat P. Treatment of unruptured tubal pregnancy by local injection of methotrexate under transvaginal sonographic control. *Fertil Steril* 1990;**54**:47–50.

7 Pansky M, Bukowsky I, Golan A *et al*. Local methotrexate injection: a non surgical treatment of ectopic pregnancy. *Am J Obstet Gynecol* 1989;**161**:393–396.

8 Fernandez H, Benifla JL, Lelaidier C, Baton C, Frydman R. Methotrexate treatment of ectopic pregnancy: 100 cases treated by primary transvaginal injection under sonographic control. *Fertil Steril* 1993;**59**:773–777.

9 Hart WR, Norris HJ. Borderline and malignant tumors of the ovary. Histologic criteria and clinical behaviour. *Cancer* 1973;**31**:1031–1045.

10 Katzenstein ALA, Mazur MT, Morgan TE, Kao MS. Proliferative serous tumors of the ovary. Histologic features and prognosis. *Am J Surg Pathol* 1978;**2**:339–355.

11 Colgan TJ, Norris HJ. Ovarian epithelial tumours of low malignant potential: a review. *Int J Gynecol Pathol* 1983;**1**:367–382.

12 Tasker M, Langley FA. The outlook for women with borderline epithelial tumours of the ovary. *Br J Obstet Gynaecol* 1985;**92**:969–973.

13 Kliman L, Rome RM, Fortune DW. Low malignant potential tumours of the ovary: a study of 76 cases. *Obstet Gynecol* 1986;**68**:338–344.

14 Hopkins MP, Kumar NB, Morley GW. An assessment of the pathologic features and treatment modalities in ovarian tumours of low malignant potential. *Obstet Gynecol* 1987;**70**:923–929.

15 Williams TJ, Symmonds RE, Litwak O. Management of unilateral and encapsulated ovarian cancer in young women. *Gynecol Oncol* 1973;**1**:143–148.

16 Webb MJ, Decker DG, Mussey E, Williams TJ. Factors influencing survival in stage I ovarian cancer. *Am J Obstet Gynecol* 1973;**116**:222–228.

17 Malkasian GD, Melton III LJ, O'Brien PC, Greene MII. Prognostic significance of histologic classification and grading of epithelial malignancies of the ovary. *Am J Obstet Gynecol* 1984;**149**:274–284.

18 Grogan RH. Accidental rupture of malignant ovarian cysts during surgical removal. *Obstet Gynecol* 1967;**30**: 716–720.

19 Einhorn N, Nilsson B, Sjovall K. Factors influencing survival in carcinoma of the ovary. Study of a well-defined Swedish population. *Cancer* 1985;**55**:2019–2025.

20 Sigurdsson K, Alm P, Gullberg B. Prognostic factors in malignant epithelial ovarian tumours. *Gynecol Oncol* 1983;**15**:370–380.

21 Sainz de la Cuesta R, Goff BA, Fuller AF, Nikrui N, Rice W. Prognostic significance of intraoperative rupture of malignant ovarian epithelial neoplasm. *Obstet Gynecol* 1994;**84**:1–7.

22 Petru E, Lahousen M, Tamussino K *et al*. Lymphadenectomy in stage I ovarian cancer. *Am J Obstet Gynecol* 1994;**170**:656–662.

23 Dembo AJ, Davy M, Stenwig AE, Berle EJ, Bush RS, Kjorstad K. Prognostic factors in patients with stage I epithelial ovarian cancer. *Obstet Gynecol* 1990;**75**:263–273.

24 Sevelda P, Vavra N, Schemper M, Salzer H. Prognostic factors for survival in stage I epithelial ovarian carcinoma. *Cancer* 1990;**65**:2349–2352.

25 Finn CB, Luesley DM, Buxton EJ *et al*. Is stage I epithelial ovarian cancer overtreated both surgically and systematically? Results of a five-year cancer registry review. *Br J Obstet Gynaecol* 1992;**99**:54–58.

26 Vergote IB, Kaern J, Abeler VM, Pettersen EO, De Vos LN, Trpé CG. Analysis of prognostic factors in stage I epithelial ovarian carcinoma: importance of degree of differentiation and desoxyribonucleic acid ploidy in predicting relapse. *Am J Obstet Gynecol* 1993;**160**:40–52.

27 Sjovall K, Nilsson B, Einhorn N. Prognostic incidence of intraoperative rupture of malignant ovarian tumour with immediate surgical treatment. In: Bruhat MA (ed) *Proceedings of the 1st European Congress on Gynecologic Endoscopy*. London: Blackwell, 1994:107–108.

28 Angstrom T, Kjellgren O, Bergman F. The cytologic diagnosis of ovarian tumors by means of aspiration biopsy. *Acta Cytol* 1972;**16**:336–341.

29 Diernaes E, Rasmussen J, Soerensen T, Hasch E. Ovarian cyst: management by puncture? *Lancet* 1987;**i**:1084.

30 Granberg S, Norstrom A, Wikland M. Comparison of intravaginal ultrasound and cytologic evaluation of cystic ovarian tumors. *J Ultrasound Med* 1991;**10**:9–14.

31 Gaetje R, Popp LW. Is differentiation of benign and malignant cystic adnexal masses possible by evaluation of cyst fluids with respect to colour, cytology, steroid hormones and tumour markers? *Acta Obstet Gynecol Scand* 1994;**73**:502–507.

32 Moran O, Menczer J, Ben-Barusch G, Lipitz S, Goor E. Cytologic examination of ovarian cyst fluid for the distinction between benign and malignant tumours. *Obstet Gynecol* 1993;**82**:444–446.

33 Andersen WA, Nichols GE, Avery SR, Taylor PT. Cytologic diagnosis of ovarian tumors: factors influencing accuracy in previously undiagnosed cases. *Am J Obstet Gynecol* 1995;**173**:457–464.

34 Maiman M, Seltzer V, Boyce J. Laparoscopic excision of ovarian neoplasms subsequently found to be malignant. *Obstet Gynecol* 1991;**77**:563–565.

35 Crouet H, Heron JF. Dissémination du cancer de l'ovaire lors de la chirurgie coelioscopique: un danger réel. *Presse Med* 1991;**20**:1738–1739.

36 Benifla JL, Hauuy JP, Guglielmina JN *et al.* Kystectomie percoelioscopique: découverte histologique fortuite d'un carcinome ovarien. Case report. *J Gynecol Obstet Biol Reprod* 1992;21:45–49.

37 Canis M, Mage G, Wattiez A *et al.* Tumor implantation after laparoscopy. In: Hunt RB (ed) *Endoscopy in gynecology AAGL 20th annual meeting proceedings.* 1993.

38 Trimbos JB, Haville NF. The case against aspirating ovarian cyst. *Cancer* 1993;72:828–831.

39 Blanc B, Nicoloso E, d'Ercole C, Cazenave JC, Boubli L. Hazards of systematic laparoscopic treatment of ovarian pathology. 2 cases. *Presse Med* 1993;22:1732–1734.

40 Hsiu JG, Given FT, Kemp GM. Tumour implantation after diagnostic laparoscopic biopsy of serous ovarian tumours of low malignant potential. *Obstet Gynecol* 1986;68 (Suppl):90S–93S.

41 Blanc B, Boubli L, D'Ercole C, Nicoloso E. Laparoscopic management of malignant ovarian cysts: a 78-case national survey. Part 1: pre-operative and laparoscopic evaluation. *Eur J Obstet Gynecol Reprod Biol* 1994;56:177–180.

42 Helawa ME, Krepart GV, Lotocki R. Staging laparotomy in early epithelial ovarian carcinoma. *Am J Obstet Gynecol* 1986;154:282–286.

43 Bonilla-Musoles F, Ballester MJ, Simon C, Serra V, Raga F. Is avoidance of surgery possible in patients with peri-menopausal ovarian tumors using transvaginal ultrasound and duplex colour doppler sonography? *J Ultrasound Med* 1993;12:33–39.

44 Dordoni D, Zaglio S, Zucca S, Favalli G. The role of sonographically guided aspiration in the clinical management of ovarian cysts. *J Ultrasound Med* 1993;12:27–31.

45 Mintz M, Bessis R, Brodaty C, Bez JP. Que deviennent les kystes para-utérins ponctionnés sous coelioscopie? Apport de l'échographie à propos d'une série de 618 cas. *Gynécologie* 1983;34:451–463.

46 Puls LE, Powell DE, Depriest PD *et al.* Transition from benign to malignant epithelium in mucinous and serous ovarian cystadenocarcinoma. *Gynecol Oncol* 1992;47:53–57.

47 Gallion HH, Powell DE, Morrow JK *et al.* Molecular genetic changes in human epithelial ovarian malignancies. *Gynecol Oncol* 1992;47:137–142.

48 Bourne TH, Whitehead MI, Campbell S, Royston P, Bhan V, Collins WP. Ultrasound screening for familial ovarian cancer. *Gynecol Oncol* 1991;43:92–97.

49 Canis M, Mage G, Wattiez A *et al.* Kystes de l'annexe: place de la coelioscopie en 1991. *Contracept Fertil Sex* 1992;20:345–352.

50 Canis M, Finkeltin F, Botchoreschvili R, Chapron C, Bruhat MA. Abdominal wall endometrioma after the laparoscopic treatment of an ovarian endometrioma. Case report. *Gynecol Endosc* (in press).

51 Cheng KK. An experimental study of mucocele of the appendix and pseudomyxoma peritonei. *J Pathol Bacteriol* 1949;61:217–225.

52 Cariker M, Dockerty M. Mucinous cystadenomas and mucinous cystadenocarcinomas of the ovary. A clinical and pathological study of 355 cases. *Cancer* 1954;7:302–306.

53 Woodruff JD, Bie LS, Sherman RJ. Mucinous tumours of the ovary. *Obstet Gynecol* 1960;16:699–712.

54 Limber GK, King RE, Silverberg SG. Pseudomyxoma peritonaei: a report of ten cases. *Ann Surg* 1973;178: 587–593.

55 Michael H, Sutton G, Roth LM. Ovarian carcinoma with extracellular mucin production: reassessment of 'pseudomyxoma ovarii et peritonei'. *Int J Gynecol Pathol* 1987;6:298–312.

56 Scully RE. Common epithelial tumours of borderline malignancy (carcinoma of low malignant potential). *Bull Cancer* 1982;69:228–231.

57 Nezhat F, Nezhat C, Welander CE, Benigno B. Four ovarian cancers diagnosed during laparoscopic management of 1011 women with adnexal masses. *Am J Obstet Gynecol* 1992;167:790–796.

58 Hauuy JP, Madelenat P, Bouquet de la Jolinière J, Dubuisson JB. Chirurgie per coelioscopique des kystes ovariens indications et limites à propos d'une série de 169 kystes. *J Gynecol Obstet Biol Reprod* 1990;19:209–216.

59 Wolf SI, Gosink BB, Feldesman M *et al.* Prevalence of simple adnexal cysts in postmenopausal women. *Radiology* 1991;180:65–71.

60 Goldstein SR, Subramanyam B, Snyder JR, Beller U, Raghavendra N, Beckman M. The postmenopausal cystic adnexal mass: the potential role of ultrasound in conservative management. *Obstet Gynecol* 1989;73:8–10.

61 Granberg S, Wikland M, Jansson I. Macroscopic characterization of ovarian tumours and the relation to the histological diagnosis: criteria to be used for ultrasound evaluation. *Gynecol Oncol* 1989;35:139–144.

62 Herrmann UJ, Locher GW, Goldhirsch A. Sonographic patterns of ovarian tumours: prediction of malignancy. *Obstet Gynecol* 1987;69:777–781.

63 Bourne TH. Transvaginal colour Doppler in gynecology. *Ultrasound Obstet Gynecol* 1991;1:359–373.

64 Eriksson L, Kjellgren O, Von Scholtz R. Functional cyst or ovarian cancer: histopathological findings during one year of surgery. *Gynecol Obstet Invest* 1989;19:155–159.

65 Potier A. Echographie et kystes de l'ovaire. Semeiologie–Doppler–Ponction echoguidée. *Contracept Fertil Sex* 1992;20:553–559.

66 Audra P, Dargent D, Akiki S, Lasne Y, Malvolti B, Rebaud A. Ponctio echoguidée des kystes de l'ovaire possibilités et limites. *Rev Fr Gynecol Obstet* 1991;86:672–675.

67 Caspi B, Zalel Y, Lurie S, Elchal U, Katz Z. Ultrasound-guided aspiration for relief of pain generated by simple ovarian cysts. *Gynecol Obstet Invest* 1993;35:121–122.

68 Ron el R, Herman A, Weinraub Z et al. Clear ovarian cyst aspiration guided by vaginal ultrasonography. *Eur J Obstet Gynecol Biol Reprod* 1991;42:43–47.

69 Timor-Tritsch IE, Lerner JP, Monteagudo A, Santos R. Transvaginal ultrasonographic characterization of ovarian masses by means of color flow-directed doppler measurements and a morphologic scoring system. *Am J Obstet Gynecol* 1993;168:909–913.

70 Schneider VL, Schneider A, Reed KL, Hatch KD. Comparison of doppler with two dimensional sonography and CA 25 for prediction of malignancy of pelvic masses. *Obstet Gynecol* 1993;81:983–988.

71 Weiner Z, Thaler I, Beck D, Rottem S, Deutsch M, Brandes JM. Differentiating malignant from benign ovarian tumors with transvaginal color flow imaging. *Obstet Gynecol* 1992;72:159–162.

72 Kawai M, Kikkawa F, Ishikawa H et al. Differential diagnosis of ovarian tumors by transvaginal color-pulse doppler sonography. *Gynecol Oncol* 1994;54:209–214.

73 Finkler NJ, Benacerraf B, Lavin PT, Wojciechowski C, Knapp RC. Comparison of CA 125, clinical impression and ultrasound in the preoperative evaluation of ovarian masses. *Obstet Gynecol* 1988;72:659–664.

74 Yedema KA, von Mensdorff-Pouilly S, Kenemans P, Verheijen RHM, Bon BG, Hilgers J. Update on the serum tumor marker CA 125. In: Bruhat MA (ed) *Ovarian Cysts*. Blackwell, 1994.

75 Malkasian GD, Knapp RC, Latvin PT et al. Preoperative evaluation of serum CA 125 levels in premenopausal and postmenopausal patients with pelvic masses: discrimination of benign from malignant disease. *Am J Obstet Gynecol* 1988;159:341–346.

76 Menczer J, Ben-Barauch G, Moran O, Lipitz S. Cyst fluid CA 125 levels in ovarian epithelial neoplasm. *Obstet Gynecol* 1993;81:25–28.

77 Dargent D, Lasne JY, Akiki S. Diagnostic de la nature des kystes de l'ovaire par le dosage dans le liquide kystique et dans le sang des stéroides et des marqueurs tumoraux. *Contracept Fertil Sex* 1990;18:1011–1016.

78 Dargent D, Audra PH, Forget E. Marqueurs intrakystiques. Abstract presented at the 3rd GEOGEM meeting in Paris, 18 December 1993.

79 Abeille JP, Moing MH, Legros R, Scholler R, Castagner M, Nahoul K. Le corps jaune kystique. Un aspect coelioscopique particulier de la pathologie fonctionelle ovarienne. *Rev Fr Gynecol Obstet* 1978;73:19–27.

80 Andolf E, Casslen B, Jorgensen C, Buchhave P, Lecander I. Fluid characteristics of benign ovarian cysts: correlation with recurrence after puncture. *Obstet Gynecol* 1995;86:529–535.

81 De Brux J, Mintz M. History, technique and results of the cytopuncture of parauterine cysts. In: Bruhat MA (ed) *The Management of Adnexal Cysts*. Oxford: Blackwell Scientific Publications, 1994:36–37.

82 Donnez J, Nisolle M, Gillerot S, Anaf V, Clerckx-Braun F, Casanas-Roux F. Ovarian endometrial cysts: the role of gonadotropin-releasing hormone agonist and/or drainage. *Fertil Steril* 1994;62:63–66.

83 Zanetta G, Lissoni A, Dalla Valle C, Trio D, Pitelli M, Rangoni G. Ultrasound guided aspiration of endometriomas: possible applications and limitation. *Fertil Steril* 1995;64:709–713.

84 Lipitz S, Seidman DS, Schiff E, Achiron R, Menczer J. Treatment of pelvic peritoneal cysts by drainage and ethanol instillation. *Obstet Gynecol* 1995;86:297–299.

85 Cole T, Corlett RC. Chronic ectopic pregnancy. *Obstet Gynecol* 1982;59:63–65.

86 Bateman BG, Nunley WC, Kolp LA, Kitchin JD, Felder R. Vaginal sonography findings and hCG dynamics of early intra-uterine and tubal pregnancies. *Obstet Gynecol* 1990;75:421–427.

87 Chambers SE, Muir BB, Haddad NG. Ultrasound evaluation of ectopic pregnancy including correlation with human chorionic gonadotrophin levels. *Br J Radiol* 1990;63:246–250.

88 Ransom MX, Garcia AJ, Bohrer M, Corsan GH, Kemmann E. Serum progesterone as a predictor of success in the treatment of ectopic pregnancy. *Obstet Gynecol* 1994;83:1033–1037.

89 Timor-Tritsch IE, Yeh MN, Peisner DB, Lesser KB, Slavik TA. The use of transvaginal ultrasonography in the diagnosis of ectopic pregnancy. *Am J Obstet Gynecol* 1989;161:157–161.

90 Bruhat MA, Manhés H, Choukroun J, Suzanne F. Essai de traitement per coelioscopique de la grossesse extra-utérine à propos de 26 observations. *Rev Fr Gynecol Obstet* 1977;72:667–669.

91 Bruhat MA, Manhés H, Mage G, Pouly JL. Treatment of ectopic pregnancy by means of laparoscopy. *Fertil Steril* 1980;33:411–414.

92 Stovall TG. Medical management of ectopic pregnancy. *Curr Opin Obstet Gynecol* 1994;6:510–515.

93 Stovall TG, Ling FW, Gray LA, Carson SA, Buster JE. Methotrexate treatment of unruptured ectopic pregnancy: a report of 100 cases. *Obstet Gynecol* 1991;77:749–753.

94 Stovall TG, Ling FW. Single dose methotrexate: an expanded clinical trial. *Am J Obstet Gynecol* 1993;168:1759–1765.

95 Ylöstalo P, Cacciatore B, Sjöberg J, Kääriäinen M,

Tenhunen A, Stenman U-H. Expectant management of ectopic pregnancy. *Obstet Gynecol* 1992;80:345–348.

96 Barnhart K, Mennuti MT, Benjamin I, Jacobson S, Goodman D, Coutifaris C. Prompt diagnosis of ectopic pregnancy in an emergency department setting. *Obstet Gynecol* 1994;84:1010–1015.

97 Darai E, Benifla JL, Naouri M *et al*. Methotrexate treatment of ectopic pregnancy by intratubal injection under echoguidance, report of a 100 cases series. (in press)

98 Egarter CH, Husslein P. Treatment of tubal pregnancy by prostaglandins. *Lancet* 1988;i:1104–1105.

99 Paris FX, Henry-Suchet J, Tesquier L, Loysel T, Loffredo V, Pez JP. Le traitement médical des grossesses extra-utérines par le RU 486. *Presse Med* 1984;13:1219–1225.

100 Pouly JL, Chapron C, Mage G *et al*. The drop in the level of hCG after conservative laparoscopic treatment of ectopic pregnancy. *J Gynecol Surg* 1991;7:211–217.

101 Lindblom B. Prediction of persistent ectopic pregnancy after laparoscopic salpingostomy. *Obstet Gynecol* 1994;84:798–802.

102 Dubuisson JB, Aubriot FX, Cardone V. Laparoscopic salpingectomy for tubal pregnancy. *Fertil Steril* 1987;47:225–228.

103 Dubuisson JB, Aubriot FX, Foulot H, Bruel D, Bouquet de Joliniére J, Mandelbrot L. Reproductive outcome after laparoscopic salpingectomy for tubal pregnancy. *Fertil Steril* 1990;53:1004–1007.

104 Klinkert J, Geldorp HJ, Chadha-Ajwani S, Huikeshoven FJM. Tubal damage after intratubal methotrexate treatment. *Fertil Steril* 1993;59:926–927.

105 Pansky M, Bukovskuy I, Golan A *et al*. Tubal patency after local methotrexate injection for tubal pregnancy. *Lancet* 1989;ii:967–968.

106 Mottla GL, Rulin MC, Guzick DS. Lack of resolution of ectopic pregnancy by intratubal injection of methotrexate. *Fertil Steril* 1992;57:685–687.

107 Timor-Tritsch IE, Monteagudo A, Madeville EO, Peisner DB, Parra Anaya G, Pirrone C. Successful management of viable cervical pregnancy by local injection of methotrexate guided by transvaginal ultrasonography. *Am J Obstet Gynecol* 1994;174:737–739.

108 Timor-Tritsch IE, Monteagudo A, Matera C, Veit CR. Sonographic evolution of cornual pregnancies treated without surgery. *Obstet Gynecol* 1992;79:1044–1049.

109 Fernandez H, Lelaidier C, Thouvenez V, Frydman R. The use of a pretherapeutic, predictive score to determine inclusion criteria for the non surgical treatment of ectopic pregnancy. *Hum Reprod* 1991;6:995–998.

Chapter 18/Pelvic masses and other interventional targets

LOTHAR W. POPP and REGINE GAETJE

Diagnosis and management of pelvic masses

Our obstetrical–gynaecological diagnoses are based, however, to a very large extent on impressions, which are, unaccessible to our eyes, exclusively mediated by palpation. A striking symbol of gynaecological diagnosis is the eye in the palpating finger. Our finger shall palpate in such sensitive manner, that the sensation shall come as close as possible to the sharpness of a visual impression [1].

Today, improvement in gynaecological diagnosis can be expected from vaginal ultrasound examination (vaginosonography) [2]. Even by using abdominal ultrasound, Andolf and Joergensen [3] found higher sensitivities for the detection of pelvic masses compared with bimanual palpation.

Vaginosonography vs. bimanual palpation in the detection of pelvic masses

The accuracy of measuring pelvic masses by vaginosonography is superior to estimation of the size of a lesion by palpation [4]. Also, the potential of vaginosonography for detecting adnexal masses is superior to that of bimanual palpation. In a multicentre prospective study, sensitivity for detecting pelvic masses by palpation was 37.6%, by vaginosonography 64.7% and by the combination of both methods 77.7% [5].

The 'normal palpation finding' requires confirmation by vaginosonography

Detection rates of adnexal masses smaller than 3 cm in diameter have been reported to be 15% by palpation compared with 97% by vaginosonography. The respective rates for masses between 3 and 5 cm in diameter were 37% vs. 96%, and for masses larger than 5 cm in diameter 51% vs. 94% (Table 18.1). As bimanual palpation frequently misses pelvic masses, including the early stages of ovarian carcinoma, the necessity of routinely checking the 'normal palpation status' by vaginosonography has been emphasized. It was also recommended that vaginosonography be routinely applied in annual preventive care examinations. It has been proposed that conventional examination together with vaginosonography be performed in one procedure and that a single-purpose vaginosonographic apparatus be installed to the right or left side of the examination couch in order to have vaginosonography available for each patient examination [5].

'Sonographic criteria of malignancy' do not exist

An analysis of vaginosonographic criteria of adnexal masses revealed disappointing results. None of the 45 criteria used was exclusively found in benign or malignant lesions (Table 18.2). The combination of three criteria (anechoic lesion, no septations and sharp outer delineation) was found in 43 of 135 benign and in 1 of 13 malignant adnexal masses. It was therefore concluded that the term 'sonographic criteria of malignancy' should be avoided [5].

Conventional management of adnexal masses

In 1991 Lehman-Willenbrock et al. [6] reported the histological examination of 1016 ovarian cysts, extirpated by laparoscopy or laparotomy; 52.3% were functional cysts or simple serous cysts and only 3.5% were malignant. The morbidity and even risk of mortality of conventional interventions, which in retrospect are unnecessary in the majority of cases, raises doubts about their beneficial role in the management of adnexal masses.

Table 18.1 Detection rates of pathological adnexal findings of different sizes: bimanual palpation vs. vaginosonography.

Preoperative estimation of size (diameter)	Detection rates of adnexal findings (correct predictions only)	
	Bimanual palpation	Vaginosonography
< 3 cm (*n* = 39)	6 (15)	38 (97)
3–5 cm (*n* = 78)	29 (37)	75 (96)
> 5 cm (*n* = 53)	27 (51)	50 (94)

Numbers in parentheses are percentages.

Modern management of 'novel adnexal findings'

There is still some uncertainty about how to draw the appropriate clinical conclusions from 'novel vaginosonographic findings'. Malignant pelvic tumours should become treatable at an earlier stage and over-treatment of non-malignant lesions should be avoided. In Table 18.3 feasible management of adnexal findings is proposed on the basis of the conventional diagnosis, which represents clinical suspicion of the histological diagnosis and, additionally, the novel vaginosonographic information [5].

If all clinical findings, including vaginosonography,

Vaginosonographic criteria	Relative occurrence (%)	
	Benign findings (*n* = 146)	Malignant findings (*n* = 13)
Outer delineation of the tumour		
Smooth	64	31
Irregular	27	69
Internal echo patterns of the tumour		
Homogeneous distribution	83	69
Inhomogeneous distribution	17	31
No internal echoes	44	24
Internal echoes present	56	77
No septations	86	83
Several chambers	14	17
Dorsal ultrasound enhancement	53	54
Echo qualities		
Intensity of the echoes		
Strong	17	15
Medium	30	23
Weak	53	62
Size of the echoes		
Fine	54	54
Medium	28	31
Coarse	19	15
Density of the echoes		
Scattered	45	39
Medium	27	15
Dense	29	46
Distribution of the echoes		
Regular	46	46
Irregular	54	54

Table 18.2 Relative occurrence of selected vaginosonographic criteria in benign and malignant adnexal tumours.

Table 18.3 Modern management of adnexal findings.

Clinical diagnosis	Management
Normal finding	Annual control examinations
No-change finding	Control examinations every 3 months for 1 year; after that annually
Functional cyst	Control examination after 6–8 weeks; in case of persistence consider laparoscopic diagnosis and therapy
Functional cyst associated with pain or recurrent functional cyst	Consider vaginosonographically guided puncture and evacuation; control examination after 6–8 weeks
Inflammatory lesion	Treat as conservatively as possible
Pelvic abscess	Consider vaginosonographically guided puncture and drainage
Benign tumour	Consider laparoscopic removal
Malignant tumour	Consider diagnostic laparoscopy: 1 in case of laparoscopic suspicion of benign tumour: laparoscopic therapy 2 in case of laparoscopic suspicion of malignant tumour: immediate laparotomy
Recurrent malignoma, metastasis or residual malignoma	Consider vaginosonographically guided sampling and vaginosonographically guided interstitial brachytherapy
Cystic tumour in an anaesthesiologically inoperable patient	Consider palliative vaginosonographically guided puncture and evacuation

reveal a normal adnexal status, annual control examinations may be recommended. However, precise criteria of what is 'normal' in the adnexa are not clearly defined so far. In future, it will be also necessary to define 'harmless no-change findings', which are slightly different from normal findings, e.g. a 2-cm anechoic ovarian cyst in a 70-year-old woman. If several 3-monthly control examinations reveal a no-change status, this type of finding may not require interventional verification and annual control examinations may be adequate.

Pelvic findings that are suspicious of functional or inflammatory lesions should be treated as conservatively as possible. Only functional cysts associated with pain, recurrent functional cysts and pelvic abscesses may be an indication for vaginosonographically guided puncture and evacuation. Adnexal findings that appear clinically and vaginosonographically as benign neoplastic lesions may be removed laparoscopically by an experienced endoscopic surgeon. In cases of suspected malignant lesions, diagnostic laparoscopy may precede conventional surgical intervention in order to avoid unnecessary laparotomies in cases of laparoscopically verified benign lesions or in cases of inoperable malignant tumours. Suspected recurrent malignomas, metastases and residual malignomas can be sampled and subsequently treated by interstitial brachytherapy under ultrasound guidance. In anaesthesiologically inoperable patients, palliative puncture and evacuation of pelvic cysts may be considered.

Sonographically guided puncture of pelvic lesions

Puncture is the establishment of a temporary tubular connection between an intracorporeal target area and outside. Ultrasound targeting has tremendously improved the accuracy of puncture procedures and, consequently, widened the spectrum of indications. Using the tubular access as a route into the body, injections of fluids, e.g. drugs, implantations of irradiating seeds and temporary therapeutic procedures, e.g. afterloading irradiation, can be performed. In the other direction, intracorporeal fluids such as blood, ascites or cyst contents, cytological or histological specimens and specific structures like the cumulus oophorus within the oocyte can be removed from the appropriate target area. For some indications permanent devices such as drains can be implanted after puncture, e.g. for repeat flushing of abscesses. For pelvic puncture procedures the transabdominal or the transvaginal route can be used. According to pelvic topography, which is hidden behind the symphysis, the transvaginal access may have obvious advantages.

The transabdominal route

In 1972 Bang and Northeved [7] introduced sonographically guided transabdominal amniocentesis and in 1974 Hahnemann [8] used ultrasound guidance for transabdominal fine-needle sampling of chorionic villi. Today, sonographically guided placentocentesis, cordocentesis and fetal sampling, as well as injection procedures, are routinely applied in prenatal diagnosis.

Sonographically guided transabdominal 'needling' of pelvic masses was used in 1971 by Angstroem *et al.* [9] and later by Sevin *et al.* [10] for fine-needle aspiration cytology of pelvic masses. Today, fine-needle aspiration cytology using needles with an external diameter of less than 1 mm is accepted in the diagnosis of recurrent or metastatic malignant tumours of many organs. Due to the risk of needle tract or peritoneal seeding it was recommended by Pasieka & Thompson [11] to avoid fine-needle aspiration in curable tumours.

Low mortality rates (0.003%) and low rates of major (0.05%) as well as minor (0.49%) complications with abdominal fine-needle aspiration procedures were reported by Livraghi *et al.* [12]. The reported sensitivities for diagnosing malignant lesions cytologically range from 70 to 95% [9,10,13,14]. Missing the target by using 'blind' puncture procedures may be the most frequent reason for false-negative results [15]. Targeting fine-needle aspiration by ultrasound improves the predictive values of negative results and also minimizes the risk of injury to adjacent organs and of bleeding. The use of slightly wider needles allows tissue biopsy that has an expected higher diagnostic accuracy.

The transvaginal route

Vaginosonographically guided puncture techniques were developed in 1984 by Popp [16,17]. Figure 18.1 shows the first puncture experiments in a water-bath using rubber balloons as targets. A needle guide was attached to an experimental vaginosonographic probe (Bruel & Kjaer, Naerum, Denmark) for free-hand puncture and an electronic puncture line was established on the screen. Also, an automatic, spring-loaded puncture device for accurate, atraumatic and almost painless puncture was developed in cooperation with Labotect, Goettingen, Germany (Fig. 18.2). After successful experiments on fresh cadavers, vaginosonographically guided puncture and evacuation of ascites and ovarian cysts was performed.

It was astonishing, at that time, how close the probe's tip could be manoeuvred towards a target area in the true pelvis and how short the puncture depths

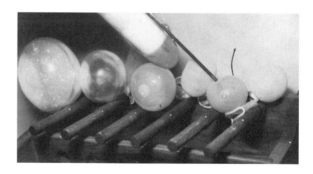

Fig. 18.1 The first vaginosonographically guided puncture experiments performed in a water-bath (1984).

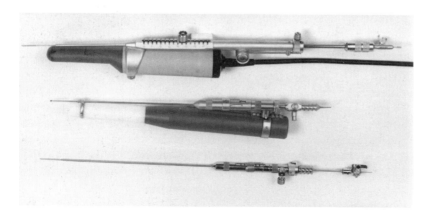

Fig. 18.2 The first spring-loaded automatic puncture devices (Labotect) (1984–87).

were. It became obvious that the vaginosonographic probe and the vaginally palpating finger were used in a similar manner: palpable pelvic findings are closely approachable by the vaginally palpating fingertip (otherwise they would not be palpable) and, correspondingly, the tip of the vaginosonographic probe can, under ultrasound vision, closely approach a sonographically identifiable pelvic finding. In January 1985 the first vaginosonographically guided follicular puncture for oocyte harvesting was done in our *in vitro* fertilization (IVF) programme (Fig. 18.3). This method spread all over the world within a few years and has today become the method of choice [16,17].

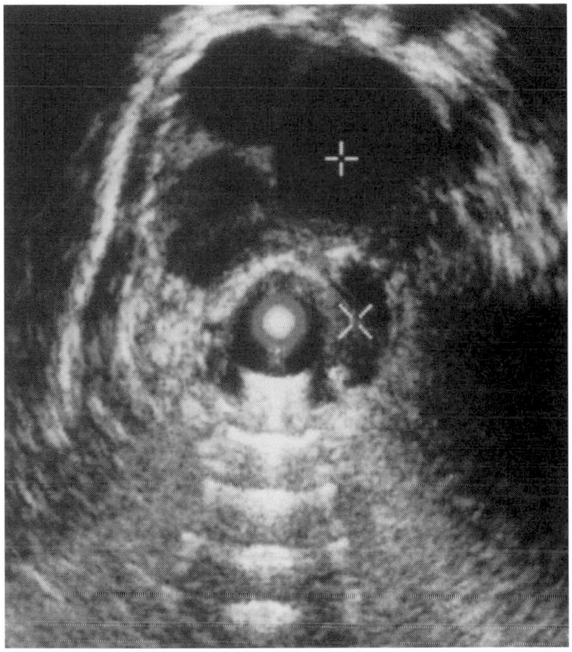

FREE-HAND VS. AUTOMATIC VAGINOSONOGRAPHICALLY GUIDED PUNCTURE

Most vaginosonographic probes are equipped with an attachable puncture device for free-hand puncture. It consists of a metal tube for guiding a needle along an electronic target line on the screen. After manoeuvring the target line into the region of interest, the examiner, who is holding the vaginosonographic probe with one hand, will push the needle forward into the target area with the other hand. By doing so, the needle tip will penetrate the vaginal wall and the parietal peritoneum and come to a stop in the target area. A sharp forward manoeuvre of the puncture needle is advantageous for hitting the target with a minimum of pain and for not pushing the organ of interest aside with the needle tip. However, even in experienced hands it is difficult to accurately coordinate needle speed and penetration depth with the forward needle movement into the target.

A spring-loaded automatic puncture device, which can be mounted on the vaginosonographic probe, provides presetting of the needle penetration depth and atraumatic high-speed puncture (Fig. 18.4). After having

Fig. 18.3 Vaginosonogram of a stimulated ovary with puncture marks for vaginosonographically guided follicular puncture (January 1985) (experimental vaginosonographic probe with a 270° panoramic sector, Bruel & Kjaer).

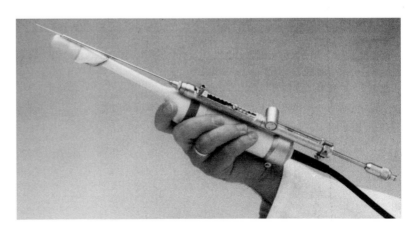

Fig. 18.4 Automatic puncture device (Labotect) mounted on a vaginosonographic probe (Siemens).

manoeuvred the target line into the target area and having measured and preset the appropriate puncture depth, automatic puncture is carried out by holding the vaginosonographic probe together with the puncture device steadily with two hands and triggering the needle-release mechanism [16].

Today, automatic puncture is the most accurate and atraumatic and also the least painful puncture

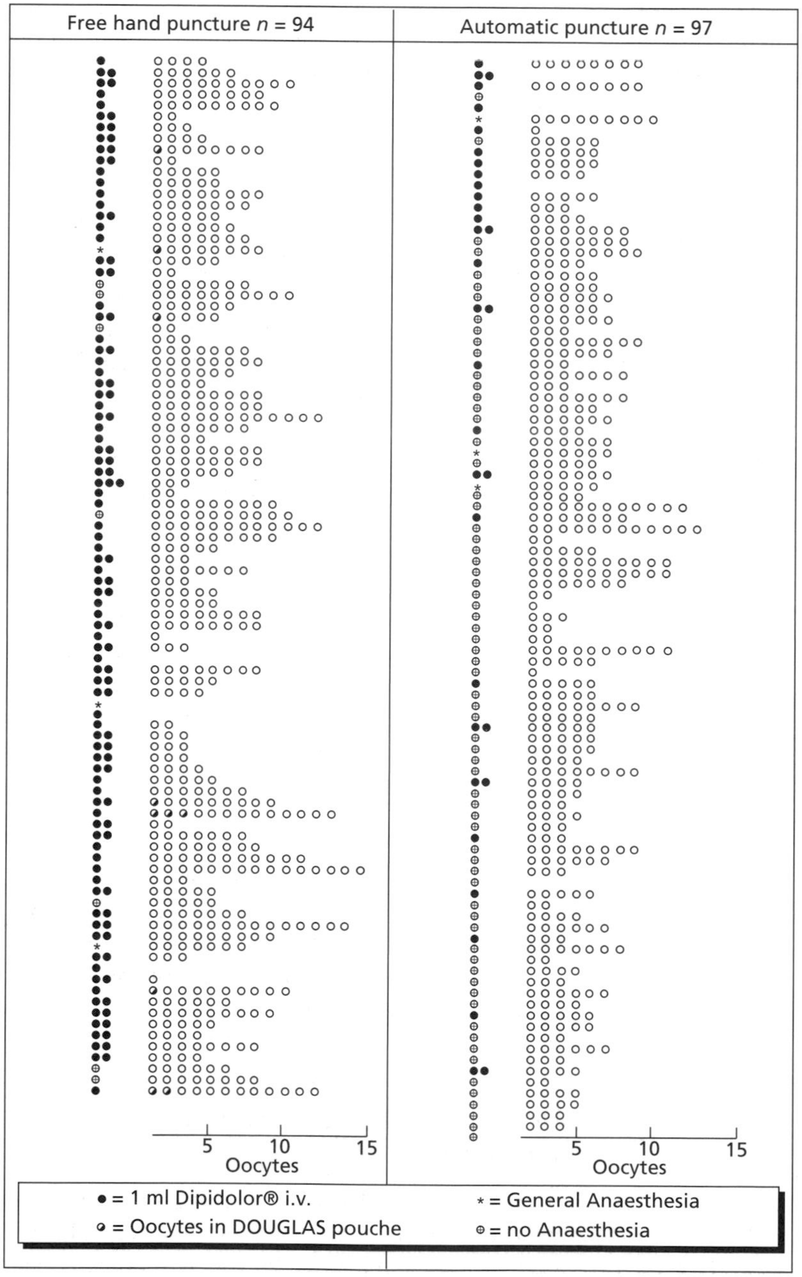

Fig. 18.5 Anaesthetic drugs used for free-hand vs. automatic follicular puncture for oocyte retrieval.

procedure. Figure 18.5 shows a comparison of the amount of anaesthetic drug used for free-hand vs. automatic follicular puncture for oocyte harvesting (Popp and Stein, unpublished data).

Evacuation of cystic adnexal masses

Evacuation of cyst fluid using vaginosonographically guided puncture is a safe, simple and almost painless method, which can be performed without anaesthesia on an outpatient basis. For removing the cyst fluid an evacuated drainage system, e.g. a Redon system, can be recommended.

Unfortunately, evaluation of cyst fluids has limited reliability in the differentiation of benign and malignant tumours. Only oestradiol levels above 1000 pg/ml may be indicative of functional cysts and carcinoembryonic antigen (CEA) levels above 10 ng/ml may be suspicious of benign as well as malignant mucinous lesions. For these reasons, vaginosonographically guided puncture and evacuation of cystic adnexal masses should be limited to suspected functional cysts associated with pain, recurrent functional cysts and palliative evacuation of cysts in anaesthesiologically inoperable patients (Table 18.3).

Evaluation of cyst fluids

COLOUR

Evaluation of 81 cyst fluids [18] from 74 benign, two borderline and five malignant cystic adnexal masses revealed the following results: water-like fluids were found in 10% of benign and in none of the malignant cysts; yellowish fluids were removed from 43% of benign and from two of five malignant cysts; bloody fluids were found in 22% of benign and in three of five malignant cysts; of 10 endometriomas six had chocolate-like, three bloody and one greenish contents.

CYTOLOGY

Well-preserved epithelial cells were found in the fluids of 5 of 74 benign cysts (7%). Three benign cystic teratomas were diagnosed by the presence of squamous cells. However, squamous cells can also originate from contamination of vaginal epithelial cells during vaginosonographically guided puncture. This phenomenon is well known from transvaginal follicular puncture for oocyte retrieval. One mucinous cystadenoma was cytologically suspected to be malignant, as epithelial cells in the cyst fluid showed pleomorphy.

Malignancy was cytologically diagnosed in two of five malignant cystic tumours. One malignant lesion was misdiagnosed as an endometrioid cyst and in the two remaining cases no epithelial cells were found in the cyst fluids. These poor results are in agreement with other reports [9,19,20].

STEROID HORMONES

Oestradiol, progesterone and testosterone levels were significantly higher in the fluids of lutein cysts and follicular cysts compared with other cystic lesions. Oestradiol levels may be the most suitable for a differential diagnosis (Fig. 18.6). A cut-off level of 1000 pg/ml, which was suggested by Ammann *et al.* [21], may be supported. Differentiation of benign and malignant ovarian blastomas by measuring steroid hormone concentrations in cyst fluids was not possible.

TUMOUR MARKERS

Fluids of non-mucinous benign cystic lesions had CEA levels below 10 ng/ml except for one endometrioid cyst with 36.2 ng/ml. CEA levels of cystic serous carcinomas ranged from 0.2 to 342 ng/ml. Elevated CEA levels, between 270 and 99 400 ng/ml, were found in the fluids of 10 benign mucinous tumours and one mucinous cystadenoma with a borderline lesion (Fig. 18.7). Therefore, CEA levels above 10 ng/ml may support the suspicion of a mucinous, a malignant and perhaps an endometrioid lesion. In contrast, the wide distributions of CA 125 (5–1 057 600 U/ml) and CA 153 levels (0.4–1700 U/ml) and a complete overlap of the levels in benign and malignant lesions did not allow for any prediction.

Vaginosonographically guided oocyte retrieval

Oocyte retrieval is the key for IVF and embryo transfer and other assisted reproduction techniques and is the most frequent indication for vaginosonographically

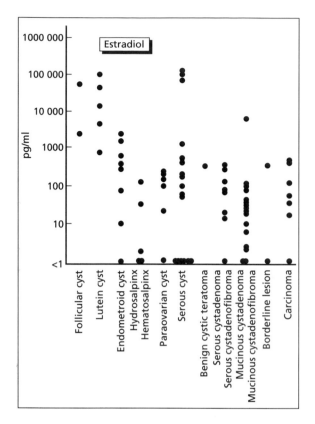

Fig. 18.6 Oestradiol levels in cyst fluids of adnexal masses.

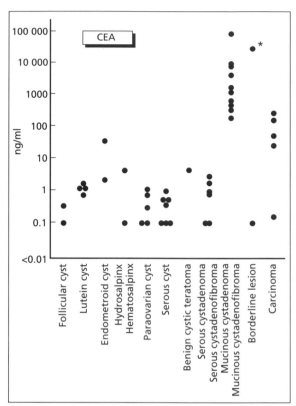

Fig. 18.7 Carcinoembryonic antigen levels in cyst fluids of adnexal masses.

guided puncture. Thin needles of about 1 mm outer diameter and an automatic puncture device are advantageous for puncture without anaesthesia. However, thick needles with a double channel or a wider lumen are mostly used because of their stiffness, which allows for multiple follicle puncture manoeuvres, 'lining the follicles up' within a stimulated ovary. This procedure is painful and traumatic, not only because of the larger needle diameter but also because of the extensive intra-ovarian injuries caused by the movements of the sharp needle tip. A thin needle, which is almost painlessly shot into each follicle, is the better alternative. For flushing the follicle, needles with a double Luer lock are equivalent to the double-channel needles [16].

As automatic follicular puncture using a thin needle is a safe and almost painless method (Fig. 18.5), thoroughly comparable to venous puncture for blood sampling, natural cycles and mildly stimulated cycles

should be considered more often for oocyte harvesting. By doing so in an appropriate case, costs of drugs and hormonal assays and complications such as ovarian hyperstimulation might be reduced. At the same time, this may give a sterile couple some relief from the desperate compulsion for the success of an expensive and troublesome stimulated cycle [22].

Evacuation of free fluid in the pouch of Douglas

Vaginosonographic detection of free fluid in the pouch of Douglas is easy, and vaginosonographically guided needle aspiration of the intra-abdominal fluid may be safer and more accurate than conventional 'blind' puncture. Echogenicity of the fluid may give a hint about serous, bloody or purulent liquids. Small amounts of fluid are frequently found and may be due to follicular rupture or retrograde menstruation. Rupture of larger cysts will result in larger amounts of free fluid in the pouch of Douglas.

Ascites may be removed safely and completely by vaginosonographically guided puncture, as the pouch of Douglas represents the deepest region of the abdominal cavity and, at the same time, the intestines are floating upwards in the intra-abdominal fluid.

Management of postoperative effusions

Vaginosonography is a simple and reliable tool for diagnosing postoperative intra-abdominal bleeding and should be one of the first diagnostic considerations. Vaginosonographic examination after hysterectomy is more reliable in detecting an effusion and estimating its size than vaginal or rectal palpation. It is therefore recommended that all patients be examined with the vaginal ultrasound probe 3–4 days after hysterectomy or other gynaecological operations.

Figure 18.8a shows a vaginosonogram of a normal right parametrial operation site 3 days after vaginal hysterectomy. In Fig. 18.8b postoperative parametrial effusion, which was punctured with a 2-mm diameter

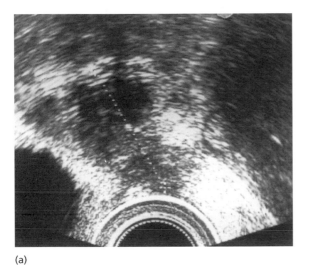

(a)

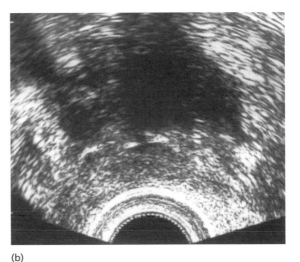

(b)

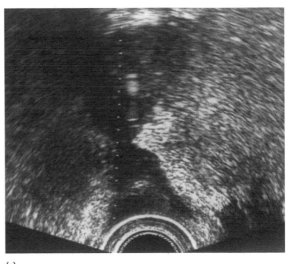

(c)

Fig. 18.8 Vaginosonograms after vaginal hysterectomy: (a) normal parametrial operation site 3 days after operation (marked is the longitudinal diameter of 3.5 cm); (b) parametrial effusion 3 days after operation; (c) vaginosonographically guided puncture of parametrial effusion 10 days after operation (note the electronic puncture line and the needle tip with echo field).

needle under vaginosonographic guidance (Fig. 18.8c) is seen. Such attempts for evacuating postoperative effusions may be unsuccessful, as the contents may not be sufficiently liquefied. Instillation of a few millilitres of physiological saline solution under ultrasound vision and subsequent aspiration may give a hint in these cases as to whether the contents are bloody, serous or putrid. For surgical drainage of postoperative effusions the vaginal route might be preferable and vaginosonographic diagnosis may indicate the most efficient site of vaginal incision.

Evacuation, drainage and flushing of pelvic abscesses

Sonographically guided puncture, evacuation and drainage of liquefied pelvic abscesses may be performed under general anaesthesia. In the literature, an 80–90% success rate has been reported for transabdominal [23,24] as well as for vaginosonographically guided catheter drainage and subsequent flushing for about 6 days [24–26]. We have used a suprapubic bladder drainage set for transvaginal abscess drainage, daily betadine flushing and systemic antibiotic therapy with good success (Fig. 18.9) [17].

Pelvic tissue biopsy

Myometrial biopsy

Many women suffer from myometrial diseases, which cause pain, bleeding and a variety of other symptoms. The basis of possible new modalities of diagnosis of adenomyosis uteri, myoma and leiomyosarcoma for example, might be myometrial biopsy [27] using an automatic cutting needle device. Morphological and immunohistochemical examination of myometrial samples may enable more specific ways of treatment. However, precise indications for myometrial biopsy still have to be defined.

TECHNIQUE AND RESULTS

For myometrial biopsy the spring-triggered Biopty device (Danimed) and Biopty-cut needles of 14 and 18 gauge were used. In fresh uterine specimens with and without adenomyosis uteri, sensitivity and specificity

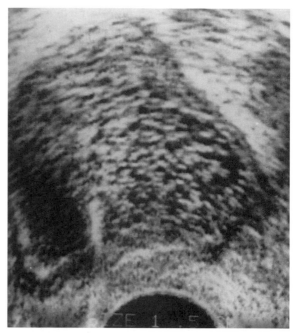

(a)

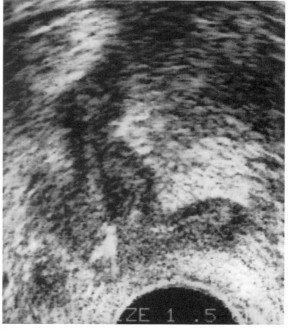

(b)

Fig. 18.9 Vaginosonographically guided puncture (a) and evacuation (b) of pelvic abscess.

for the detection of adenomyosis uteri was evaluated. When 10 samples were taken from a uterus, sensitivity ranged from 40 to 70%, depending on the the the grade of adenomyosis uteri. For one sample, the respective sensitivities ranged from 8 to 19%. For clinical application it is therefore proposed that several samples are obtained from one uterus. Specificity of the method was 100%.

In 34 patients, one to five myometrial biopsies were taken at laparoscopy using a 14-gauge needle. After removal of the puncture needle from the myometrium, bleeding occurred for more than 10-min observation time. Injection of 3–5 ml of an ornipressin solution (2.5 IU of POR 8, Sandoz, dissolved in 50 ml of physiological saline solution) around the puncture site was used to stop the bleeding. Bleeding was prevented in six further patients by injecting 2–3 ml of the ornipressin solution into the biopsy cannula after having removed the mandrin together with the specimen (Fig. 18.10).

Using the new, bloodless sampling method, 14 vaginosonographically guided myometrial sampling procedures were performed in six patients with suspected adenomyosis uteri. A Bruel and Kjaer 7-MHz vaginosonographic probe type 8538 with an attached puncture device type 0875 was used (Fig. 18.11). Repeat vaginosonographic examinations after biopsy did not show evidence of intra-abdominal bleeding. No adenomyotic foci were found in the specimens.

Prophylactic injection of ornipressin solution may also be used for Trucut biopsy of other organs known for bleeding after biopsy, e.g. the parametrium.

Chorionic villous sampling

Chorionic villous sampling under abdominal ultrasound guidance can be performed either transcervically using flexible instruments (catheters, forceps, brushes) or by

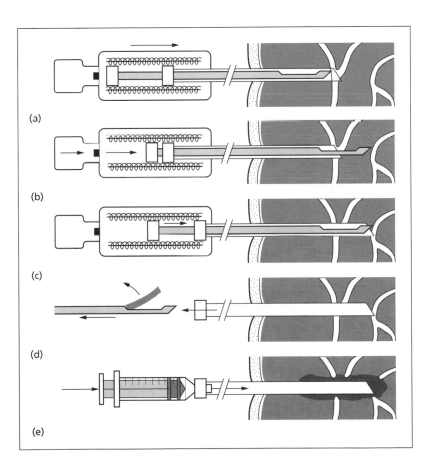

Fig. 18.10 Automatic Trucut biopsy with injection of ornipressin solution to prevent bleeding.

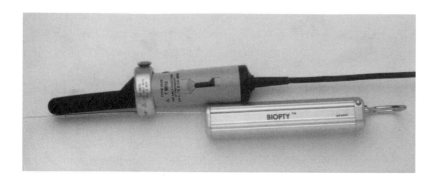

Fig. 18.11 Vaginosonographic
Trucut biopsy system.

transabdominal fine-needle aspiration. Vaginosonographically guided chorionic villous sampling was first done by Ghirardini and Popp in 1983 [28,29]. Even though vaginosonographically guided chorionic villous sampling has obvious advantages, the method did not catch on in a large way.

Preoperatively, all the different chorionic villous

Fig. 18.12 Vaginosonographically guided chorionic villous sampling: (a) schematic drawing; (b) vaginosonographic needle placement in the chorion frondosum at 8 postmenstrual weeks.

sampling procedures require a detailed vaginosonographic evaluation of the viability of the pregnancy and localization and sonomorphological structure of the chorion frondosum [28]. In most cases the electronic puncture line can be manoeuvred into the chorion frondosum area, parallel to the uterine wall. Consequently, vaginosonographic puncture can be carried out, taking the shortest possible puncture distance (Fig. 18.12).

Ovarian biopsy

Large ovarian tumours require operative treatment

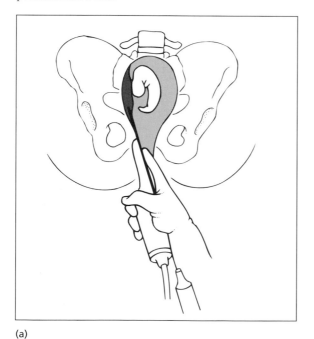

(a)

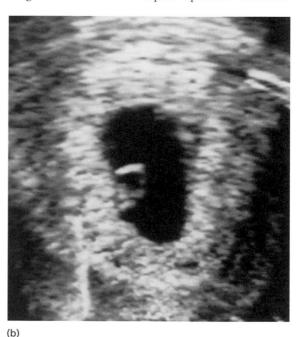

(b)

and preoperative biopsy may be unnecessary. Small tumours might be considered for vaginosonographically guided ovarian biopsy. However, it can be difficult to define the target area within the sonomorphological complexity of many ovarian tumours and high rates of false-negative results must be expected. Also, the risk of needle tract seeding in case of a malignant tumour is unknown. Therefore, criteria for ovarian biopsy still have to be defined.

Parametrial biopsy and biopsy of recurrent or metastatic pelvic tumours

For obtaining samples for histological evaluation from an infiltrated parametrium or a suspected recurrent or metastatic pelvic tumour, Trucut biopsy as described for myometrial biopsy may be recommended.

Injection procedures

Intrachorionic injection for ectopic pregnancy treatment

Vaginosonography allows for the detection of 62% of viable ectopic pregnancies during the seventh postmenstrual week (Fig. 18.13) [30]. With diameters of 1–2 cm at that time [30], chorionic cavities of viable ectopic pregnancies are convenient targets for vaginosonographically guided puncture, comparable to follicular puncture (Fig. 18.14). The automatic puncture technique is advisable, as the very mobile pregnant tube may escape from the needle tip when the needle speed is too slow.

Vaginosonographically guided intrachorionic injection of antitrophoblastic substances has been performed since 1987 [31] using methotrexate [32], potassium chloride [33], hyperosmolar glucose solution [34] and other substances. In a multicentre prospective study, 1 of 18 injected ectopic pregnancies required laparoscopic operation in spite of slightly decreasing serum β human chorionic gonadotrophin (β-hCG) levels. Decrease of serum β-hCG levels below 10 mIU/ml took a minimum of 1 week and a maximum of 9 weeks [35].

Fetal reduction

Multiple pregnancies may create the dilemma of aborting all embryos as against reducing the number of pregnancies to a singleton or a twin pregnancy. Reduction procedures are performed at about seven postmenstrual weeks by intrachorionic injection of potassium chloride solution [36] or by aspirating the chorionic fluid [37] under abdominal or vaginal ultrasound guidance. The use of an automatic puncture device is recommended [36].

Endometrial, or intracavitary embryo, or gamete implantation

Transmural intraendometrial embryo or gamete transfer was proposed by Popp in 1986 [22]. The embryo or the gametes should be implanted, preferably protected by an absorbable capsule, into the endometrium in the fundus area using a vaginosonographically guided puncture technique (Fig. 18.15). By doing so, the site of implantation would be chosen by the operator and flotation of the embryo within the uterine cavity and perhaps even loss of an embryo by cervical leakage would be avoided. *In vitro* experiments with transmural intraendometrial implantation were promising. However, the method was never practically used. Transmural intracavitary embryo transfer under vaginosonographic guidance was occasionally done in cases of an obstructed cervical canal.

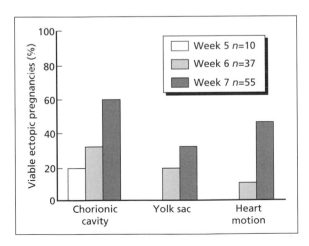

Fig. 18.13 Vaginosonographic detection rates of embryological structures in viable ectopic pregnancies.

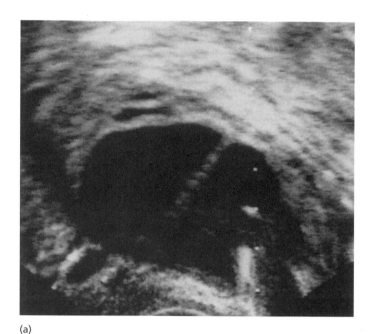

(a)

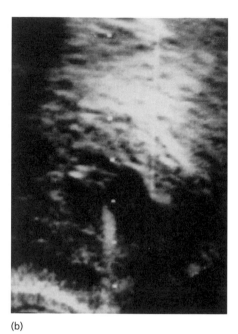

(b)

Fig. 18.14 Vaginosonograms of (a) follicular puncture for oocyte retrieval and (b) therapeutic intrachorionic injection of viable ectopic pregnancy at 7 postmenstrual weeks.

Interstitial brachytherapy

Brachytherapy plays an increasingly important role in the treatment of gynaecological malignancies. Recurrent, metastatic or residual tumours can be treated by interstitial brachytherapy using irradiating implants (seeds) or afterloading needles. They can be brought into position by abdominal, rectal or vaginal ultrasound guidance. Correct positioning is critical for the therapeutic distribution of the isodoses.

Hoetzinger [38] has used rectosonographic guidance for transvaginal positioning of afterloading needles, 2.2 mm in outer diameter, into recurrent pelvic tumours. In a 2-year follow-up, 5 of 32 patients were free of disease and 17 patients experienced a partial response.

Non-invasive, vaginosonographically guided hyperthermia treatment of ectopic pregnancy

In 1853 Bacchetti [39,40] reported on a non-invasive

treatment of ectopic pregnancy using electric current. His technique spread, with different modifications, to France and North America [41]. In 1993, Popp *et al.* [42] reported on successful experiments using a rabbit

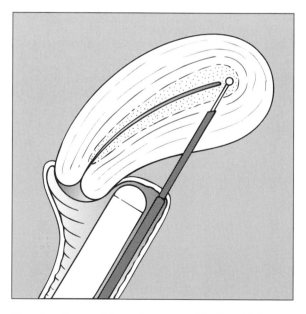

Fig. 18.15 Proposal for vaginosonographically guided endometrial embryo or gamete implantation.

model for induction of demise of pregnancy by the application of hyperthermia (42–45 °C). On this basis, non-invasive treatment of ectopic pregnancy in humans by vaginosonographically guided application of local hyperthermia was proposed (Fig. 18.16). This new therapeutic principle has not been clinically applied so far.

Outlook

Acceptance and further improvement of interventional ultrasound in the true pelvis has technical, practical and clinical aspects. Technical improvement is desirable with respect to:

1 appropriate design of the vaginosonographic probes, which should allow for puncture (free-hand and automatic) and other devices (e.g. for hyperthermia);

2 further refinement of automatic puncture devices, mainly for tissue biopsy; and

3 development of hyperthermic devices for vaginosonographic application.

The practical and clinical aspects are closely related: as vaginosonography in gynaecological examinations is more and more accepted, the demand for interventional vaginosonographic procedures will increase. The clinical applications aim to minimize the invasiveness of diagnostic and therapeutic procedures. They are, however, still under development or even in experimental stages. More clinical applications, e.g. vaginosonographically guided interruption of early pregnancy, and the application of other technological principles, e.g. vaginosonographically guided thermotherapy, may be expected in the near future. Their clinical acceptance is dependent on a variety of factors, not the least

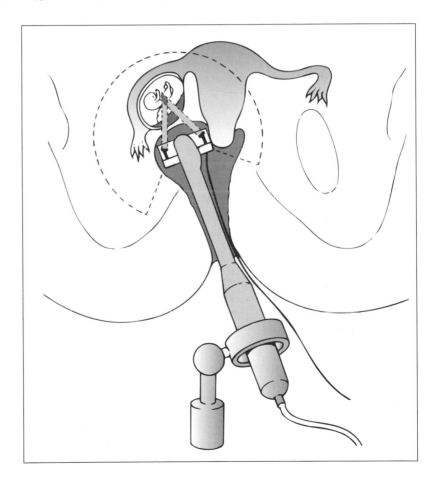

Fig. 18.16 Proposal for vaginosonographically guided local hyperthermia treatment of ectopic pregnancy.

of which is the psychological dimension. Common sense, inventiveness and a sure eye for simplification of procedures are necessary to meet patients' needs on the one hand and reasonable medical progress on the other.

References

1 Schultze B. Bildliche Darstellung des gynaekologischen Tastbefundes. *Dtsch Med Wochenschr* 1890;**16**:821–822.

2 Popp LW, Lucken RP, Mueller-Holve W, Lindemann HJ. Gynaekologische Endosonographie: Erste Erfahrungen. *Ultraschall* 1983;**4**:92–97.

3 Andolf E, Joergensen C. A prospective comparison of clinical ultrasound and operative examination of the female pelvis. *J Ultrasound Med* 1988;**7**:617–620.

4 Popp LW, Gaetje R, Stoyanov M. Accuracy of bimanual palpation versus vaginosonography in determination of the measurements of pelvic tumours. *Arch Gynecol Obstet* 1993;**252**:197–202.

5 Popp LW, Gaetje R. Die Rolle der Vaginosonographie bei der gynaekologischen Untersuchung. *Frauenarzt* 1994;**35**: 819–826.

6 Lehmann-Willenbrock E, Mecke H, Semm K. Pelviskopische Ovarialchirurgie: eine retrospektive Untersuchung von 1016 operierten Zysten. *Geburtshilfe Frauenheilkd* 1991;**51**: 280–287.

7 Bang J, Northeved A. A new ultrasonic method for transabdominal amniocentesis. *Am J Obstet Gynecol* 1972;**114**:599–601.

8 Hahnemann N. Early prenatal diagnosis: a study of biopsy technique and cell culturing from extraembryonic membranes. *Clin Genet* 1974;**6**:294.

9 Angstroem T, Kjellgren O, Berbman F. The cytologic diagnosis of ovarian tumours by means of aspiration biopsy. *Acta Cytol* 1972;**26**:336–341.

10 Sevin BU, Greening SE, Nadji M, Ng ABG, Averette HE, Staffan SRB. Fine needle aspiration cytology in gynecologic oncology. *Acta Cytol* 1979;**23**:277–281.

11 Pasieka JL, Thompson NW. Fine-needle aspiration biopsy causing seeding of a carcinoid tumour. *Arch Surg* 1992;**127**: 1248–1251.

12 Livraghi T, Damascelli B, Lombardi C, Spangnoli I. Risk in fine-needle abdominal biopsy. *J Clin Ultrasound* 1983;**11**:77–81.

13 Nash JD, Burke TW, Woodward JE, Hall KL, Weiser ER, Heller PB. Diagnosis of recurrent gynecological malignancy with fine-needle aspiration cytology. *Obstet Gynecol* 1988;**71**:333–337.

14 Imachi M, Tsukamoto N, Shigematsu T, Saito T, Kamura T, Nakano H. Fine needle aspiration cytology in patients with gynecologic malignancies. *Gynecol Oncol* 1992;**46**: 309–312.

15 Sevin BU, Saks M, Nadji M. Feinnadelaspiration in der gynaekologischen Onkologie. *Gynaekologe* 1986;**19**: 116.

16 Popp LW. Vaginosonographisch gezielte Punktion (1). *Gynaekol Prax* 1989;**13**:695–708.

17 Popp, LW. Vaginosonographisch gezielte Punktion (2). *Gynaekol Prax* 1990;**14**:79–87.

18 Gaetje R, Popp LW. Is differential diagnosis of cystic adnexal masses possible by evaluation of cytology, steroid hormones, and tumour markers in cyst fluid? *Acta Obstet Gynecol Scand* 1994;**73**:502–507.

19 Dienares E, Rasmussen J, Soerensen T, Hasch E. Ovarian cysts: management by puncture. *Lancet* 1987;**i**:1084.

20 Stanley MW, Horwitz CA, Frable WJ. Cellular follicular cyst of the ovary: fluid cytology mimicking malignancy. *Diagn Cytopathol* 1991;**7**:48–52.

21 Ammann M, Haenggi W, Baumann U, Keller PJ. Differentialdiagnostik zystischer Ovarialtumoren durch Bestimmung von Oestradiol im Zystenpunktat. *Geburtshilfe Frauenheilkd* 1991;**51**:481–483.

22 Popp LW. Moeglichkeiten der vaginosonographisch gezielten Punktion in einem In-vitro Fertilisationsprogramm. In: Popp LW (ed) *Gynaekologische Endosonographie.* Quickborn: Ingo Klemke Verlag, 1986:153–162.

23 Shulman A, Maymon R, Shapiro A, Bahary C. Percutaneous catheter drainage of tubo-ovarian abscesses. *Obstet Gynecol* 1992;**80**:555–557.

24 Casola G, van Sonnenberg E, d'Agostino HB, Harker CP, Varney RR, Tavior B. Percutaneous drainage of tubo-ovarian abscesses. *Radiology* 1992;**182**:399–402.

25 van Sonnenberg E, d'Agostino HB, Casola G, Goodacre BW, Sanchez RB, Tavior B. US-guided transvaginal drainage of pelvic abscesses and fluid collections. *Radiology* 1991;**181**:53–56.

26 van der Kolk HL. Small, deep pelvic abscesses: definition and drainage guided with an endovaginal probe. *Radiology* 1991;**181**:283–284.

27 Popp LW, Schwiedessen JP, Gaetje R. Myometrial biopsy in the diagnosis of adenomyosis uteri. *Am J Obstet Gynecol* 1993;**169**:546–549.

28 Ghirardini G, Popp LW, Gualerzi C, Spreafico L, Fochi F, Agnelli P. Chorionskopische und vaginosonographisch gezielte Trophoblastbiopsie. In: Popp LW (ed) *Gynaekologische Endosonographie.* Quickborn: Ingo Klemke Verlag, 1986:133–141.

29 Popp LW, Ghirardini G. The role of transvaginal sonography in chorionic villi sampling. *J Clin Ultrasound* 1990;**18**:315–322.

30 Popp LW, Colditz A, Gaetje R. Diagnosis of intrauterine and ectopic pregnancy at 5–7 postmenstrual weeks. *Int J Obstet Gynecol* 1993;**44**:33–38.

31 Feichtinger W, Kemeter P. Conservative treatment of ectopic pregnancy by transvaginal aspiration under sonographic

control and methotrexate injection. *Lancet* 1987:381–382.

32 Popp LW, Mettler L, Weisner D, Mecke H, Freys I, Semm K. Ectopic pregnancy treatment using pelviscopic or vaginosonographically-guided intrachorionic injection of methotrexate and POR 8. *Ultrasound Obstet Gynecol* 1991;1:136–143.

33 Timor-Tritsch IE, Baxi L, Peisner DB. Transvaginal salpingocentesis: a new technique for treating ectopic pregnancy. *Am J Obstet Gynecol* 1989;160:459–461.

34 Lang PF, Tamussino K, Hoenigl W, Ralph G. Treatment of unruptured tubal pregnancy by laparoscopic instillation of hyperosmolar glucose solution. *Am J Obstet Gynecol* 1992;166:1378.

35 Popp LW, Colditz A, Gaetje R. Management of early ectopic pregnancy. *Int J Gynecol Obstet* 1994;44:239–244.

36 Timor-Tritsch IE, Peisner DB, Monteagudo A. Puncture procedures utilizing transvaginal ultrasonic guidance. *Ultrasound Obstet Gynecol* 1991;1:144–150.

37 Itskovitz J, Boldes R, Thaler I, Bronstein M, Erlik Y, Brandes JM. Transvaginal ultrasonography-guided aspiration of gestational sacs for selective abortion in multiple pregnancy.

Am J Obstet Gynecol 1989;160:215–217.

38 Hoetzinger H. Endosonography in gynecology: hysterosonography, rectosonography, vaginosonography: comparison with CT and MRI, applications with radiotherapy. In: Feifel G, Hildebrandt U, McMortensen NJ (eds) *Endosonography in Gastroenterology, Gynecology, and Urology.* Berlin: Springer, 1990:153–214.

39 Bacchetti O. Nuova applicazione dell'ago-elettro-puntura in un caso giudicato di gravidanza extrauterina tubarica. *Gazz Med It Feder Toscana* 1853;5:137–140.

40 Ghirardini G, Popp LW. Bacchetti (1853) and the first electro-puncture: a milestone in the non-surgical therapy of extrauterine pregnancy. *Clin Exp Obstet Gynecol* 1992;14:203–205.

41 Brothers A. The treatment of extra-uterine pregnancy by electricity. *Am J Obstet Dis Women Children* 1888;21:474–484.

42 Popp LW, Gaetje R, Staus S, Lierse W. A rabbit model for the evaluation of minimal access treatment of ectopic pregnancy in humans, using intrachorionic injection and local hyperthermia. *Clin Exp Obstet Gynecol* 1993;20:226–235.

Chapter 19/Transvaginal sonographic puncture procedures for the management of ectopic pregnancies

ANA MONTEAGUDO, JODI P. LERNER and
ILAN E. TIMOR-TRITSCH

Introduction

The aim of this chapter is to present the reader with another option, besides surgery, for the treatment of ectopic pregnancies. Non-surgical management of ectopic pregnancies includes systemic administration of methotrexate or RU 486 (mifepristone), or local injection of methotrexate, potassium chloride or prostaglandins under laparoscopic or sonographic guidance [1,2]. We concentrate on the transvaginally guided local injection of either potassium chloride or methotrexate.

Most obstetricians and gynaecologists in the world first became familiar with transvaginal sonography (TVS) after it was successfully used in *in vitro* fertilization/embryo transfer (IVF/ET) programmes. Punctures performed under ultrasound guidance may be used as diagnostic as well as therapeutic tools. The rationale behind using ultrasound-guided punctures as therapy is twofold: first, it saves the patient from a more complicated surgical procedure, usually under general anaesthesia; second, it renders treatment at least as good as with conventional surgery.

The advantages of performing transvaginal punctures are numerous. Among these advantages the important ones are:

1 the needle is placed in an accurate fashion within the target organ or site;

2 there is almost no injury to the neighbouring organs since the procedure is carried out under real-time sonography;

3 the technical skills to perform the puncture procedures are easy to master;

4 the ultrasound equipment is portable and therefore the diagnostic test and treatment can be offered in a variety of settings;

5 it has a relatively low cost per procedure;

6 the risks to the patient from the procedure itself are minimal.

When one engages in transvaginally directed puncture procedures one should be familiar with the term 'slice thickness'. Obviously, due to its physical properties, there is a third dimension to the ultrasound plane. This is the 'slice thickness', and even though this thickness is negligible and decreases with increasing frequency, it still has to be taken into account. This is the reason that at times, although the tip of the needle is seen within the desired structure, in reality it may be in front or behind the target structure.

Another important aspect is the 'free-hand' approach to puncture procedures. Transabdominally, it is easy to use the free-hand approach, which is dependent on the operator's eye–hand coordination. It is easy to readjust the tip under sonographic control. However, there is extremely limited mobility of the probe and the needle when performing transvaginal punctures. It is therefore much easier to 'force' the entire length of the needle into the scanning plane. This can readily be done, by using a needle guide, thus giving perfect visual control over the exact placement of the tip of the needle.

In this chapter there will be ample reference to an automated spring-loaded puncture device (Labotect, Göttingen, Germany) that is mated to the vaginal probe (Fig. 19.1). This automated puncture device (APD), which was first used in assisted reproduction [3], uses a dotted double line that is displayed on the monitor and is generated by the software program of the ultrasound machine. This directional line measures depth for accurate needle penetration. The APD is equipped with a depth setting, which is then adjusted according to the depth measured on the screen. In addition to its accuracy, needle penetration is virtually painless due to the high velocity of the needle. Very little or no analgesia

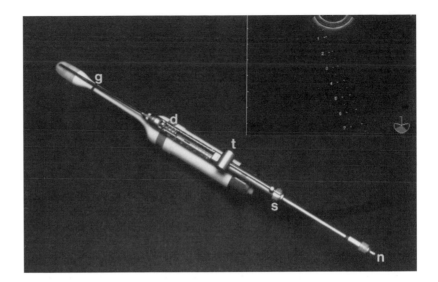

Fig. 19.1 The automated puncture device (APD) mated to the Siemens transvaginal probe. g, needle guide; d, depth setting and housing of the spring; t, trigger; s, safety; n, needle within the device. Inset: the directional and depth markers. The needle penetrates and is visible between the dotted double line.

is needed. Almost all puncture procedures performed in our centre are performed using this ingenious and highly accurate device [4–8]. We determined the accuracy of APD needle placement *in vitro* and found this to be within ± 1–2 mm (I.E. Timor-Tritsch, unpublished data).

Several of the punctures used in the diagnosis and treatment of ectopic pregnancies are now discussed.

Puncture procedures

Culdocentesis

Before the advent of sonography, culdocentesis was the 'gold standard' diagnostic test to identify a ruptured ectopic pregnancy. Transabdominal sonography increased the detection rate of ectopic pregnancies, but as recent as the early 1980s culdocentesis continued to play a key role in the diagnosis of tubal pregnancy. More recently, with the increasing availability of TVS and its high sensitivity in imaging the cul-de-sac and any fluid that it may contain, the indications to perform a diagnostic culdocentesis have significantly decreased. Currently, in our institution the indications to perform culdocentesis are changing and its use in the diagnosis of a ruptured ectopic pregnancy is declining fast. We perform culdocentesis mostly to drain pelvic fluid collections such as peritoneal inclusion cysts and inflammatory processes resulting in abscess formation.

There are several problems with the diagnostic value of culdocentesis in the work-up of ectopic pregnancies. In one study Vermesh *et al.* [9] concluded that culdocentesis is an invasive and painful procedure with very little value in the clinical setting where TVS and rapid pregnancy testing are available. Patients in whom the ectopic gestation cannot be ruled out by means of ultrasonography and pregnancy testing are probably best managed by laparoscopy rather than culdocentesis. It is easy to understand this statement since TVS can readily detect the smallest amounts of pelvic fluid and even, at times, distinguish between completely sonolucent pelvic contents and particulate matter containing fluid in the pelvis. In the right clinical setting, fluid containing particulate matter strongly suggests the presence of blood.

If there is still a need to perform analysis of pelvic fluid, we strongly suggest the use of sonographically directed transvaginal puncture, which enables an accurate needle insertion and avoids dry taps or inserting the needle into unwanted structures such as dilated blood vessels.

The technique of culdocentesis

Culdocentesis classically has been performed blindly, but using TVS it can be performed under real-time sonographic guidance. A needle guide or APD can be employed in order to optimize needle placement.

The technique of 'blind' culdocentesis is as follows. The patient is placed in the lithotomy position in reversed Trendelenburg. A speculum is inserted and the vagina and cervix are cleaned with Betadine solution. A 16–18-gauge spinal needle is attached to a 20-ml syringe. The syringe is filled with air. The anterior lip of the cervix is grasped with a tenaculum and the patient is asked to cough or bear down as the cul-de-sac is entered with the needle. If non-clotted blood or fluid is present in the cul-de-sac, it would be aspirated with the syringe.

Culdocentesis guided by TVS is similar to the above-described technique but the important differences are that there is no need to place a tenaculum, the needle is introduced under real-time sonography and the fluid pocket can be very precisely targeted, no air is injected into the abdominal cavity and finally all of the fluid present can be removed (this is important if the indication for the culdocentesis was drainage of a peritoneal inclusion cyst).

Treatment of ectopic pregnancies

Since the introduction of TVS, it has become clear that the entity of 'ectopic pregnancy' contains a large number of diseases with different manifestations requiring different treatment. The classic approach to ectopic pregnancies has always been surgical: the diseased tube, ovary or cornual area was resected. In the case of a cervical pregnancy, hysterectomy was the rule.

The possibility of classifying the different clinical patterns of the disease has enabled the consideration of different therapeutic approaches to this disease [10]. The introduction of high-frequency TVS, as well as the knowledgeable use of local or systemic administration of methotrexate, has opened new frontiers for the treatment of ectopic pregnancies.

It is not by chance that the first transvaginally guided puncture procedure performed to treat a tubal ectopic pregnancy by injecting methotrexate was developed by a group proficient in assisted reproductive technologies and IVF. This group took the skills acquired for performing ovum aspiration and applied them to the non-surgical treatment of ectopic pregnancy [11,12].

Three kinds of ectopic gestations and their puncture treatment are discussed: (i) tubal pregnancies (salpingocentesis), (ii) cornual pregnancies and (iii) cervical pregnancies.

TUBAL ECTOPIC PREGNANCIES (SALPINGOCENTESIS)

The diagnosis of a tubal ectopic pregnancy is made when a patient presents with a positive β human chorionic gonadotrophin (β-hCG) and on TVS has an empty uterus as well as the typical adnexal 'ring' or 'bagel sign'. Viable tubal ectopic pregnancies may be present in up to one-third of all ectopic gestations. Cases of tubal ectopic pregnancies to be considered for transvaginally guided puncture must meet several criteria: the ectopic gestational sac must contain a viable fetus with a menstrual age of less than 8.5 weeks' gestation, and the tubal diameter should not exceed 2.5–3 cm.

We reviewed over 100 cases of tubal ectopic pregnancies published in the literature that were treated by transvaginally directed injection of prostaglandin, potassium chloride and/or methotrexate. Table 19.1 summarizes these cases [4,5,12–27].

The reported complication rates of salpingocentesis at this time are about 15%. However, it is hard to compare the success rate between different groups since there is no agreed basis for comparison. In the literature, different kinds of ectopic pregnancy, non-viable and viable with different gestational ages and different sizes, have been treated by injection. Careful evaluation of these reports reveal that, due to lack of understanding of the natural course of the disease after the injection, some of the reported cases do not match the strict definition of a failed treatment. Some of the authors, including our group, were quick to consider a case a failure and thus institute additional treatment because of findings that now are considered part of the natural sequence of events after injections are performed [28]. Only recently has this sequence of events been elucidated. The most important signs and symptoms of the post-puncture convalescent period include the following.

1 *A relatively slow decrease of serum β-hCG levels.* The slope of the decay curve for serum β-hCG levels after salpingocentesis depends upon which substance (potassium chloride or methotrexate) was injected during the procedure. When potassium chloride is injected during salpingocentesis it takes 30–80 days for the

Table 19.1 Reported cases of salpingocentesis.

Reference	Year	No. of cases	Success rate no. (%)
Feichtinger & Kemeter [11,12]	1987, 1989	11	8 (72)
Robertson *et al.* [13,14]	1987	12	5 (42)
Leeton & Davison [15]	1988	2	2 (100)
Timor-Tritsch *et al.* [4,5]	1989, 1991	10	6 (60)
Ribic Paucelij *et al.* [16]	1989	2	0
Menard *et al.* [17]	1990	17	13 (76)
Aboulghar *et al.* [18]	1990	1	1 (100)
Fernandez *et al.* [19]	1990	21	14 (66)
Tulandi *et al.* [20]	1991	12	10 (83)
Popp *et al.* [21]	1991	4	4 (100)
Shalev *et al.* [22]	1991	12	9 (75)
Venezia *et al.* [23]	1991	5	5 (100)
Jehng *et al.* [24]	1992	2	2 (100)
Atri *et al.* [25]	1992	25	19 (76)
Bider *et al.* [26]	1992	2	0
Caspi *et al.* [27]	1992	1	1 (100)
Total		139	

β-hCG to become negative [5]. On the other hand, when methotrexate is injected, the β-hCG levels fall more abruptly, taking only 10–35 days to reach non-pregnant levels [4,11,12,21–23,25].

2 *Lower abdominal cramping or pain.* Between 3 and 7 days after puncture the patient may experience lower abdominal pain or cramping [28]. The possible cause of this pain is either uterine contractions as the decidual cast is being expelled from the uterus or tubal abortion with varying degrees of intra-abdominal bleeding. If the patient's vital signs and the amount of free fluid (blood in the pelvis) is not significant, the patient may be followed up conservatively.

3 *Transvaginal sonographic and colour Doppler findings.* These include increasing distension of the haematosalpinx, increasing colour vascularity and increasing venous spaces [25].

The technique of salpingocentesis

First we consider patient and probe preparation. Generally, the punctures are performed after the patient is informed and extensively counselled about her treatment options. During the counselling session the procedure, the risks and complications, and the nature of the post-procedure follow-up are described to the patient; lastly, the patient is asked to sign an informed consent form. Before describing the technique, we would like to stress that treatment of ectopic pregnancies with these procedures should still be considered experimental, and require the signing of the above-mentioned informed consent form. In our institution a specially worded consent approved by our Institutional Review Board is used.

We perform the puncture employing a 5–7.5 MHz transvaginal probe (Siemens, Isaqua). The high-frequency vaginal probe is covered with a sterile plastic sheath. A needle guide should be used to ensure accurate and steady placement of the needle. We prefer to use the previously described APD; however other needle guides mated to the vaginal probe can serve the same function. The thinnest possible needle should be used; usually a 21-gauge needle is preferred.

The patient is placed in the lithotomy position. The perineum is cleaned with a Betadine (iodine) solution. A speculum is placed in the vagina and the vagina and cervix are thoroughly cleaned using Betadine. Sterile drapes are employed to create a sterile field. Sterile gel is used for good sonic contact.

A software-generated fixed line is displayed on the monitor by which the exact depth of the ectopic pregnancy is located. If the APD is employed, the depth of needle penetration is controlled by the centimetre scale located on the shaft of the APD (Fig. 19.1). The patient is asked to stop breathing to prevent any movement during normal inspiration/expiration and the needle is released. If a standard needle guide is used, the needle should be inserted in a rapid fashion otherwise the ectopic pregnancy may be pushed away from the field of view rather than penetrated. Before the needle is inserted the location of the uterine artery and vessels of the adnexa should be carefully established and care should be taken not to puncture these vessels during insertion of the needle (Fig. 19.2). The target area is located near the fetal heart and either methotrexate or potassium chloride is injected once the needle is in place to stop cardiac activity. As the needle is withdrawn, methotrexate may also be injected into the area of the placental bed. Care must be exercised not to overly distend the already compromised tube.

Procedures are usually documented by still images and/or by videotape recordings. It is important to observe the pelvic structures and the cul-de-sac following the withdrawal of the needle. Patients recover and are rescanned after 2–3 hours for possible complications. Complications we have encountered while performing such puncture procedures include immediate bleeding from the puncture site as soon as the needle is withdrawn, as well as slowly enlarging haematomas over several hours.

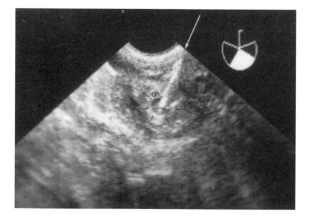

Fig. 19.2 Tubal ectopic pregnancy during the process of salpingocentesis. Arrow points to the needle. GS, gestational sac.

CORNUAL/INTERSTITIAL ECTOPIC PREGNANCIES

Approximately 2–4% of all tubal ectopic pregnancies are located in the cornual/interstitial area of the uterus [29]. The rupture of a cornual pregnancy brings about severe haemorrhage, exposes the patient to significant morbidity and carries with it a maternal mortality rate of up to 2.5% [29]. The procedure of choice to treat these patients is cornual resection. Cornual resection is feasible in over 50% of cases. However, in the remainder of the patients hysterectomy is unavoidable [29].

Using TVS the diagnosis of a cornual ectopic pregnancy is made when: the patient presents with a positive β-hCG; an empty uterine cavity; eccentrically placed or very lateral chorionic sac seen separately and at least 1 cm from the most lateral edge of the uterine cavity; thin myometrium covering the gestational sac; myometrium present between sac and uterine cavity; and no gestational sac visible above the level of the internal os in the longitudinal plane of the uterus [6,30]. Another useful sonographic sign is the interstitial line described by Ackerman *et al.* [31], which is a thin echogenic line extending directly to the centre of the interstitial gestational sac. In their hands this line had an 80% sensitivity, 98% specificity and 96% positive predictive value for accurate detection of interstitial pregnancy. Care must be taken not to mistake a bicornuate uterus with a cornual ectopic pregnancy. To be candidates for TVS-guided puncture pregnancy must have a viable pregnancy with a gestational age of less than 12 weeks. To date, we have treated 12 patients with cornual ectopic pregnancy using an injection of either potassium chloride or methotrexate. We believe that puncture injection of the very early (6–8.5 menstrual weeks) gestation using the guidance of TVS is a valid alternative to a more extensive surgical procedure. In the subsequent pregnancy, after cornual resection, the patient is exposed to the risks of uterine rupture and/or Caesarean section.

We have reported on the successful injection of cornual pregnancies [6] (Fig. 19.3). It is important to emphasize that non-viable cornual pregnancies with stable or declining β-hCG levels can be followed by TVS, with or without parenteral methotrexate treatment. There is no need to inject them or to take them to the operating room for cornual resection [6].

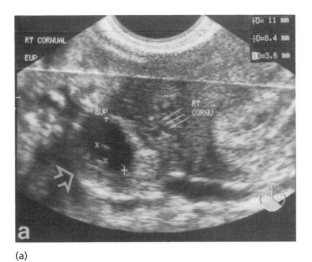

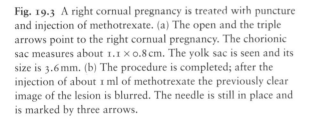

(a)

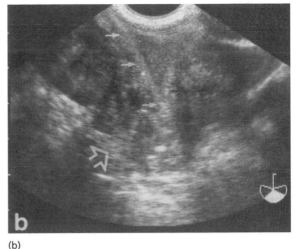

(b)

Fig. 19.3 A right cornual pregnancy is treated with puncture and injection of methotrexate. (a) The open and the triple arrows point to the right cornual pregnancy. The chorionic sac measures about 1.1 × 0.8 cm. The yolk sac is seen and its size is 3.6 mm. (b) The procedure is completed; after the injection of about 1 ml of methotrexate the previously clear image of the lesion is blurred. The needle is still in place and is marked by three arrows.

Another publication dealing with the long-term non-surgical management of non-viable cornual/interstitial pregnancies is a case report by Zalel *et al.* [32]. In both of these publications long-term non-surgical follow-up of non-viable cornual/interstitial pregnancy was carried out using serial β-hCG levels and transvaginal sonographic evaluation.

Karsdorp *et al.* [33] reported on the successful treatment of five interstitial pregnancies using methotrexate. One of five interstitial pregnancies initially was punctured transvaginally, the contents aspirated and subsequently injected with methotrexate and Leucovorin. Due to the limited number of viable cornual ectopic pregnancies treated with transvaginal puncture at present, the post-injection complication rates have not been elucidated. Similarly, as in salpingocentesis, the most feared complication would probably be bleeding from the site of the puncture.

Based on the present data, some preliminary post-puncture convalescent information is available.

1 The serum level of β-hCG returns slowly to non-pregnant levels (and initially may even increase). In cornual ectopic pregnancies treated with methotrexate, similar to the salpingocentesis experience, β-hCG returns faster to non-pregnant levels than when potassium chloride is used or when followed expectantly without treatment (12 weeks, 15 weeks and up to 23 weeks respectively).

2 Most importantly, the sonographic 'lesion' and rich vascular supply, as imaged with colour Doppler, persists for a prolonged period of time [6,33]. In our original report, in two patients who returned for follow-up 64 weeks after the puncture, the sonographic lesion (the chorionic cavity) was still evident and measured over 1 cm in size.

Due to our experience in injecting cornual/interstitial pregnancies, we developed a certain technique for the needle placement. In order to avoid rupturing the bulging chorionic sac, covered only by a thin myometrial layer, using a lateral approach, we now advocate reaching the sac containing the live embryo through a medial approach. This way the needle traverses first a thicker muscular layer which at the extraction of the needle prevents rupture or bleeding [34].

More information is desired, although these observations point toward the possibility of treating selected cases of cornual pregnancy using transvaginal puncture and local injection of potassium chloride and/or methotrexate. The technique for this kind of puncture procedure is identical to the one performed for tubal salpingocentesis.

CERVICAL ECTOPIC PREGNANCIES

The rare occurrence of cervical pregnancy is in clear contrast with the severity of the complications seen in other locations. Because of under-reporting, the true incidence of cervical pregnancy is largely unknown. There is usually severe bleeding and improvised, unplanned emergency treatment. These sometimes unorthodox treatment regimens have given rise to a significant body of short communications. However, a general consensus has not yet been developed regarding the detection and prevention of the sometimes unavoidable hysterectomies [35].

We evaluated the feasibility of transvaginal methotrexate injection of viable cervical pregnancies as a means to avoid the complications of the more classic surgical procedures and to preserve fertility [7] (Fig. 19.4). The first task of the obstetrician is to rule out the possibility of a non-viable pregnancy in the process of passing through the cervix from the uterine cavity, this being the main differential diagnosis of a cervical pregnancy. Only viable cervical pregnancies should be considered. In addition, our group suggests new sonographic diagnostic criteria for a cervical pregnancy.

1 The placenta and the entire chorionic sac containing the live fetus should be below the internal os. The level of the internal os on a coronal view is considered to be at the level of the insertion of the uterine arteries (using Doppler or colour Doppler sonography).

2 The uterine cavity should be empty.

3 The cervical canal is barrel-shaped and significantly dilated.

We have published data on five viable cervical pregnancies that were treated by transvaginal injection of methotrexate [7]. In three, the APD was employed. All five cases were successful. No complications were noted and the more extensive surgical procedure was avoided. Four additional cases of viable cervical pregnancy were also injected with potassium chloride [36]. These were also successful, and the highest gestational age was 7 weeks and 1 day. This new treatment modality should be considered as an additional therapeutic modality when cervical pregnancies are diagnosed early in gestation. Centini *et al.* [37] published a case report of a cervical pregnancy diagnosed by TVS and successfully treated at 6 weeks and 4 days by needle aspiration of the products of conception and curettage of the cervical canal and uterus.

Lately we published on the successful transvaginal puncture and injection using KCl in two heterotopic pregnancies targeting the cervical embryos [38]. Both pregnancies ended with delivery (Caesarean sections) of the intrauterine fetus. The cervix returned to normal size and appearance several months later.

The technique of puncture of cervical pregnancy is similar to that described for tubal ectopic pregnancy. The most feared complication in this group of patients is once again bleeding, either at the time of puncture or several days after the procedure. In our group of

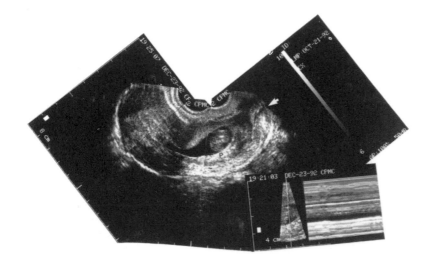

Fig. 19.4 A composite sagittal section of an empty uterus with a live cervical pregnancy. P, cervical pregnancy; arrow points to the external cervical os. Inset: M-mode tracing of the cardiac activity. (From Timor-Tritsch *et al.* [7], with permission.)

five treated cervical ectopic pregnancies, a slow and continuous discharge of small amounts of tissue was observed over the first 2 weeks after the procedure.

Conclusions

It is our belief that an early, and maybe compulsory, transvaginal sonographic examination of all pregnant patients, especially the high-risk population for ectopic pregnancy, should be considered and scientifically tested to identify and classify ectopic gestations, and this must take place when they do occur, in order to be able to apply the best and most efficient therapeutic approach, which leads to fewer complications and a better distribution of funds.

The advantages and disadvantages of transvaginally performed puncture procedures to treat the different types of ectopic pregnancy have been described and summarized. It is clear that the transvaginal route provides us with a simple and accurate way of inserting a thin needle into the desired structure. These puncture procedures enable diagnostic and therapeutic options. In most cases, abdominal and vaginal surgery can be avoided. There is a very low procedure complication rate, and the technical simplicity and the ease with which it can be performed renders it a desirable outpatient procedure. The use of the APD has to be considered as the most accurate and least painful needle insertion to date.

A final statement should be made about the gradual decrease of levels of β-hCG after the puncture and injection of the different kinds of ectopic pregnancy. After an initial rise or sometimes a plateau of the titres, the values usually decrease and return to non-pregnant levels within 3–13 weeks.

The experience brought to the reader in this chapter should also raise the possibility of performing some of the more simple transvaginal puncture procedures in the office or in the emergency room.

References

1 Pansky M, Golan A, Bukovsky I, Caspi E. Nonsurgical management of tubal pregnancy. Necessity in view of the changing clinical appearance. *Am J Obstet Gynecol* 1991;**164**:888–895.

2 Kooi S, Kock HCLV. A review of the literature on nonsurgical treatment in tubal pregnancies. *Obstet Gynecol Surv* 1992;**47**:739–749.

3 Kemeter P, Feichtinger W. Transvaginal oocyte retrieval using a transvaginal sector-scan probe combined with an automated puncture device. *Hum Reprod* 1986;**1**:21–24.

4 Timor-Tritsch IE, Baxi L, Peisner DB. Transvaginal salpingocentesis: a new technique for treating ectopic pregnancy. *Am J Obstet Gynecol* 1989;**160**:459–461.

5 Timor-Tritsch IE, Peisner DB, Monteagudo A. Puncture procedures utilizing transvaginal ultrasonic guidance. *Ultrasound Obstet Gynecol* 1991;**1**:144–150.

6 Timor-Tritsch IE, Monteagudo A, Matera C, Veit CR. Sonographic evolution of cornual pregnancies treated without surgery. *Obstet Gynecol* 1992;**79**:1044–1049.

7 Timor-Tritsch IE, Monteagudo A, Mandeville EO, Peisner DB, Anaya GP, Pirrone EC. Successful management of viable cervical pregnancy by local injection of methotrexate guided by transvaginal sonography. *Am J Obstet Gynecol* 1994;**170**:737–739.

8 Timor-Tritsch IE, Montcagudo A, Peisner DB. Puncture procedures using the transvaginal probe in obstetrics and gynecology. *Ultrasound Quarterly* 1993;**11**:41–57.

9 Vermesh M, Graczykowski JW, Sauer MV. Reevaluation of the role of culdocentesis in the management of ectopic pregnancy. *Am J Obstet Gynecol* 1990;**162**:411–413.

10 Rottem S, Thaler I, Timor-Tritsch IE. Classification of tubal gestations by transvaginal sonography. *Ultrasound Obstet Gynecol* 1991;**1**:197–201.

11 Feichtinger W, Kemeter P. Conservative treatment of ectopic pregnancy by transvaginal aspiration under sonographic control and methotrexate injection. *Lancet* 1987;**i**:381.

12 Feichtinger W, Kemeter P. Treatment of unruptured ectopic pregnancy by needling of sac and injection of methotrexate or PGE2 under transvaginal sonography control: report of 10 cases. *Arch Gynecol Obstet* 1989;**246**:85–89.

13 Robertson DE, Smith W, Moye MAH *et al.* Reduction of ectopic pregnancy by injection under ultrasound control. *Lancet* 1987;**i**:974–975.

14 Robertson DE, Smith W, Craft I. Reduction of ectopic pregnancy by ultrasound methods. *Lancet* 1987;**ii**:1524–1525.

15 Leeton J, Davison G. Nonsurgical management of unruptured tubal pregnancy with intra-amniotic methotrexate: preliminary report of two cases. *Fertil Steril* 1988;**50**:67–69.

16 Ribic Paucelij M, Novak-Antolic Z, Urhovec I. Treatment of ectopic pregnancy with prostaglandin E$_2$. *Clin Obstet Gynecol* 1989;**16**:106–109.

17 Menard A, Crequat J, Mandelbrot L, Hauuy JP, Madelanat P. Treatment of unruptured tubal pregnancy by local injection of methotrexate under transvaginal sonographic control. *Fertil Steril* 1990;**54**:47–50.

18 Aboulghar MA, Mansour RT, Serour GI. Transvaginal injection of potassium chloride and methotrexate for the treatment of tubal pregnancy with a live fetus. *Hum Reprod* 1990;5:887–888.

19 Fernandez H, Baton C, Lelaidier C, Frydman R. Conservative management of ectopic pregnancy: prospective randomized clinical trial of methotrexate versus prostaglandin sulpostrone by combined transvaginal and systemic administration. *Fertil Steril* 1991;55:746–752.

20 Tulandi T, Bret PM, Atri M, Senterman M. Treatment of ectopic pregnancy by transvaginal intratubal methotrexate administration. *Obstet Gynecol* 1991;77:627–643.

21 Popp LW, Mettler L, Weisner H, Mecke I, Freys I, Semm K. Ectopic pregnancy treatment using pelviscopic or vaginosonographically guided intrachorionic injection of methotrexate. *Ultrasound Obstet Gynecol* 1991;i:136–143.

22 Shalev E, Zalel Y, Bustan M, Weiner E. Ectopic pregnancy: sonographically guided transvaginal reduction. *Ultrasound Obstet Gynecol* 1991;i:127–131.

23 Venezia R, Zangara C, Comparetto G, Cittadini E. Conservative treatment of ectopic pregnancies using a single echo-guided injection of methotrexate into a gestational sac. *Ultrasound Obstet Gynecol* 1991;i:132–135.

24 Jehng CH, Ng Ky, Jou HJ, Jenh AL, Lien YR. Successful treatment of two viable tubal pregnancies by two-step local injection. *J Formos Med Assoc* 1992;91:823–827.

25 Atri M, Bret PM, Tulandi T, Senterman MK. Ectopic pregnancy: evolution after treatment with transvaginal methotrexate. *Radiology* 1992;185:749–753.

26 Bider D, Oelsner G, Admon D *et al.* Unsuccessful methotrexate treatment of a tubal pregnancy with a live embryo. *Eur J Obstet Gynecol Reprod Med* 1992;46:154–157.

27 Caspi B, Barash A, Friedman A, Appelman Z, Pausky M, Borenstein R. Aspiration of ectopic pregnancy under guidance of vaginal ultrasonography. *Eur J Obstet Gynecol Reprod Biol* 1992;46:51–52.

28 Carson SA, Buster JE. Ectopic pregnancy. *N Engl J Med* 1993;329:1174–1181.

29 Thompson JD, Rock JA (eds) *TeLinde's Operative Gynecology*. Philadelphia: JB Lippincott, 1992:428–430.

30 deBoer CN, van Dongen PWJ, Willemsen WNP, Klapwijk CWDA. Ultrasound diagnosis of interstitial pregnancy. *Eur J Obstet Gynecol Reprod Biol* 1992;47:164–166.

31 Ackerman TE, Levi CS, Dashefsky SM *et al.* Interstitial line: sonographic finding in interstitial (cornual) ectopic pregnancy. *Radiology* 1993;189:83–87.

32 Zalel Y, Caspi B, Insler V. Expectant management of interstitial pregnancy. *Ultrasound Obstet Gynecol* 1994;4:238–240.

33 Karsdorp VHM, Van der Veen F, Schats R *et al.* Successful treatment with methotrexate of five vital interstitial pregnancies. *Hum Reprod* 1992;7:1164–1169.

34 Timor-Tritsch IE, Monteagudo A, Lerner JP. A 'potentially safer' route for puncture and injection of cornual ectopic pregnancies. *Ultrasound Obstet Gynecol* 1996;7:353–355.

35 Yankowitz J, Leake J, Huggins G, Gazaway P, Gates E. Cervical ectopic pregnancy: review of the literature and report of a case treated by single-dose methotrexate therapy. *Obstet Gynecol Surv* 1990;45:405–414.

36 Frate MC, Benson CB, Doubilet PM, DiSalvo DN, Laing FC, Brown DL. The sonographic diagnosis and nonsurgical treatment of cervical ectopic pregnancy. *J Ultrasound Med* 1994.

37 Centini G, Rosignoli L, Severi F. A case of cervical pregnancy. *Am J Obstet Gynecol* 1994;171:272–273.

38 Monteagudo A, Tarricone NJ, Timor-Tritsch IE, Lerner JP. Successful transvaginal ultrasound-guided puncture and injection of a cervical pregnancy in a patient with simultaneous intrauterine pregnancy and a history of a previous cervical pregnancy. *Ultrasound Obstet Gynecol* 1996;8:381–386.

Chapter 20/Ultrasound-guided transcervical metroplasty

DENIS QUERLEU

Introduction

Sectioning of uterine septa may be performed hystero-scopically with low morbidity and good surgical outcome [1,2]. Using this technique, in order to prevent uterine perforation during division of the upper part of a uterine septum, both laparoscopic or ultrasonic monitoring have been proposed [3]. The aim of this chapter will be to present our experience with the first 24 patients operated by the transcervical section of uterine septa under ultrasonographic control without the concomitant use of hysteroscopy or laparoscopy [4,5]. All these ultrasound-guided transcervical metroplasty procedures were performed between June 1984 and June 1989. Ohl *et al.* [6], using the same ultra-sonographically guided technique, reported their results in 1991. Their post-operative results were excellent in 19 out of 37 patients. In five cases, the result was judged unsatisfactory and required a repeat metroplasty. At the time of publication, 18 pregnancies had occurred in 15 patients: two early and one late miscarriage, one ectopic pregnancy, eight term pregnancies and four ongoing pregnancies.

Operative technique

The operation is performed under general anesthesia or neuroleptanalgesia. The bladder is filled with 250 ml of saline isotonic solution through a balloon catheter. An assistant places the transducer of a real time ultra-sound scanner in longitudinal or transverse position according to the needs of the surgeon.

The uterine fundus is checked, and the differential diagnosis from bicornuate uterus is made. The septum is measured in width and in length (Fig. 20.1). A pair of 4-mm diameter endoscopic scissors (26 175 MS, Karl Storz, Tuttlingen, Germany) generally employed

for laparoscopic surgery are used (Fig. 20.2). The scissors are introduced into the uterine cavity through the cervix without any cervical dilation. The entire operation is performed under ultrasound imaging of the position of the instrument (Figs 20.3–6). The tip of the scissors comes into contact with the lower edge of the septum. The scissors are opened, and the blades are placed respectively on the right and on the left side of the septum. The septum is divided at an equal distance from the anterior and posterior surface of the uterus. The posterior serosal wall is always seen, without necessitating the placement of liquid in the cul-de-sac. The procedure is considered complete when the distance between the upper limit of the section and the serosal surface of the uterine fundus is 10 mm. The operating time is in some cases, less than 10 minutes. Since the efficacy of this procedure in maintaining the uterine shape is still under investigation, no intrauterine device is inserted [5]. Although day care surgery is a reasonable choice, in our series all patients remained hospitalized for 24 hours. Patients were given cyclic hormonal therapy for a period of three months (ethinyl estradiol 100 mg daily for 21 days and norethisterone acetate 1 mg daily during the final 7 days of estrogen therapy). The goal of this hormonal therapy is to help endometrial regeneration. Since the efficacy of such treatment is considered controversial, a second look hysteroscopy is proposed following the withdrawal bleeding three months after the operation (Fig. 20.7). The result was documented by hysterography only at the beginning of our experience, but we believe that control radiography is no longer justified.

Patient selection

The uterine septum was diagnosed in every case by hysterography and/or ultrasonography. Twelve of the

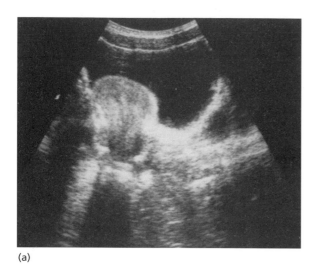

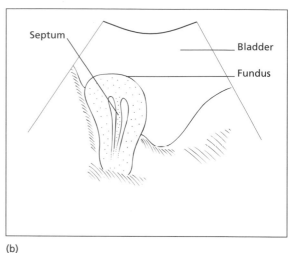

(a)

(b)

Fig. 20.1 Sonographic picture of a septate uterus.

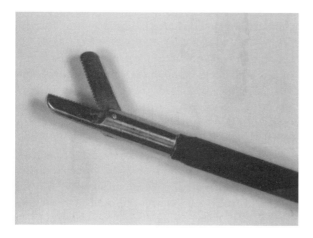

Fig. 20.2 The 4-mm endoscopic scissors.

salpingography, endometrial biopsy, postcoital test, and sperm analysis. A male factor was diagnosed in one case. Three patients registered in our *in vitro* fertilization (IVF) program, because of tubal infertility. Five patients presented with unexplained infertility. In the last three patients, uterine septa were asymptomatic, and metroplasty was performed as an additional procedure during section of a vaginal septum. All three patients had a complete division of cervix and corpus diagnosed by clinical examination and ultrasonography. No additional evaluation of fertility was done in this group.

Of the entire series, 18 patients had a complete septum including the internal (*n*:11) or external os (*n*:7). Six patients had a partial septum reaching the lower third of the uterine cavity. Patients with an arcuate uterus were excluded.

Post surgical evaluation

No significant bleeding or intraoperative complications were encountered in any of the 24 cases. Uterine perforation was never observed and the postoperative period was uneventful.

Eighteen patients had a morphological evaluation of the uterine cavity. In eleven patients, the results were considered excellent and no significant indentation of

patients had previously suffered two or more spontaneous first or second trimester losses. Complete work-up included hysterosalpingography, endometrial biopsy, parental karyotype, plasma/thyroid stimulating hormone (TSH) and 17-hydroxy-progesterone. Uterine septum was the only factor of recurrent abortion in all cases. Nine patients presented with primary infertility of at least 18 months duration. The mean age of these patients was 29 years. Work-up included hystero-

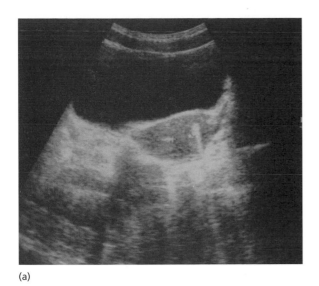

(a)

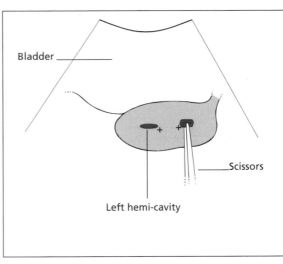

(b)

Fig. 20.3 (a) Transverse ultrasound section. (b) Scissors are placed in the right hemi-cavity.

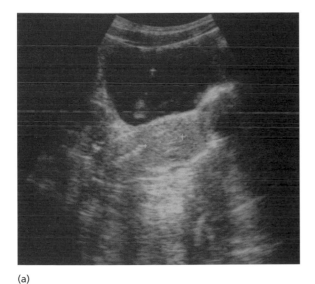

(a)

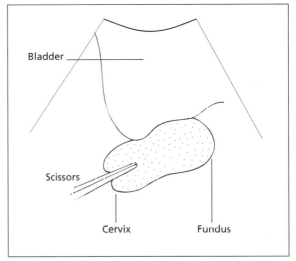

(b)

Fig. 20.4 (a) Sagittal ultrasound section. (b) Scissors are placed at the lower end of the septum.

the uterine fundus was detected at the time of the second look hysteroscopy. The persistence of an arcuate fundus, without clinical significance, was noted in four patients. In two instances, a residual septum measuring 10–20 mm was divided under hysteroscopic control (these two patients had initially a complete septum to the external os). In the last case, the result was judged unsatisfactory because of the occurrence of an extensive synechia. However, after hysteroscopic division of the adhesion, the patient became pregnant.

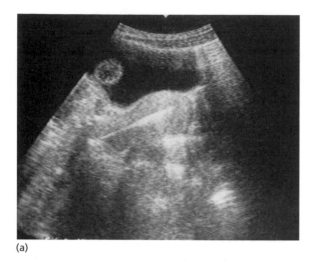

(a)

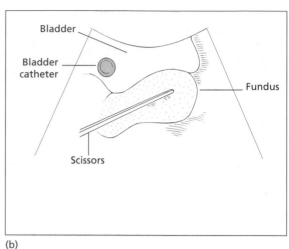

(b)

Fig. 20.5 (a) Sagittal ultrasound section. (b) Scissors are placed at the uterine fundus, showing the thickness of the uterine wall.

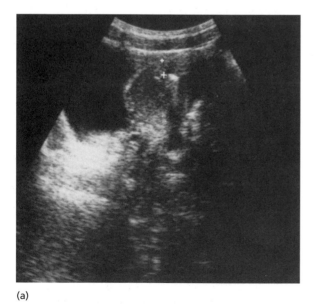

(a)

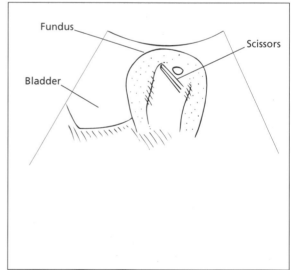

(b)

Fig. 20.6 Sonographic picture of opened scissors.

Long-term obstetrical outcome

Two patients did not want to become pregnant and

obstetrical outcome will be presented for the remaining 22 patients. Of these, 20 conceived. One spontaneous first-trimester abortion occurred in a patient with history of recurrent abortions and who presented to us with a partial uterine septum, and in whom the post operative hysteroscopy showed a residual arcuate uterus. One

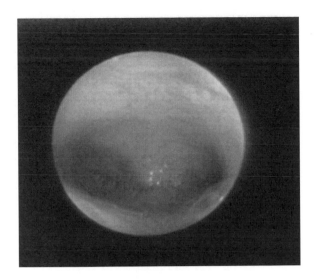

Fig. 20.7 Hysteroscopic follow-up, 3 months after ultrasound-guided metroplasty.

no technical limitations to the procedure and wide uterine septa can be incised in the majority of cases in a single operation. Numbers of myometrial scars or pelvic adhesions resulting from the ultrasound guided metroplasty are comparable to those obtained after hysteroscopic procedures [7]. Finally, since this procedure is performed without an additional laparoscopy, the morbidity and potential mortality of the metroplasty is also reduced when done under ultrasound guidance.

Conventional indications for surgical treatment of a septated uterus include the history of one or more spontaneous abortions [8]. In this series, 20 of 22 patients desired pregnancy and 92% had a successful pregnancy. It seems reasonable to propose that ultrasound-guided metroplasty may reduce the risk of miscarriage. Some investigators have advised against the incision of the cervical septum, so as to minimize the risk of creating a single incompetent cervix from two single cervices [8]. In seven patients of our series, surgical incision of the cervical septum at the external os was followed by ultrasound-guided division of the remaining cervical and uterine septum. Six out of these patients then became pregnant: one of them suffered a second-trimester abortion, and later had a term pregnancy with the help of a cervical cerclage. The hypothesis of iatrogenic cervical incompetence in this case must be raised [9,10].

ectopic pregnancy occurred and one patient aborted a twin pregnancy at 22 weeks. Despite a history of cervical incompetence, her obstetrician did not consider a cervical cerclage. This patient conceived soon after this loss, underwent a Shirodkar suture, and had a term delivery. Eighteen patients delivered, including the case described above. Fourteen patients were delivered vaginally, and four Caesarean sections were performed. The indications for Caesarean section were: cephalopelvic disproportion, premature rupture of the membranes with intra-amniotic infection and prematurity, pre-eclampsia, breech presentation and fetal macrosomia. Three premature deliveries occurred, all in the infertile patients' group. Two patients are still not cured. One patient from the infertility group had an additional cause of infertility due to a tubal factor. One additional patient has persistent unexplained infertility.

Discussion

Asymptomatic patients with a septate uterus do not need any surgical treatment. However, if surgery is indicated in these patients to correct a vaginal septum, division of the uterine septum may be proposed since there is low additional risk, time and cost involved if done under ultrasonographic control. Furthermore, there are

Conclusion

Transcervical metroplasty is at this time the procedure of choice for the treatment of septate uteri with reproductive failure. Ultrasound scanning enhances the safety of the procedure, as it allows precise checking of the thickness of myometrium left intact. Progress in ultrasound imaging has led us to investigate the possibility of performing metroplasty without hysteroscopic vision. In our preliminary study, the absence of complications and the observation of results comparable with those obtained by abdominal as well as hysteroscopic metroplasty provides evidence that ultrasound guided transcervical approach is feasible and with a satisfactory pregnancy outcome. Although some authors advocate the use of radiologic monitoring [11], we feel that ultrasound guidance is simpler and safer. It may be used alone or to monitor an hysteroscopic procedure.

References

1 Edstrom KGB. Intra-uterine surgical procedures during hysteroscopy. *Endoscopy* 1979;**6**:175–181.

2 Fayez JA. Comparison between abdominal and hysteroscopic metroplasty. *Obstet Gynecol* 1986;**68**:399–402.

3 Lin BL, Iwata Y, Myamoto N, Hayashi S. Three contrast method: an ultrasound technique for monitoring transcervical operations. *Am J Obstet Gynecol* 1987;**156**: 469–472.

4 Querleu D, Decocq J, Boutteville C, Locquet F, Crepin G. Section rctrograde de cloison uterine sous controle echographique. *Presse Med* 1988;**42**:2253–2255.

5 Querleu D, Leroy-Brasme T, Parmentier D. Ultrasound guided transcervical metroplasty. *Fert Ster* 1990;**54**:995–998.

6 Ohl J, Nisand I, Dellenbach P. Section sous controle echographique des cloisons uterines. *J Gynecol Obstet Biol Rep* 1991;**20**:538–540.

7 Daly DC, Maier D, Soto-Albors C. Hysteroscopic metroplasty: six years' experience. *Obstet Gynecol* 1989;**73**: 201–205.

8 Rock JA, Jones HW. The clinical management of the double uterus. *Fert Ster* 1977;**28**:798–806.

9 Rock JA, Murphy AA, Cooper WH IV. Resectoscopic technique for the lysis of a class V: complete uterine septum. *Fert Ster* 1987;**48**:495–496.

10 Fedele L, Arcaini L, Parazzini F, Vercellini P, De Nola G. Reproductive prognosis after hysteroscopic metroplasty in 102 women: life-table analysis. *Fert Ster* 1993;**59**:768–772.

11 Valle JA, Lifchez AS, Moise J. A simpler technique for reduction of uterine septum. *Fert Ster* 1991;**56**:1001–1003.

Chapter 21 / Laparoscopic ultrasound technology

CEANA NEZHAT, FARR NEZHAT and CAMRAN NEZHAT

Introduction

Operative laparoscopy has revolutionized the approach to surgery within many disciplines, and although few can argue with the remarkable benefits of this technique [1], there are limitations. Most notable is the absence of tactile feedback. The introduction of laparoscopic direct contact ultrasound is proving effective in overcoming many aspects of this drawback. As laparoscopic ultrasonography develops, we look forward to its use in the diagnosis of intramural leiomyoma or small intraovarian cystic or solid masses; identifying a ureter behind an adherent ovary; identifying intraluminal pathology in the appendix; and precisely defining the bladder during laparoscopic hysterectomy, Burch or Marshall–Marchetti–Krantz procedures. When utilizing Doppler, retroperitoneal blood vessels can be identified easily. Our own experience with this new technology in identifying ovarian remnants has been positive [2].

A laparoscopic ultrasound probe contains a transducer array that is placed in contact with tissue to form a real-time ultrasound image. Figure 21.1 is a simplified representation of such an array and the type of image it produces. Typically these arrays have 96–144 individual piezoelectric transducers, each of which is both a transmitter and receiver of ultrasound. Each small transducer element is connected to the imaging system and its own processing electronics through a miniature coax cable. Every element of the array can be the origin of a line in the ultrasound image. To form an image, a group of 32–64 elements is combined electronically to make both a transmitting and receiving acoustic lens.

In the transmit mode, a group of elements is fired by driving them with a short electrical burst. There are small time differences between the bursts going to the elements that create a converging acoustic field, as shown schematically in Fig. 21.1. This focused acoustic field propagates through tissue reflecting off tissue interfaces and those reflections are detected by the same group of elements.

The returning acoustic echoes are detected by each element in the array and are in turn focused electronically, creating a single line of data representing the echo interfaces along that line. The electronic array system then shifts this group of elements by one and repeats the process to form the next acoustic line. These lines are then interpolated to form the two-dimensional image shown in the screen on the right side of Fig. 21.1.

The resolution in an ultrasound image is determined by the frequency of the piezoelectric crystals that make up the array and by the line spacing in the image. Higher frequencies produce shorter pulses but are more rapidly absorbed in tissue. As described above, the line spacing in the image is determined by the width of the individual array elements. To resolve small structures, lines must be close together and hence the elements must be narrow. For the work reported here, the array frequency was 10 MHz and there were 128 elements each 200 μm wide. Thus, the line spacing is 200 μm and the width of the image is 128 × 0.2 mm = 25.6 mm. Table 21.1 lists specifications for other arrays used in laparoscopic ultrasound.

First-generation laparoscopic ultrasound arrays have been built into 10-mm diameter rigid and articulated probes. Obviously, the packaging of large numbers of transducers and their cables is a difficult task. With further development, however, arrays with comparable imaging capability will be built into 5-mm and smaller diameter laparoscopic devices that are more suitable for gynaecology.

Gynaecological case histories

We have used laparoscopic ultrasound to detect ovarian

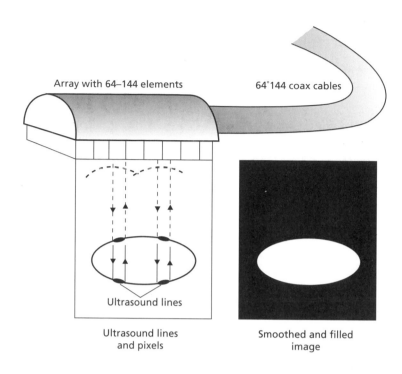

Array with 64–144 elements   64°144 coax cables

Ultrasound lines

Ultrasound lines
and pixels

Smoothed and filled
image

Fig. 21.1 A representation of a transducer array and the type of image it produces.

Table 21.1 System specifications.

Typical system specifications	10 MHz linear	7.5 MHz linear	6 MHz linear
Line spacing (mm)	0.2	0.3	0.41
Resolution: average of axial and lateral (mm)	0.3	0.4	0.5
Image depth (typical) (mm)	30	75	120
Array width/image width (mm)	25	35	52
Typical clinical application (organ)	Ovaries, fallopian tubes	Uterus, pancreas, liver	Liver

remnants in a 41-year-old woman who presented with chronic pelvic pain. She had previously undergone an abdominal hysterectomy and bilateral salpingo-oophorectomy. A pelvic examination revealed extreme vaginal cuff tenderness and transvaginal ultrasound demonstrated a right cystic structure, but both examinations were limited by the patient's discomfort. A CT scan with intravenous contrast indicated a smooth,

non-septated cystic mass in the right pelvis, most likely of ovarian origin. Ovarian hormone profile revealed follicle-stimulating hormone and oestradiol levels within the premenopausal, follicular phase range.

At videolaparoscopy, we found extensive pelvic adhesions between the rectosigmoid colon and the vagina, pelvic side wall and bladder. Because the pelvic mass was not readily apparent on laparoscopic examination, a 10-MHz, two-way articulating laparoscopic ultrasound probe (Tetrad Corporation, Englewood, Colorado) was introduced through a 10-mm suprapubic trocar (Fig. 21.2). Coupling of the ultrasound beam to the tissues was accomplished by introducing 20-ml of sterile saline solution into the pelvic cavity. The surface of the probe was placed on the bowel and systematic sweeps of the pelvic contents were performed on both sides. Articulation of the linear-array probe was used to direct the ultrasound beam into small lateral spaces and between adhesions.

There was a sonolucent (echo-free) cystic mass measuring approximately 8×5 cm on the right, which did not appear to have internal echoes, septations or

Fig. 21.2 (a) TETRAD Model 8A transabdominal probe and (b) shows the probe's control unit. (c) Shows its data entry panel.

debris, and was positioned over the right external iliac artery and vein and the right ureter. It extended from the pelvic brim to the bladder and was severely attached to the bladder, ureter and rectosigmoid colon.

Ultrasound examination of the left adnexa revealed a smaller, sonolucent, cystic mass measuring 3×3 cm that also seemed free of internal debris and septations. It was located in the pelvic brim and was attached to the left external iliac artery and vein, left ureter and rectosigmoid colon. This mass had not been imaged on CT.

Both masses were resected at laparoscopy. Pathology revealed that ovarian tissue was removed from the left and right sides. The operation lasted approximately 4 hours and blood loss was less than 100 ml. A postoperative hormone profile indicated that the patient was postmenopausal. One year later, she is doing well and reports significant improvement in her pain.

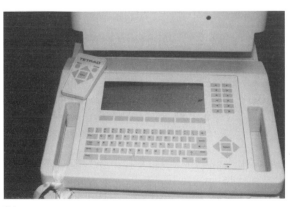

(a)

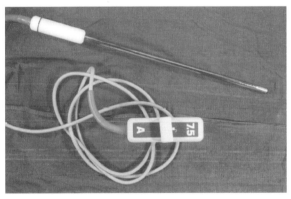

(b)

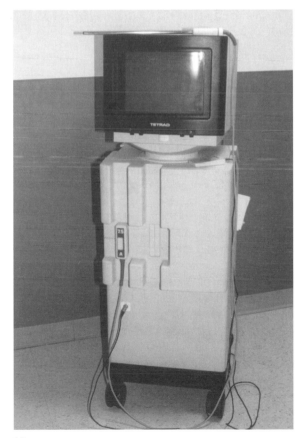

(c)

In another gynaecological study, laparoscopic ultrasound was used to identify a previously undetected uterine myoma and accurately show the size and location in relation to the myometrium and endometrial cavity. Laparoscopic ultrasound is also useful in evaluating the ovary, as internal cystic structure can be clearly defined. In some cases, invasive ovarian exploration by aspiration, biopsy or excision may be precisely directed or avoided based on intraoperative ultrasound findings [3].

Other clinical applications

We expect an increase in the use of laparoscopic ultrasound through the remainder of this decade. Two current examples are laparoscopic ultrasound for screening the common bile duct (CBD) for stones [4,5] and abdominal cancer staging [6,7].

Ultrasound imaging of the CBD during laparoscopic cholecystectomy

Cholecystectomy is the most common general surgery procedure. Over 600 000 are performed each year in the USA, over 90% at laparoscopy. Stones typically accumulate in the gallbladder but can also lodge in the CBD. The established X-ray procedure for detecting stones in the CBD is cholangiography.

A recent prospective study compared the accuracy of laparoscopic ultrasound and cholangiography in detecting CBD stones [4]. Laparoscopic ultrasound scans were done with a rigid, 7.5-MHz, linear-array probe. Cholangiography was done with a C-arm digital fluoroscopy unit that records a real-time image of the dye being injected into the CBD. Results of the 95-patient trial are compared in Table 21.2, and are similar to those published in other studies [5,8].

To perform cholangiography, a small catheter, typically less than 3 mm in diameter, is threaded into the cystic duct. This is technically challenging and cannot be done safely in roughly 5% of cases. In a small percentage of patients, ultrasound scanning of the CBD cannot be accomplished. Some small CBDs collapse entirely and are difficult to image. The average time difference between the ultrasound scan and cholangiography is significant, for the cholangiogram can take up to 30 min of expensive operating room time. Both techniques

Table 21.2 Comparison of laparoscopic ultrasound and cholangiography for detecting common bile duct (CBD) stones.

	Ultrasound	Cholangiography
Procedures successfully completed	93/95	90/95
Average time of procedure (min) (mean + SD)	8 ± 3	14 ± 6
Observation of entire CBD	84/93	86/90
Observation of cystic duct	87/93	80/90
Detection of duct stones	12/93	5/90

allow good visualization of the duct. There is a difference in the rate of stone detection because ultrasound reveals stones less than 2 mm, which may be missed on a cholangiogram but are not considered clinically significant. The five large stones that were significant were apparent on both scans. Ultrasound imaging of the CBD compares favourably with cholangiography. Regarding operating room cost, ultrasound is shorter, eliminates X-ray contrast agents and disposable catheters, and the equipment costs less. If surgeons are comfortable with the real-time, high-resolution, cross-sectional scans versus the single global view provided by the cholangiogram, ultrasound may become the preferred method for screening the CBD for stones.

Laparoscopic cancer staging

Laparoscopic cancer staging is effective in determining the resectability of tumours before initiating open surgery [6,7]. This may reduce exploratory laparotomy, benefiting both the patient and payer. Patients who are not surgical candidates can avoid open exploratory surgery and receive chemotherapy immediately, rather than after a long postoperative recovery. This approach for cancer staging is being studied for use in gynaecology.

Minimally invasive surgery (MIS) cancer staging is a hybrid consisting of a minimally invasive procedure and a diagnostic imaging examination. The surgeon has a magnified view of internal organs combined with direct, organ-contact ultrasound. This is superior to non-invasive imaging and provides an accurate and safe guide

Table 21.3 Summary of results of a laparoscopic staging procedure on patients selected for tumour resection based upon diagnostic imaging and clinical data.

	No. (%)
No. of surgical candidates	50
Unresectable	22 (44)
Determined by laparoscopy alone	11 (22)
Determined by laparoscopic ultrasound alone	11 (22)
Resectable at laparoscopic staging	28 (56)
Successful resection	26 (96)

for tissue biopsy. An extensive diagnostic imaging work-up that includes CT, angiography and CT portography, examinations typically performed for staging cancer, can be more expensive than this MIS procedure without providing the level of detail or the quality of tissue samples.

Over 40% of hepatobiliary and pancreatic cancers that are deemed surgically resectable based on extensive diagnostic studies are found to be unresectable during open surgery [6,7]. In nearly half of patients with metastatic lesions of the liver, additional lesions are found during surgery with direct organ-contact ultrasound imaging.

In a recent report [6], 50 patients with tumours of the liver ($n - 7$), biliary tract ($n = 11$) and pancreas ($n = 32$) were diagnosed as having surgically resectable lesions, based on an average of 2.7 diagnostic studies per patient. Studies included CT (96%), retrograde cholangiography (72%), arterioportography (22%) and magnetic resonance imaging (14%).

These patients underwent a laparoscopic staging procedure that included ultrasound scans. The results are summarized in Table 21.3. At laparoscopic staging, only 56% were still found suitable for resection, meaning that 44% would have had unnecessary laparotomy.

References

1 Nezhat C, Nezhat F, Luciano AA, Siegler AM, Metzger DA, Nezhat CH. *Operative Gynecologic Laparoscopy: Principles and Techniques.* New York: McGraw Hill, 1995.
2 Nezhat F, Nezhat C, Nezhat CH, Sly E, Seidman DS. The use of laparoscopic ultrasonography to detect ovarian remnants. *J Ultrasound Med* 1996;**15**(6): 487–488.
3 Hurst BS, Tucker KE, Caleb AA, Schlaff WD. Endoscopic ultrasound: a new instrument for laparoscopic surgery. *J Reprod Med* 1996;**41**:67–70.
4 Teefey SA, Soper NJ, Middleton WD *et al.* Imaging of the common bile duct during laparoscopic cholecystectomy: sonography vs. cholangiography. *Am J Radiol* 1995;**165**: 847–851.
5 Stiegmann GV, McIntyre RC, Pearlman NW. Laparoscopic intracorporeal ultrasound: an alternative to cholangiography? *Surg Endosc* 1994;**8**:167–172.
6 Callery MP, Doherty GM, Norton JA, Soper NJ, Strasberg SM. Staging laparoscopy with laparoscopic ultrasonography: optimizing resectability in hepatobiliary and pancreatic (HBP) malignancy. Abstract presented at American Association for Study of Liver Diseases, November 1995.
7 John TG, Greig JK, Crosbie JL, Miles WF, Garden OJ. Superior staging of liver tumors with laparoscopy and laparoscopic ultrasound. *Ann Surg* 1994;**220**:711–719.
8 Jakimowicz JJ, Rutten H, Jurgens PJ, Carol EJ. Comparison of operative ultrasonography and radiography in the screening of the common bile duct for calculi. *World J Surg* 1987;**11**(5):628–634.

Chapter 22/Techniques for assisted reproduction

MOSHE D.FEJGIN and ISAAC BEN-NUN

Introduction

Sonography was introduced to the field of infertility in the early 1970s, for the evaluation of the ovaries [1] as part of the infertile woman's work-up. Several years later, when a good correlation between the ultrasonic and endocrine assessment of the developing follicle had been shown [2], sonography became an integral part of ovulation induction.

In vitro fertilization (IVF) has emerged as an important technique in the treatment of infertile couples. This method, which was originally used in patients with mechanical factors of infertility, has been recently broadened to other indications such as endometriosis, male and unexplained infertility. During the early years of IVF, aspiration of the follicles was performed via laparoscopy during the middle of a normal cycle. Later on, it was shown that following controlled stimulation of the ovaries the follicles could be successfully accessed and aspirated under ultrasonic guidance. The improvements in ultrasonic imaging, combined with the fact that the procedure is less costly and does not require general anaesthesia, made ultrasound-guided ovum pick-up the preferred technique.

This chapter deals with the use of ultrasonography in the various techniques of assisted reproduction. In addition to the description of the procedures, we suggest approaches to special situations as well as hints for the prevention and management of complications.

Ovulation induction–ovarian stimulation

In an effort to increase the number of retrieved oocytes and to improve the success rate, most assisted reproductive technologies use some form of ovarian stimulation. The use of clomiphene citrate, human menopausal gonadotrophins (hMG) and human chorionic gonado-trophins (hCG) with or without gonadotrophin-releasing hormone (GnRH) agonist have been extensively reported. Serial blood hormone assessments of oestradiol (E2) and progesterone, combined with transvaginal sonographic follow-up of follicular growth, are effective for estimating follicular/oocyte degree of maturity. Ovulation is induced by administration of hCG when one or more of the follicles reaches 16mm or more in size, combined with E2 levels of 150–200 pg/ml per large follicle. Follicular aspiration is scheduled 33–36 hours following hCG administration.

Ovum recovery

Over the years, different approaches to ultrasonic-guided ovum recovery have been suggested. Transabdominal recovery can be performed while ultrasound imaging is applied transabdominally or transvaginally. Transvaginal recovery can also use either transabdominal or trans-vaginal ultrasonic imaging. Other alternative approaches for follicular aspiration are transvesical and perurethral. Since transvaginal imaging and ovum recovery is the method most commonly used, it is described in detail, while the alternative methods are discussed briefly.

Transabdominal ovum recovery

This technique was first described in 1981 by Lenz *et al.* [3]. The success of ultrasonic-guided ovum pick-up was met with enthusiasm, and raised doubts about the place of laparoscopy in IVF [4].

ANALGESIA/ANAESTHESIA

One of the shortcomings of percutaneous ovum retrieval procedures is the fact that it may be painful and cause a great deal of discomfort to the patient. A good proportion of the patients do not tolerate the procedure with just local anaesthesia and tranquilizers and require general or epidural anaesthesia.

EQUIPMENT

The most useful ultrasound transducer is a high-resolution 3.5-MHz sector or convex scanner. A biopsy guide is also very helpful; however a free-hand technique is possible for abdominal puncture.

Larger needles may increase the rate of ovum recovery, but are associated with a more painful procedure. A 25-cm long, 16- or 18-gauge single-channel needle is effective for most clinical situations and ovarian locations. A disposable needle is recommended, since the blunt tip of a reusable needle may make the procedure very difficult and painful.

PROCEDURE

The ultrasound machine is covered with a sterile plastic sheet and the transducer is placed in a sterile bag. The abdomen is prepared and draped. The location and accessibility of the ovaries may be changed by filling and emptying of the bladder. Following the scanning process a puncture site is selected. It is infiltrated with 1% lignocaine to the depth of the abdominal wall. The needle is inserted into the most superficial follicle in a brisk single motion, and the follicular fluid is aspirated using an aspiration pump with controlled suction of up to 100mmHg. The follicle is flushed using a flushing medium and the collected fluid is inspected for the presence of the oocyte. The adjacent follicle is then punctured and the procedure is repeated until all follicles of the ovary have been aspirated. The same procedure is performed with the other ovary. Transabdominal aspiration may be performed under transvaginal ultrasonography.

Transabdominal ovum retrieval is the procedure of choice for ovaries adherent to the abdominal and pelvic side walls, but is quite impossible when the ovaries are adherent to the cul-de-sac or the posterior wall of the uterus.

Perurethral aspiration

This technique was first described by Parsons *et al.* [5] in 1985. The procedure is performed with the patient in the lithotomy position. The needle is placed in a side opening at the tip of a no. 14 Foley catheter. The catheter with the needle are inserted into the bladder, which is filled with saline. The needle is then advanced through the posterior wall of the bladder into the designated follicle and the aspiration performed as previously described.

It was initially felt that this approach improved the visualization of the needle compared with the transabdominal route. However, since the development of the transvaginal technique the perurethral route has been practically abandoned, because of the relative increased discomfort it causes to patients.

Transvaginal ovum recovery

Ultrasonic-guided transvaginal follicular puncture has evolved into the most popular method for oocyte retrieval, due to its simplicity, ease of replication and the avoidance of deep general anaesthesia. The procedure is performed in the operating room under strict antiseptic conditions, with the patient in the lithotomy position.

EQUIPMENT

We have used one of the following ultrasound machines: Elscint 1000 (Elscint Ltd, Haifa, Israel) (Fig. 22.1) with a mechanical 5-MHz vaginal probe and a needle biopsy guide attachment (Fig. 22.2); or Aloka 650 with a 7-MHz vaginal probe with a needle biopsy guide attachment. We use the Jan Craft suction pump (Rocket of London, model 29.699) with a floor control (Fig. 22.3).

Disposable equipment includes: 16-ml tubes for follicular fluid (Falcom, USA, catalogue no. 2037); heating blocks for follicular fluid temperature preservation (DRI-Bath modular elements; Thermolyne Corp., Debuque, Iowa, USA) (Fig. 22.4); Wallace catheter for embryo transfer (HG Wallace, UK); Teflon tubing system for follicular aspiration (Kemeter–Feichtinger, Vienna, Austria) (Fig. 22.5); and 16-gauge 25–30-cm long needles for follicular puncture (Echo-Tip, Cook, Spencer, Indiana, USA catalogue no. KSDN-163001) (Fig. 22.5).

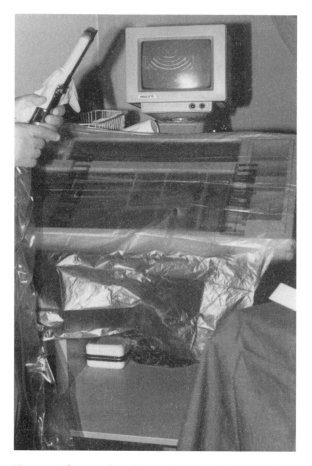

Fig. 22.1 Ultrasound machine and vaginal probe covered with a sterile plastic sheet.

VAGINAL PREPARATION

Proper vaginal preparation is an integral part of a successful IVF procedure. Meticulous cleansing helps reduce the risk of pelvic infection as well as the risk of contamination of the follicular fluid. Betadine solution (povidone iodine) is commonly used for disinfection of the vaginal mucosa and perineum. A self-retaining vaginal speculum is used; in order to expose the vaginal mucosa entirely, it must be rotated. The Betadine is then washed off by sterile saline. At this point the bladder is emptied by catheter.

PROCEDURE

The instruments are handled only after the glove powder has been rinsed off. The ultrasound machine control panel and the cord of the transducer are covered with sterile plastic sheets (Fig. 22.1). A small amount of viscous gel is applied to the tip of the probe, which is placed in a sterile condom or glove from which the powder has been rinsed off. The aspiration set and the needle are flushed with a small amount of flushing medium. The probe is placed into the vagina, firmly pressed against the fornix (Fig. 22.6) and the ovaries are visualized. The target follicle is punctured by a short swift motion, while the other hand keeps the probe firmly applied to the vaginal fornix. As soon as the follicle has been entered, the pump is activated by the foot pedal producing negative pressure. As the follicular

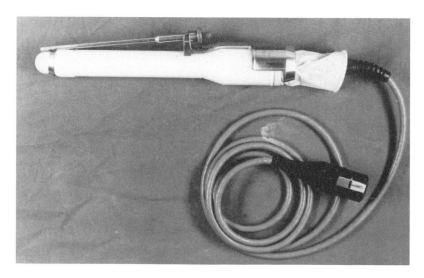

Fig. 22.2 Vaginal probe covered with a condom, with biopsy guide attached.

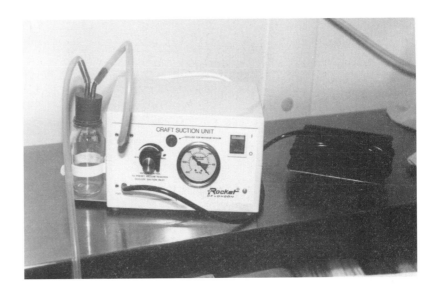

Fig. 22.3 Jan Craft suction pump.

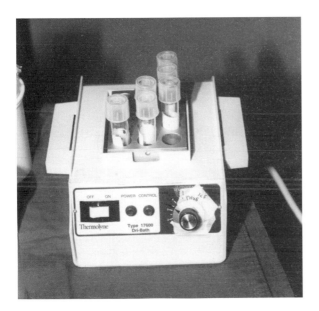

Fig. 22.4 Thermolyne heating blocks.

fluid is being aspirated, the collapsing follicle is viewed on the screen. By proper manipulation of the probe, all or most follicles of the same ovary can be aspirated without the need to withdraw the needle. However, in order to reach the contralateral ovary, the needle usually must be withdrawn and the procedure repeated.

During follicular aspiration, special attention must be devoted to the prevention of accidental puncture of large vessels. These can be positively identified by rotating the transducer and achieving a longitudinal view of the vessel, in contrast to the follicle which remains round-shaped and virtually unchanged. In patients where the ovaries are adherent to bowel, accidental aspiration of bowel contents can be avoided by simply watching for peristalsis.

The tubes containing the follicular fluid are immediately placed on the heated block and transferred to the laboratory.

CHOICE OF ANAESTHESIA/ANALGESIA

Different kinds of anaesthesia and analgesia have been used for transvaginal follicular aspiration. One is 'superficial' general anaesthesia using short-acting barbiturates in combination with nitrous oxide and halothane. This type of anaesthesia has the benefits of a short induction time and provides complete pain alleviation. Unfortunately, this combination of drugs is suspected of having a toxic effect on the oocytes [6,7]. Paracervical block with 1% lignocaine and vaginal mucosal infiltration at the puncture site, in combination with a sedative drug, may be sufficient in most patients. Epidural block is an excellent choice for this procedure; however it is costly and time-consuming and therefore cannot be used routinely.

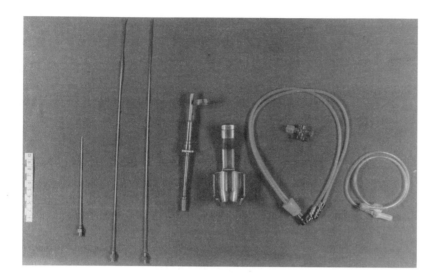

Fig. 22.5 Table set-up: Teflon tubings, needles and biopsy guide.

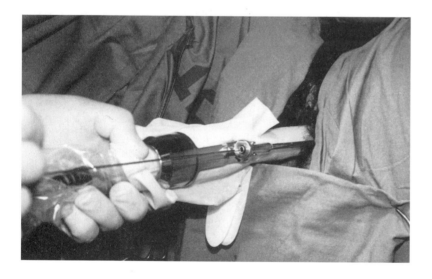

Fig. 22.6 Handling of the probe and the needle during a transvaginal ovum pick-up procedure.

PROBLEMS AND COMPLICATIONS

Highly positioned ovaries, distantly located from the fornices, may be difficult to puncture vaginally. Placing the patient in the Fowler position and applying slight external pressure to the abdomen may make the ovaries accessible. Ovaries located behind the uterus can also create technical problems. In order to avoid puncturing the uterus or cervix, an attempt is made to reposition the ovaries. This is done with the patient in the Fowler position and by sweeping the ovary to the desired location with a firmly applied probe.

Following the completion of the procedure it is advisable to aspirate blood from the cul-de-sac and observe for a minute or two whether any intra-abdominal bleeding can be detected. Inspection through the speculum for possible bleeding points in the vagina is also advisable. Such bleeding sites can be controlled by applying pressure or leaving a vaginal pack for several hours. Active bleeding can be sutured with chromic catgut.

Several reports of life-threatening peritonitis or pelvic abscesses following vaginal egg retrievals have appeared in the literature [8]. Surgical drainage may be required in such cases. Although transvaginal follicular aspiration is considered a safe procedure, intra-abdominal complications have been reported by several authors. In one large series of 3656 ovum retrievals, Dicker *et al.* [9] described 14 cases (0.38%) of acute abdomen. Of those, nine patients had pelvic and/or ovarian abscesses, three had severe intraperitoneal bleeding and two had ruptured endometriomas. Eight of the 14 patients required laparotomy or surgical laparoscopic interventions, while the other six underwent culdocentesis drainage. Therefore, the use of prophylactic antibiotics has been adopted by many groups. Our group, after encountering two such cases of tubo-ovarian abscess, choose to administer 1 g of cefonicid (Smith Kline) intravenously 45–60 min prior to the procedure. Since this policy was adopted, we have had no other case of infectious complication in over 500 procedures.

Transcervical embryo transfer

Transcervical embryo transfer is by far the most popular technique today. Prior to the transfer, the catheter in an open envelope and with a tuberculin syringe attached to it are warmed in a CO_2 incubator at 37 °C for about 1 hour. The patient is placed in the lithotomy position. A self-retained speculum is used to expose the cervix, which is cleaned with a sponge soaked with flushing medium. In order to explore the conditions for the transfer, an empty transfer catheter is gently passed through the cervical canal until it reaches the uterine fundus. Failure to enter the uterus may be caused by a sharply anteverted or retroverted uterus. In such a case, the outer sheet of the catheter is bent to adapt to the uterine shape. Another option is to grasp the anterior lip of the cervix with a single-tooth tenaculum and apply a gentle pull on it. A less traumatic option for solving the problem of a sharply anteverted uterus is filling the bladder with 300 ml of sterile saline. In patients with known cervical stenosis, lamminaria tents may be used 5–6 hours prior to the scheduled embryo transfer. The selected embryos are put in a dish containing the patient's serum. The catheter is also flushed with the serum and then emptied. The syringe is filled in the following order: 0.1–0.15 ml of air, serum, air bubble,

embryos, air bubble, serum. The volumes must be kept to a minimum, in order to prevent uterine contractions following the embryo replacement. After touching the uterine fundus with the tip of the catheter, it is pulled back approximately 1 cm and the embryos are injected into the uterine cavity. After waiting for about 20 s, the catheter is withdrawn and taken to the laboratory for inspection. A small amount of medium is used to flush the catheter into a dish without creating bubbles (which may make it impossible to identify an embryo). If bubbles do occur, they may be punctured with a fine needle. Following the completion of the procedure the patient is kept on bed rest for several hours before discharge.

Since the majority of the oocytes aspirated (70–80%) become fertilized, while only 10% implant, alternative techniques for embryo transfer were attempted, such as ultrasound-guided transfer. An abdominal transducer is used to follow the catheter as it is being advanced through the uterine cavity until it reaches the fundus. Strickler *et al.* [10] compared this method with the blind one and felt it was easier and more accurate. In cases with severe cervical stenosis, surgical ultrasound-guided embryo transfer has been described [11], in which the embryos are replaced through a 16-gauge needle that is inserted through the uterine wall, using the same needle guide used for ovum pick-up. A small amount of medium is injected. Lack of resistance to the injection and its identification in the uterine cavity confirms the location of the tip of the needle, and the embryos are replaced. Again, this technique is reserved for special cases in which transcervical replacement is impossible.

Another option, in which the embryos are passed through the cervix and uterine cavity and into the tubes, was described by Jansen *et al.* [12]. Transcervical zygote intrafallopian transfer (ZIFT) is limited to patients with normal fallopian tubes. The device used for this technique consists of a flexible 5.5 French Teflon outer cannula with a metal obturator, which is used to pass through the cervix, and a 3.0 French inner cannula (William Cook, Australia). Following the insertion of the outer catheter into the uterine cavity, an endovaginal probe is introduced. The inner catheter is then advanced into the isthmic portion of the tubes under ultrasonic guidance.

This approach allows access to the fallopian tubes without the need for laparoscopy and general anaesthesia.

Nevertheless, it is sometimes technically difficult to reach the tubal isthmus, and during the manipulation mucosal trauma and bleeding may occur. As a result, since the pregnancy rate did not increase with the use of transcervical ZIFT, this technique has not been widely adopted.

Expected results

Transvaginal ovum retrieval is an effective technique. In our unit, we have performed 2050 such retrievals. Only in two cases were no oocytes obtained. A total of 21 430 follicles larger than 15 mm plus many smaller ones were aspirated, yielding a total of 27 332 eggs. Of these, 13 377 embryos were obtained and 343 pregnancies were achieved.

References

1 Kratchowil A, Urban G, Friedrich F. Ultrasonic tomography of the ovaries. *Ann Chir Gynaecol Fenn* 1972;**61**: 211–214.

2 Hackeloer BJ, Fleming R, Robinson HP *et al*. Correlation of ultrasonic and endocrinologic assessment of human follicular development. *Am J Obstet Gynecol* 1979;**135**: 122–128.

3 Lenz S, Lauritsen JG, Kjellow M. Collection of human oocytes for *in vitro* fertilization by ultrasonic guided follicular puncture. *Lancet* 1981;i:1163–1164.

4 Feichtinger W, Kemeter P. Laparoscopic or ultrasonic guided follicle aspiration for *in vitro* fertilization? *J In Vitro Fert Embryo Transf* 1984;1:244–249.

5 Parsons J, Riddle A, Booker M *et al*. Oocyte retrieval for *in vitro* fertilization by ultrasonic guided needle aspiration via the urethra. *Lancet* 1985;i:1076–1077.

6 Rowland AS, Baird DD, Weinberg CR, Shore DL, Shy CM, Wilcox AF. Reduced fertility among women employed as dental assistants exposed to high levels of nitrous oxide. *N Engl J Med* 1992;**327**:993–997.

7 Chetrowski R, Nass T. Isoflourane inhibits early mouse embryo development *in vitro*. *Fertil Steril* 1988;**49**:171–173.

8 Ben-Nun I, Kaneti H, Fejgin M, Goldberger S, Ghetler Y, Beyth Y. Ovarian abscesses following transvaginal follicular aspiration for *in vitro* fertilization treatment. *Isr J Obstet Gynecol* 1991;2:181–182.

9 Dicker D, Ashkenazi J, Feldberg D *et al*. Severe abdominal complications after transvaginal ultrasonographically guided retrieval of oocytes for *in vitro* fertilization and embryo transfer. *Fertil Steril* 1993;**59**:1313–1315.

10 Strickler RC, Christianson C, Crane JP *et al*. Ultrasonic guidance for human embryo transfer. *Fertil Steril* 1985;**43**: 54–61.

11 Parsons JH, Bolton VN, Wilson L, Campbell S. Pregnancies following *in vitro* fertilization and ultrasound-directed surgical embryo transfer by perurethral and transvaginal techniques. *Fertil Steril* 1987;**48**:691–693.

12 Jansen RPS, Anderson JC, Sutherland PD. Nonoperative embryo transfer to the fallopian tube. *N Engl J Med* 1988;**319**:288–291.

Chapter 23 / Urogynaecology

JACQUES BECO

Introduction

Until recently, the role of ultrasonography in exploring urinary incontinence in women has been limited to studying post-voiding residue and measuring the descent of the bladder neck under stress [1,2]. New approaches, now possible with the advent of high-resolution endocavitary probes, have advanced this technique to the point where it will soon be indispensable in carrying out efficient exploration. Ultrasonography is easily integrated into classical urodynamic exploration. It provides very useful morphological information and clarifies the meaning of manometric curves [3,4].

Materials and methods

As in any other exploration technique, final results depend upon the choice of material and the method used to carry out the examination.

Urodynamic ultrasonography may theoretically be carried out using six different methods of approach: transperineal, transparietal, transrectal, transvaginal, introital and intraurethral. The transperineal [5] and transparietal [1] pathways use low-frequency emissions (3.5 MHz), since the structures to be studied are already located beyond the exploratory range of high-frequency probes. Image definition will be weak at a greater depth. Due to the proximity of the structures to be studied, endocavitary probes can use high-frequency emissions, which offer excellent structural definition at a shallow depth of exploration. Transrectal ultrasound mostly uses linear probes emitting at 5 MHz [6–8]. Transvaginal ultrasound may use either linear [9,10] or sector probes (5 or 7.5 MHz). Depending on the depth of sector probe insertion into the vagina, the ultrasonography technique is termed introital [11–13] or transvaginal [14,15].

Intraurethral ultrasonography using a 20 MHz, 3-mm diameter probe (360° cross-sectional scan) is still experimental [16].

Choice of methodology

CHOICE OF APPROACH PATHWAY AND PROBE

Linear probe use via the vaginal pathway offers advantages over other techniques.

1 Visualization of the sphincteral zone and its contents (urethral pulse, manometric catheter, echostructure, suburethral sling) is without doubt the most effective. This is due both to the proximity of the urethra and the bladder base, allowing optimal high-definition probe (7.5 MHz) utilization, as well as to the fact that the axis of the urethra is perpendicular to the ultrasonic beam, offering better definition of the structures compared with the introital pathway (in ultrasonography, axial definition is always much better than transverse definition).

2 Patient discomfort is almost nil, in contrast to the endorectal pathway.

3 No effort need be exerted to keep the probe in the examination position. Therefore, simultaneous urodynamic exploration by a single operator is facilitated. This is not the case for perineal and introital techniques. In fact, obstruction of the probe disturbs simultaneous examination in the case of perineal ultrasonography. Quality introital imagery necessitates great technical skill on the part of the operator, who must take care to maintain the probe at the threshold of disconnection while maintaining a perfect section plane. To obtain a quality image, this type of probe necessitates intimate contact with, and therefore pressure on, the structure to be studied. The greater the pressure, the greater the increase in the number of artefacts, and the more

the extremity of the probe runs the risk of becoming displaced towards the interior of the vagina during exploration [17].

4 The probe is placed in the vagina and on an external support in a perfectly horizontal plane, which directly gives a horizontal reference plane without requiring technical tricks. During introital or vaginal sector ultrasound, this plane can be derived with the aid of a guide line echoguiding a biopsy, as long as the probe is kept horizontal [14], or with an 'ultrasonographic level', i.e. filling the balloon of the Foley catheter half-full with liquid and the other half with air [18].

5 The difficulties encountered in transrectal ultrasonography under the stress of coughing or pushing, due to the interposition of air or faeces, does not exist when the vaginal pathway is chosen.

6 The artefacts induced by this technique are known and have been controlled [19]. Two types of artefact are induced by transvaginal linear ultrasonography: an increase in the posterior urethro-vesical angle (revealed by simultaneous transparietal ultrasonography) and a reduction in the urethral angulation (measured with the aid of a cotton swab and an orthopaedic goniometer) at rest and during the stress of coughing. The first type of artefact also exists if the linear probe is introduced into the rectum. The second one is constant, and well controlled by linear regression, and therefore without clinical impact. Unlike introital sonography [17], no significant modification of classical urodynamic parameters has been revealed.

7 Among the different possible approaches, transvaginal ultrasonography is the only one (with endorectal ultrasound) usable at any time during the urodynamic exploration.

CHOICE OF PATIENT POSITION

The lithotomy position offers ideal comfort for the patient and the operator, permitting better repeatability of the measurements thanks to the quality of the image. In addition, dorsal decubitus is the true rest position of the urethro-vesical unit. In fact, Vierhout and Jansen [8] have observed that, at rest, the bladder neck is located lower in a sitting position that in the dorsal decubitus position. Nevertheless, under the maximum stress of coughing, the neck is located at the same level in both positions. This means that the passage from

dorsal decubitus to the sitting position is already an effort that modifies the position of the neck and that the maximum displacement is therefore measured in dorsal decubitus. The study of micturition is perhaps an exception, since miction is easier in the sitting position [20].

UTILITY OF A MANOMETRIC CATHETER

A fine manometric catheter with continuous perfusion is preferred, since it does not rigidify the urethra, as a cotton swab does, and generates few artefacts. In addition, it permits simultaneous measurement of bladder and urethral pressures. This catheter must be visualized along the full length of its supra-symphysary portion to confirm the quality of the section plane. In the absence of this catheter, the position of the bladder neck and the urethra is very difficult to locate. This is particularly true under the stress of coughing. The bladder neck is, under these conditions, often confused with the bladder base in a parasagittal plane.

In practice

Ideally, the probe is a linear array emitting at 7.5 MHz, slight in diameter (1 cm diameter maximum) with a minimum length of 4.5 cm. The non-emitting distal extremity of the probe must be as short as possible (1 or 2 mm). To obtain a repeatable image, the patient is installed in the dorsal decubitus position with the knees half-bent and the feet on the level of the buttocks (standard gynaecological position). The ultrasonographic probe is positioned in the vagina in a perfectly horizontal plane (resting on an external support), without exerting any pressure, in such a way that the manometric catheter (ideal diameter 2 mm) is visible along the full length of the supra-symphysary urethra, and the thickness of the arcuate ligament of the pubis is maximum. If the section plane is slightly parasagittal, the arcuate ligament becomes thinner (Fig. 23.1).

If it is offset by several millimetres (wrong section plane), the point of reference becomes 'too clear'. This reference point is the pubic bone, which appears in the form of a hyperechogenic line with a posterior convexity. The extremity of the probe must be introduced without effort barely a few millimetres beyond the bladder neck. If the visualization of the bladder neck is impossible

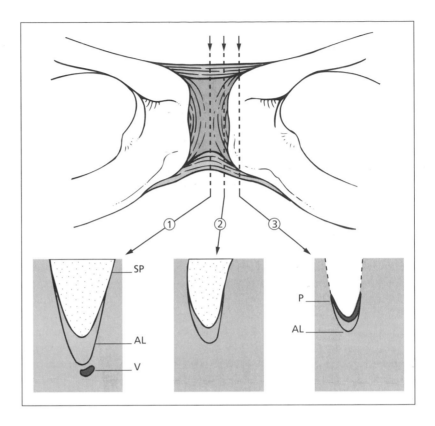

Fig. 23.1 Ideal section plane.
1, *Ideal sagittal section plane*: the arcuate ligament (AL) is the thickest. Its echogenicity is equivalent to that of the Retzius space. A small vein often underlines its posterior contour (V).
2, *Slightly parasagittal section plane*: the arcuate ligament becomes thinner but no hyperechogenic line is visible. The section plane remains in the space between the pubic bones (SP, symphysis pubis).
3, *Wrong section plane*: it is offset by several millimetres. The point of reference becomes 'too clear'. This point is the pubic bone (P) which appears in the form of a hyperechogenic line with a posterior convexity.

under these conditions (short vagina), the transrectal pathway must be preferred. The exploration is videotaped. This reference technique is not exclusive and can, in certain applications, be replaced by other methodologies with excellent results.

The classical sagittal section

Some anatomical structures are well visualized in the classical sagittal section imaged with linear endovaginal ultrasonography (Fig. 23.2).
1 The sphincteral zone and its content: this fusiform hypoechogenic structure corresponds to the totality of muscular, elastic and vascular tissues surrounding the urethral vent. The urethral pulse corresponds to a hyperechogenic beating located along the manometric catheter at the spot where the sphincteral zone is the thickest.
2 The lower part of the bladder with anechogenic content: its anterior wall is well individualized in comparison with the Retzius space. The air bubble introduced during bladder catheterization may be visualized when the bladder is not very full. If the section level is parasagittal, the hyperechogenic ureteral 'squirts' localize the position of the ureteral meatus. To study the bladder completely (and the posterior urethro-vesical angle), it is necessary to use the introital or transparietal pathways.
3 The pubic symphysis and the arcuate ligament of the pubis: the symphysis appears in the form of a slightly hyperechogenic line with posterior convexity. It is doubled backwards by the arcuate ligament of the pubis, whose posterior extremity is an essential reference point. This ligament is difficult to visualize, since its echogenicity is equivalent to that of the Retzius space. A small vein often underlines its posterior contour, but it is revealed quite precisely by small backward and forward movements with the ultrasonographic probe maintained horizontally (compression–decompression of the space between the probe and the arcuate ligament).

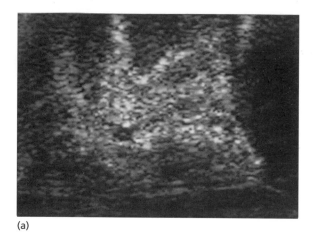

(a)

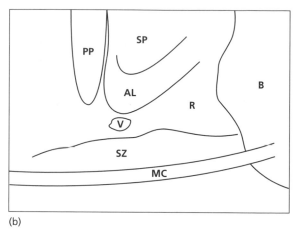

(b)

Fig. 23.2 Classical sagittal section (transvaginal linear ultrasound). SP, symphysis pubis; AL, arcuate ligament; MC, manometric catheter; B, bladder; PP, 'prepubien'; R, Retzius space; SZ, sphincteral zone; V, vein.

These movements cause a relative displacement of soft tissues in relation to the arcuate ligament, which should then be easily located. To be perfectly sagittal, the section plane must pass through the zone where the arcuate ligament is thickest (5–10 mm).

4 The 'prepubien' structure is a small hypoechogenic contractile structure 6 mm thick on average, located in the space between the clitoris and the external urethral meatus. This structure is involved in micturition and urethral instability.

Ultrasound as an aid for urodynamic exploration

Urodynamic exploration is divided into different steps: urethrocystometry, urethral pressure profile at rest, during coughing and holding, uroflowmetry, and electromyography. In each of these steps ultrasound could contribute some information to classical urodynamics.

Urethrocystometry

Obviously, ultrasound is an aid in searching for the cause of bladder or urethral instability (stone, diverticulum, polyp, foreign body) but recently has become the best

way to study the anatomical changes associated with these manometric modifications.

Thus, bladder instability is well visualized in endovaginal ultrasonography. If the urethra remains closed, a centrifugal displacement of the vesical walls is observed, with an opening of the bladder neck. During involuntary urination, the urethra opens and the vesical walls move in the opposite direction [4]. More recently, linear endovaginal ultrasonography has revealed the existence of three movements associated in a characteristic manner to the urethral pressure drops of urethral instability [4,10,21]. A muscular activity seems to correspond to each of these movements. The first of these is a shortening of the sphincteral zone, which occurs when the striated sphincter relaxes. The second, linked to a relaxation of the levator anii muscles, is revealed by an increase in the distance separating the posterior edge of the arcuate ligament from the ultrasonographic probe. The last movement is called 'contraction of the prepubien structure'. This is a forward displacement of the well-delimited hypoechogenic structure located in the interclitorido-meatic space. This activity causes traction on the anterodistal part of the sphincteral zone and is associated with a drop in urethral pressure (Fig. 23.3). The 'prepubien' structure very probably corresponds to the bulbo-cavernosus muscles and the fibrous tissue which joins them on the median line at this level.

Ultrasonography can therefore confirm the existence of urethral instability by breaking it down into different muscular activities. It also allows echoguided infiltration

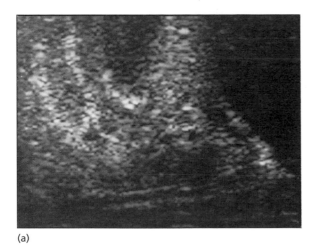

(a)

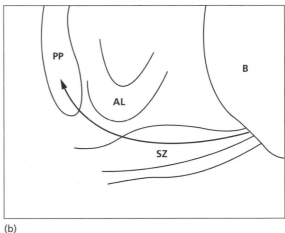

(b)

Fig. 23.3 'Contraction of the prepubien'. The 'prepubien' (PP) moves toward the clitoris inducing traction on the anterodistal part of the sphincteral zone and a rapid drop in urethral pressure. AL, arcuate ligament; SZ, sphincteral zone; B, bladder.

Fig. 23.4 Total urethral length (TUL) is the distance between the bladder neck (BN) and the upper edge of the hyperechogenic line created by the calcified cursor (CC) of the urethrometer (external urethral meatus). AL, arcuate ligament; B, bladder; SZ, sphincteral zone.

with lignocaine [22] or electromyography of the striated sphincter of the urethra (see Fig. 23.8).

Finally, when the contraction of the prepubien structure occurs together with urethral instability, digital compression of this structure under ultrasound control inhibits the instability and the urge to urinate in 75% of all cases. This observation, and the absence of therapeutic alternatives in some cases of symptomatic instability, have been at the basis for the perfection of the 'section of the prepubien structure' technique, which gives good results in 68% of all cases overall [21].

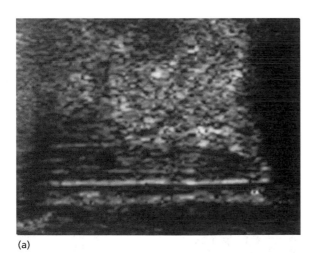

(a)

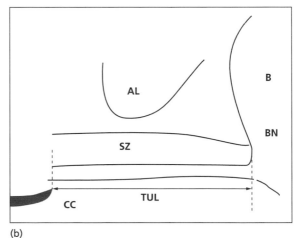

(b)

Resting urethral pressure profile

The resting urethral pressure profile (UPP) qualifies certain distances (functional profile length, total profile length) and pressures (maximum urethral closure pressure, bladder pressure and maximum urethral pressure) that characterize the female urethra [23].

With ultrasound it is possible to study the urethra itself and its position with respect to other anatomical structures. By correlating the manometric and ultrasonographic parameters, it is possible to understand why a pressure is low or high. Moreover, because the urethral pressure sensor is clearly visualized on the screen, it is easy to locate the different key points of the UPP curve with regard to the urethra [11].

ULTRASOUND PARAMETERS

Total urethral length

The total urethral length (TUL) can only be obtained by linear endocavitary ultrasonography [4]. The distal quarter of the urethra cannot be studied using sectorial probes [11,12]. Because the external urethral meatus is barely visible using ultrasound, the TUL is measured with the aid of a urethrometer with a calcified cursor. The stem of this tool is introduced into the urethra and the cursor placed against the meatus without exerting any pressure. The latter creates a hyperechogenic line that exactly locates the external urethral meatus (Fig. 23.4). The TUL is the distance between the bladder neck (defined by the junction between the sphincteral zone and the anterior bladder wall) and the external urethral meatus (upper edge of the hyperechogenic line). The TUL is 36 mm on average.

Thickness of the urethra (sphincteral zone)

Because the sphincteral zone is a well-defined oblong hypoechogenic structure, its maximum thickness is easy to measure. The maximum thickness of the anterior half of the sphincteral zone is 7 mm on average [4,11]. The sphincter cross-sectional area can be studied using intraurethral ultrasonography [16].

Ultrasonographic urethral pulse

In urodynamics, the urethral pulse appears as an

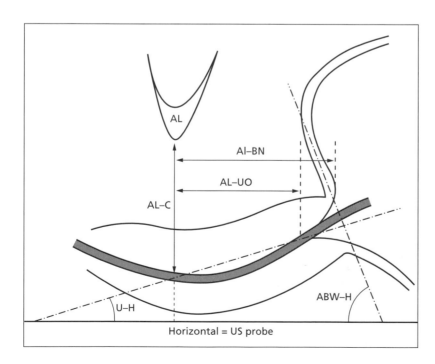

Fig. 23.5 Ultrasonographic parameters. AL, arcuate ligament of the pubis; AL–BN, arcuate ligament–bladder neck distance; AL–UO, arcuate ligament–urethral opening distance; AL–C, arcuate ligament–anterior border of the manometric catheter; ABW–H, anterior bladder wall–horizontal angle (use the 2 cm of the bladder wall near the bladder neck); U–H, urethra–horizontal angle (the axis of the urethra is the line between the extremity of the urethral opening and the manometric catheter at the level of the posterior border of the arcuate ligament). This angle is positive if the bladder neck is backward the mid-urethra and negative in the other case.

oscillation of the urethral pressure curve synchronous with the heart beat. The ultrasonographic urethral pulse (UUP) appears as a hyperechogenic beating located near the manometric catheter [24]. With transvaginal colour Doppler sonography, the submucosal vascular plexus (location of the pulse) and its pulsatility can be visualized. Its thickness and length are easily measurable.

Position of the urethro-vesical unit

Some reference points are indispensable for measuring the parameters that define the position of the urethrovesical unit. Three of them are usable: the posterior edge of the arcuate ligament of the pubis (often confused with the symphysis or even the pubic bone), the horizontal plane and the axis of the symphysis. A system of reference including the anterior inferior border of the symphysis and a perpendicular line passing through its lower edge is used exclusively in transperineal ultrasonography [5].

At the present time, authors use their own parameters. While some of them are common to several teams, there is no standardization. In practice, the measurements must be easy, useful, precise and repeatable. The position of the bladder wall in relation to the urethra, of the urethra in relation to an orthogonal reference system (including the arcuate ligament and the horizontal or symphysis axis) and the size of the bladder neck opening must appear in the data collected; if not, one

runs the risk of underusing the ultrasonographic technique. Limiting ultrasound to locating the bladder neck in relation to the posterior edge of the pubic symphysis is obviously insufficient.

As an example, our system of reference includes the horizontal axis, defined by the plane of the probe and the posterior edge of the arcuate ligament of the pubis. The five parameters chosen are described in Fig. 23.5. The average value of these parameters in a population of female patients who have never been operated and their evolution depending on age, parity and urethral closure pressure are described in Table 23.1. Interobserver and intraobserver repeatability of these measurements is excellent. All the measurements are made with the bladder filled with 250 ml water.

CORRELATIONS BETWEEN MANOMETRIC AND ULTRASONOGRAPHIC PARAMETERS

Total profile length

The TUL measured with ultrasound is 5 mm longer on average than the total profile length. This difference is dependent on the length of the functional bladder neck opening and on the distal zone of the urethra, while exerting no pressure. The functional bladder neck opening is the distance between the point where the urethral pressure sensor is located just before the urethral pressure rise and the bladder neck (junction of

Table 23.1 Ultrasonographic parameters: values and correlations. These values and correlations have been obtained in a population of 91 female patients who have never been operated (59 are incontinent during stress). The average age is 47.3 years and average urethral closure pressure (MUCP) is 53.4 cmH$_2$O.

Parameters	Mean	Min.	Max.	Pearson correlation coefficient		
				Age	MUCP	Parity
AL–BN (mm)	16	−5	32	−0.58	0.51	NS
AL–UO (mm)	14.4	−5	31	−0.56	0.55	NS
AL–C (mm)	9.4	3	24	0.30	−0.34	NS
ABW–H (°)	86.6	36	137	0.61	−0.46	NS
U–H (°)	−0.6	−35	116	0.38	−0.38	NS
BN descent (mm)	10.6	2	32	NS	NS	NS

AL–BN, arcuate ligament–bladder neck distance; AL–UO, arcuate ligament–urethral opening distance; AL–C, arcuate ligament–anterior border of the manometric catheter; ABW–H, anterior bladder wall–horizontal angle; U–H, urethra–horizontal angle; BN descent, descent of the anterior edge of the bladder neck in relation to the posterior edge of the arcuate ligament of the pubis during a maximum cough (see Fig. 23.5 and 23.6).

the sphincteral zone with the anterior bladder wall). The radiological length is also shorter than the TUL when there is a cervical opening. This difference is due to the fact that the bladder neck is poorly defined using X-rays under such a condition.

Maximum urethral closure pressure

The TUL is poorly correlated with the maximum urethral closure pressure (MUCP) and the thickness of the urethra is not correlated at all [4]. Thus the size of the sphincteral zone has quite a weak effect on the MUCP. Actually, a small muscle can be strong and vice versa. Nevertheless, a correlation was found between the sphincter cross-sectional area and the degree of continence [16].

The submucosal vascular plexus is like a sponge surrounded by a fibromuscular sheath. This vascular sponge seems to play a more important role in MUCP. Thus, the amplitude of the urodynamic pulse and the MUCP are closely correlated. The percentage of ultrasonographic visualization of the pulse increases with the amplitude of the latter, measured urodynamically. A pulse of more than $3\,cmH_2O$ is always visualized in ultrasonography. In practice, if one observes an ultrasonographic pulse, it means that the MUCP is normal or high ($78\,cmH_2O$ on average; never under $30\,cmH_2O$). If there is no ultrasonographic pulse the MUCP is lower ($43\,cmH_2O$ on average) [24]. With transvaginal colour Doppler sonography the pulse in the submucosal vascular plexus is frequently visualized even when no pulse can be measured in urodynamics. The thickness of the submucosal vascular plexus measured with this technique is well correlated with the amplitude of the urodynamic pulse. There is a reverse correlation of this parameter with the age of the female patient. The role of this vascular 'sponge' in MUCP has already been emphasized [25]. Ultrasound seems to confirm this hypothesis.

The position of the urethro-vesical unit also plays an important role in MUCP [26]. In our practice, all the parameters we use to define this position are correlated with MUCP (Table 23.1). These correlations mean that when the urethra is well supported, the MUCP tends to be high, and vice versa.

It is possible to estimate MUCP by using some of these parameters, selected by discriminant analysis,

in addition to the visualization of a UUP. Using a mathematical formula including these parameters, the estimate is correct if the UUP is visible (Pearson's coefficient $r^2 = 0.58$) and poor if the UUP is not visible [26].

There are significant differences between all the resting parameters measured in continent patients compared with those measured in incontinent patients. In patients presenting with urinary stress incontinence, the neck is located lower and further back from the arcuate pubic ligament. However, there is no discriminating threshold [9,26].

Functional profile length

The functional profile length is best correlated to the arcuate ligament–urethral opening distance (AL–UO from Fig. 23.5).

UPP during coughing

The urodynamic parameter normally used to study the urethra during coughing is the pressure transmission ratio (PTR). This ratio is the increment in urethral pressure under stress as a percentage of the simultaneously recorded increment in intravesical pressure. Unfortunately, this ratio and all the measurements associated with this parameter are not reliable. In the same patient, it depends on the type of manometric catheter used, on the cough magnitude, on the position of the urethral sensor in the urethra and on certain other factors. More recently, a new parameter called the 'critical pressure' (CP) has been introduced by Schick [27]. This parameter is defined as the minimal vesical hyperpressure that induces urine leakage. The CP is a constant value for a given patient provided the bladder volume is kept constant and the position of the patient during the examination is unchanged. Another name was given to this parameter by McGuire *et al.* in 1993: the 'leak point pressure' [28]. It has to be compared with the 'maximum cough bladder hyperpressure' [29], which reflects the bladder solicitation during everyday activities, to better approach the importance of the lack of continence. Given the MUCP and the CP measured with cough efforts, it is easy to obtain a more precise pressure transmission ratio: PTR = 1 – MUCP/CP [19].

During abdominal hyperpressure, there is a backward and downward displacement of the bladder neck. This movement is significantly greater in stress-incontinent patients than in continent patients. Nevertheless, there is no real threshold, because the bladder neck is sometimes fixed in a stress-incontinent patient with low MUCP or after surgery and sometimes hypermobile in a continent patient with high MUCP [9,26].

While ultrasound does not play a determinant role in the diagnosis of stress urinary incontinence, which is better approached by simple clinical (stress test) or other complementary examinations (distal urethral electric conductance, ambulatory urodynamics, etc.), it is very useful in measuring the descent of the bladder neck under stress. It is important to be familiar with this parameter, since a slight displacement of the neck is, like a very weak closure pressure or 'leak point pressure', synonymous with a high rate of failure in classical surgery [28].

In linear endovaginal ultrasonography, the measurement consists of evaluating the cephalo-caudal displacement of the anterior edge of the bladder neck (junction between the sphincteral zone and the anterior bladder wall) in relation to the posterior edge of the arcuate ligament during the effort of maximum coughing [4,10,19,26]. The probe must move freely along the horizontal plane while nevertheless preventing the neck from leaving the field of exploration. Initial measurement of the cephalo-caudal distance between the arcuate ligament and the neck is taken in rest position (Fig. 23.6). Then the patient is asked to cough with maximum force. The ultrasonographic image will be instantly captured at the peak of bladder pressure induced by the effort of coughing, using a specially designed software package (Geyre Electronique). A second measurement is then taken, for calculation of the bladder neck descent. To obtain a precise measurement, without disturbing vagueness, the number of images per second characterizing the equipment must be as high as possible (at least 25 images/s). For the same reason, a single focus must be used and the autocorrelation system on the device must be disabled.

Under these conditions, while the endovaginal linear probe reduces the tipping of the urethra (a known and controllable artefact), it only slightly reduces the descent of the neck, which is produced along the axis of the probe. Other possibilities exist to evaluate the descent of the neck under effort [3,5–9,11,13,14]. Nevertheless, none of them uses only anatomical landmarks as structures of reference. The bladder neck is either confused with the opening of the urethra, or located indirectly by the extremity of a cotton swab or the balloon of the Foley catheter. Other techniques using no fixed anatomical reference point are even less precise [6]. As for those which are carried out keeping the ultrasonographic probe totally immobile, they inevitably diminish the descent of the neck [9,30].

Bladder neck descent is correlated with MUCP only if the patient is incontinent during stress (the bladder neck descent of patients with very low MUCP is usually very small).

UPP during holding

The effort of retention produces an upward and forward displacement of the bladder neck in relation to the arcuate ligament. If the levator anii contraction is weak (no movement of the bladder neck), it is possible to be sure that the patient is making an effort of retention by looking at the prepubien structure. In such a situation the prepubien structure moves toward the back (the opposite of movement during urethral instability). To obtain repetitive measurement using ultrasound, the patient must remain with the buttocks on the table and the probe must be kept horizontal.

Ultrasound is able to quantify the anatomical effect of the perineal contraction. This effect is therefore compared before and after re-education to make an objective assessment of its efficacy. While the use of ultrasound in biofeedback is theoretically possible, this application necessitates costly material and a patient capable of deciphering the ultrasonographic image.

In practice, it is not so much the amplitude of the movement of the sphincteral zone as its position during the effort of maximum retention that has an impact on MUCP. The best two ultrasonographic parameters correlated to the increase in MUCP measured during the effort of maximum retention are the distances from the arcuate ligament to the anterior edge of the manometric catheter and to the ultrasonographic probe under maximum effort [19]. The shorter these distances, the greater the increase. Apparently, the sphincteral zone is being crushed by the levators against the arcuate ligament, which acts as an abutment.

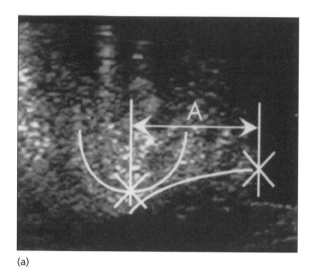

(a)

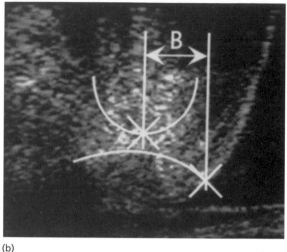

(b)

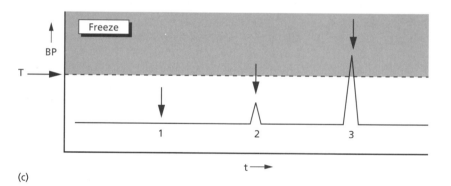

(c)

Fig. 23.6 Descent of the bladder neck under stress. Parts (a)
and (b) refer to points 1 and 3 respectively in part (c). (c) 1,
At rest, the bladder neck (junction between the anterior
bladder wall and the sphincteral zone) is located at a
distance 'A' from the posterior edge of the arcuate ligament.
2, During a small cough, the bladder neck movement is
clearly visible. The imagery is not frozen because the bladder
pressure (BP) remains under the threshold (T). The latter is
set a level corresponding to the bladder hyperpressure
induced by a maximum cough, $-10\,cmH_2O$. 3, During a
maximum cough (if the bladder pressure goes beyond the
threshold), the imagery is instantly fixed at the peak of
bladder pressure thanks to a software package provided
(Geyre Electronique). The bladder neck is located at a
distance 'B' from the arcuate ligament. The descent of the
bladder neck is the distance A–B.

Uroflowmetry

On a continuous urine flow recording, the four recommended International Continence Society parameters
[23] studied are: the maximum flow rate, the time to
maximum flow, the flow time and the voided volume.
It is also possible to measure the detrusor and bladder
pressures during voiding and to construct a pressure–
flow relationship to classify micturition in three groups:
obstructed, unobstructed and equivocal.

The study of micturition using ultrasound demands
much patience on the part of the practitioner, who must
often employ various tricks to obtain urination. We
usually use the dorsal decubitus position. Others prefer
the sitting position because it favours urination [20].
The bladder is filled until the patient feels a strong desire
to void (sometimes with cold water). Then the filling

catheter is removed, a paper ball is set on the probe in front of the urethral meatus to protect the practitioner from urine and the patient is asked to urinate. Care must be taken to remain in the axis of the urethra to avoid false obstacle images due to oblique section planes (a small manometric catheter is helpful).

SOFT TISSUE MOVEMENTS

The study of the soft tissues during urination can only be carried out by ultrasound [4,11,12,31]. Thus, the three movements characteristic of urethral instability may be visualized during the drop in urethral pressure initiating urination. Bladder contractions present the same characteristics as those described in the context of vesical instability. In addition to these movements, abdominal pressure may intervene at any point during urination producing a downward and backward displacement of the bladder neck in relation to the arcuate ligament.

URETHROGRAPHY DURING URINATION

Information concerning the appearance of the urethral conduit during urination is equivalent to that obtained by X-rays, but without radiation (Fig. 23.7). If uroflowmetry and detrusor pressure measurements suggest an obstacle, endovaginal ultrasonography often allows its visualization [4,11,12,31]. It is frequently

Fig. 23.7 (a) Classical aspect during urination. (b) AL, arcuate ligament; U, urethra; B, bladder.

located at the posterior edge of the bladder neck. Verification may be completed by an echoguided electromyography (if dyssynergy is suspected) or by withdrawal under ultrasonographic examination of a 'bougie à boule'.

POST-MICTURITION RESIDUE

Transparietal ultrasonography has been used for several years to measure post-voiding residue [2]. This application is particularly useful in men, children and neurological patients.

Electromyography (EMG)

Muscle action potentials may be detected either by surface electrodes or by needle electrodes. Surface electrodes detect the action potentials from a group of adjacent motor units underlying the recording surface. It permits study of the degree of contraction or relaxation of the levator anii muscles or of the anal striated sphincter. Needle electrodes are placed directly into the muscle mass and permit visualization of the individual motor unit action potential. Needle EMG is necessary to search for denervation of the urethral intrinsic striated sphincter.

After proper disinfection, the EMG needle is introduced at 12 o'clock, 5 mm in front of the external meatus. Care must be taken to avoid contact with the symphysis pubis or with the arcuate ligament, which is very painful. The movement of the needle in the urethral musculature is followed on the screen until it reaches

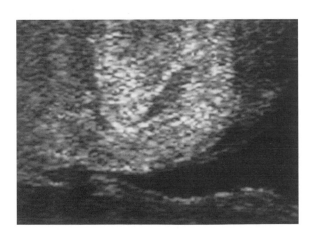
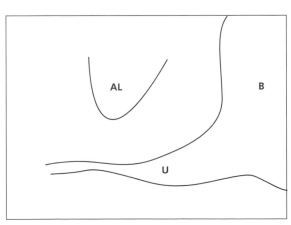

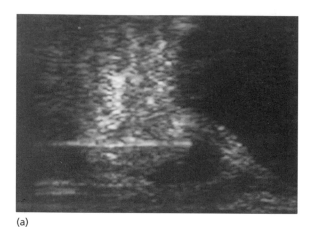

(a)

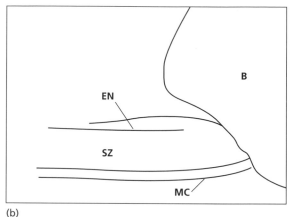

(b)

Fig. 23.8 EMG needle guiding. (a) The movement of the EMG needle is followed on the screen until it (b) reaches the intrinsic striated sphincter in the anterior layer of the sphincteral zone (at this level the striated sphincter is the thickest). EN, EMG needle; B, bladder; MC, manometric catheter; SZ, sphincteral zone.

the intrinsic striated sphincter in the anterior layer of the sphincteral zone (Fig. 23.8). At this point, typical EMG tracing and a 'motorbike-like' noise appear.

To facilitate needle guiding, the ultrasound probe must be held parallel to the needle. This method decreases patient pain by avoiding the useless and blind movements that are otherwise necessary to insert the needle in the right place without ultrasound guiding.

Urinary stress incontinence surgery and ultrasound

Theoretically, ultrasonography can be used for preoperative assessment, during surgery and for postoperative assessment.

Preoperative assessment

This assessment must be used to confirm the stress incontinence diagnosis, to evaluate the elements of a possible prolapsus, to look for surgical contra-indications and to help the surgeon in the choice of appropriate surgery.

STRESS INCONTINENCE DIAGNOSIS

This diagnosis is chiefly clinical and anamnestic. Ultra-

sonography is not very useful in this application: if urine loss is visible by ultrasonography, usually it can also be assessed clinically. Furthermore, some insignificant losses during stress tests cannot be observed by ultrasonography. Moreover, none of the static or dynamic ultrasonographic parameters, alone or in association, can ensure valid discrimination between continence and incontinence. There are significant differences between the two populations, but crossovers are such that the use of this technique offers no new elements compared with clinical examinations [9,26].

EVALUATION OF PROLAPSES

The different elements of prolapses and the efficiency of the continence mechanism can be clearly evaluated clinically, using a valve to push back the vaginal wall opposite the element to be studied. Without the valve, the prolapsed elements can support each other, which could lead to an underestimation of the extent of the prolapse or of stress incontinence. Traction on the uterine neck allows evaluation of the degree of uterine descent. Ultrasonography helps to show hidden prolapsed elements. By using endovaginal or introital ultrasonography, enterocele diagnosis is easily obtained if a rectal examination is performed during the Valsalva effort. A pocket, often containing the small intestine, infiltrates between the finger and the vaginal wall. More rarely, ultrasonography will discriminate between a cystocele and a prolapsus of the furthermost part of the uterus, subsequent to a subvesical surgical basculation of this structure (obsolete technique for stress incontinence treatment). A significant lengthening of neck beyond the vagina or a 'sliding cystocele' (bladder sneaking between the vaginal wall and the urethra) can also be easily diagnosed by ultrasonography.

DETECTION OF SURGICAL CONTRA-INDICATIONS

Symptomatic urethral or bladder instability, the existence of an obstructive uroflowmetry (especially in the presence of bladder hypocontractility), major sphincter insufficiency and the absence of bladder neck descent at the moment of the leak are the four classical surgical contra-indications. Ultrasonography is indispensable to detect a fixed bladder neck but it can also be used to assess urethro-vesical instability (a 'prepubien section' can eventually be associated with the stress incontinence treatment) and to search for an obstacle to urination.

OPERATIVE PROGNOSIS

The purpose of the preoperative examination of an incontinent patient is theoretically to choose the most appropriate operation, and to define the percentage chance of cure for this operation. Thus, in the case of Mouchel's operation [32], by using discriminant analysis on the preoperative ultrasonographic and urodynamic parameters, it is possible to select seven parameters which, introduced in a mathematical formula ('first canonical variable'), permit correct prediction of the result of this operation in 96% of cases [19,33]. The most effective parameter is without question the descent of the bladder neck under maximum cough (see Fig. 23.6). The second parameter is the maximum urethral pressure. The next four parameters are the static parameters of Fig. 23.5 excluding the AL–BN distance. The last parameter is the maximum cough pressure measured in the bladder. When only urodynamic data are used, the effectiveness of the prediction falls to 40%. This approach, using the preoperative urodynamic and ultrasonographic parameters, once extended to other operations should permit a rational choice, depending on the surgeon, of the most effective and the least harmful operation for a given patient. Ultrasonography allows urodynamics to graduate from a purely descriptive or dissuasive technique to a predictive technique.

Measurement of TUL and the search for an intestinal interposition in front of the bladder are part of the ultrasonic preoperative assessment.

Use of ultrasonography during surgery

There are five potential objectives of the technique: control of the suspension's position; assessment of the tension of the vesical neck suspension; monitoring of a tool in the Retzius space; injection of autologous or heterologous material into the sphincter; placing a cystocatheter.

1 The control of the suspension's position is easier using a Mouchel surgical urethrometer [32]. Since the TUL is known, after preoperative ultrasonography the cursor of the urethrometer must simply be placed at a certain distance from its extremity, corresponding to the TUL. The shaft of the instrument must then be introduced into the urethra until the cursor reaches the external urethral meatus. At that point, it is sufficient to touch the extremity of the urethrometer to know the exact position of the neck. If surgery is performed through the vagina, the instrument can also be used to tilt the urethra, which significantly facilitates placement of the strip under the urethra.

2 The tension of the suspension is considered as optimal when it allows long-term healing of the patient without uncomfortable dysuria or significant residue. This ideal tension can vary greatly according to the type of surgery, the severity of incontinence, and vesical contractility. As of today, no study has been able to prove the utility of ultrasonography for this indication.

3 The passage of an instrument into the Retzius space can, theoretically, be monitored by ultrasonography. The clinical utility of this application has not been proven.

4 When urinary stress incontinence is observed in the presence of a perfectly fixed vesical neck and a very low MUCP, only two surgical solutions can be contemplated to treat the patient: placing an artificial sphincter or performing an intrasphincterial injection of autologous or heterologous material. These injections are currently performed under urethroscopic monitoring by the intraurethral or periurethral pathway. According to our experience, linear endovaginal ultrasonography can be used to easily guide an infiltration needle under the urethral mucous membrane at the level of the vesical neck. The method is identical to the one described for electromyography, but here the needle does not remain

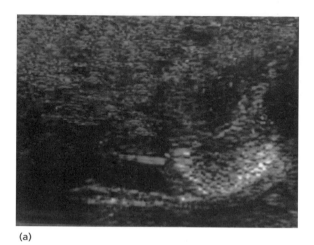

(a)

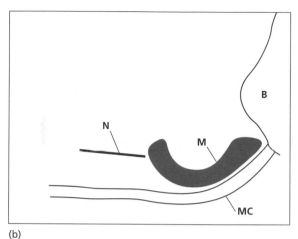

(b)

Fig. 23.9 Injection of heterologous material. The needle must penetrate as far as just beneath the mucous membrane (1 or 2 mm from the manometric catheter) in the area of the bladder neck. The distribution of the substance injected is evaluated by changing the orientation of the ultrasonic probe. N, needle; B, bladder; MC, manometric catheter; M, substance injected (Macro-plastique).

in the superficial layer of the urethra but penetrates as far as just beneath the mucous membrane (1 or 2 mm from the intraurethral catheter). The distribution of the substance injected is easily evaluated by changing the orientation of the echographic probe (Fig. 23.9). The products that can be injected are numerous, from fat taken from the abdomen to different types of heterologous material (Teflon, Macro-plastique, collagen). The operation can be performed under local anaesthesia. A preoperative effectiveness test can be performed by injecting physiological serum at the same point. However, these recent techniques should be validated before they become routine surgery.

5 The use of a suprapubic vesical catheter facilitates the treatment of the patient who underwent surgery for incontinence or the patient who suffers from retention [34,35]. The placement of this type of catheter is usually easy. The risks are even lower if, during preoperative assessment, transparietal ultrasonography on a full bladder is performed to make sure there is no intestinal interposition in front of the bladder and to locate the ideal puncture area. In case of difficulty, monitoring of

the trocar will be performed classically (as for amniotic liquid puncture). Although theoretically monitoring by ultrasonography can help avoid some incidents due to the fact that puncture is performed blindly, the low complication rate of the classical technique does not justify the systematic use of ultrasonography.

Postoperative assessment

ANATOMICAL MODIFICATIONS

Used after the operation, ultrasonography can help control the effectiveness and the position of the suspension. Practically, static parameters (see Fig. 23.5), vesical neck descent (see Fig. 23.6) and the urethrography performed during urination are compared before and after the operation. Furthermore, with the help of a urethrometer with calcified cursor (see TUL), it is possible to measure the distance between the suspension and the external meatus. After a successful Burch anterior colposuspension, the neck is usually located in front and on top of the posterior edge of the arcuate pubic ligament [4]. The urethra is bent from bottom to top and from back to front. During effort, it remains completely closed and the neck scarcely moves (max. 5 mm). During urination, a 'spur' is frequently observed on the posterior edge of the neck (Fig. 23.10). Comparison between various types of operation is possible. Thus, the bladder neck is fixed more efficiently and in a higher position after a Burch than after a Stamey or a Gittes procedure [30].

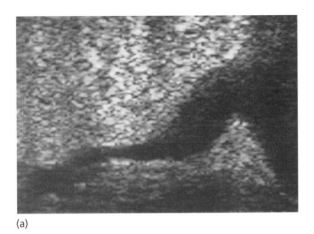

(a)

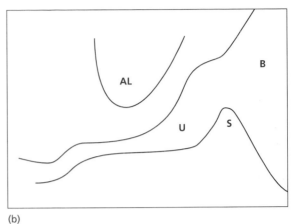

(b)

Fig. 23.10 Classical aspect during urination after a Burch colposuspension (compare with Fig. 23.7). S, 'spur' induced by colposuspension; AL, arcuate ligament; B, bladder; U, urethra.

Ultrasonography associated with urodynamics can help explain failure by insufficient traction or a collapse of the assembly (excessive mobility of the neck), by an alteration of the sphincter zone (collapse of urethral closing pressure; opening of the urethra without displacement of the neck), or by an excessive vesical solicitation (very large 'maximal cough pressure').

Fig. 23.11 Polytetrafluoroethylene (PTFE) sling. The sling appears in the form of two hyperechogenic lines with marked attenuation of the echo towards the rear. PS, PTFE sling; AL, arcuate ligament; B, bladder.

The postoperative obstacle to urination is investigated classically (see p. 233).

VISUALIZATION OF THE EXOGENOUS TISSUES

The position of exogenous implanted tissue as well as its behaviour under coughing and during urination can easily be studied. Thus, a polytetrafluoroethylene (Gore Tex) sling appears in the form of two hyperechogenic lines with marked attenuation of the echo towards the rear (Fig. 23.11) [4,32]. A polyacrylamide hydrogel implant is a well-delimited hypoechogenic structure [36]. Macro-plastique (see Fig. 23.9), Teflon, artificial collagen [37] or sphincter can also be studied.

The movements of the implant and modifications over time can be monitored by ultrasonography.

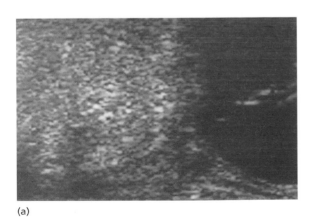

(a)

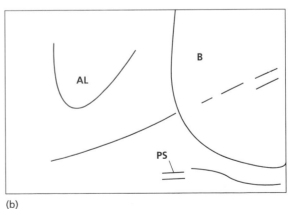

(b)

Conclusions

Urodynamic ultrasonography offers the practitioner, at a reasonable cost and without radiation, valuable morphological information on the female urethrovesical unit.

It perfectly completes urodynamic exploration and should find its proper place among other methods of investigation in the near future.

References

1 Bhatia NN, Ostergard DR, McQuown D. Ultrasonography in urinary incontinence. *Urology* 1987;**29**:90–94.

2 Hakenberg OW, Ryall RL, Langlois SL, Marshall VR. The estimation of bladder volume by sonocystography. *J Urol* 1983;130:249–251.

3 Koelbl H, Hanzal E, Bernaschek G. Sonographic urethrocystography: methods and applications in patients with genuine stress incontinence. *Int Urogynecol J* 1991;2:25–31.

4 Beco J. Echographie endovaginale en urologie. In: Perrott N, Boudghene B (eds) *Echographie Endovaginale, Collection d'Imagerie Radiologique.* Paris: Masson, 1991:107–128.

5 Clark AL, Creighton SM, Pearce JM, Stanton L. Localisation of the bladder neck by perineal ultrasound: methodology and applications. Proceedings of the International Continence Society, 20th annual meeting, Aarhus 1990.

6 Bergman A, Ballard CA, Platt LD. Ultrasonic evaluation of urethrovesical junction in women with stress urinary incontinence. *J Clin Ultrasound* 1988;16:295–300.

7 Richmond DH, Sutherst JR. Clinical application of transrectal ultrasound for the investigation of the incontinent patient. *Br J Urol* 1989;63:605–609.

8 Vierhout ME, Jansen H. Supine and sitting rectal ultrasound of the bladder neck during relaxation, straining and squeezing. *Int Urogynecol J* 1991;2:141–143.

9 Weil EHJ, van Waalwijk van Doorn ESC, Heesakkers JPFA, Meguid T, Janknegt RA. Transvaginal ultrasonography: a study with healthy volunteers and women with genuine stress incontinence. *Eur Urol* 1993;24:226–230.

10 Beco J, Sulu M, Schaaps JP, Lambotte R. Une nouvelle approche des troubles de continence chez la femme: l'échographie urodynamique par voie vaginale. *J Gynecol Obstet Biol Reprod* 1987;16:987–998.

11 Lemery D. *Echo-anatomie morphologique et fonctionnelle du bas appareil urinaire feminin normal.* Mémoire pour le diplome d'études et de recherches en biologie humaine, Paris, 1989.

12 Jacquetin B, Lemery D, Decamps C, Suzanne F. Normal ultrasonic anatomy of the female lower urinary tract with vaginal endosonography. Proceedings of the 1st World Congress of the International Society of Ultrasound in Obstetrics and Gynaecology, London, 7–10 January 1991.

13 Koelbl H, Bernaschek G, Deutinger J. Assessment of female urinary incontinence by introital sonography. *J Clin Ultrasound* 1990;18:370–374.

14 Quinn MJ, Beynon J, McMortensen NJ, Smith PJB. Transvaginal endosonography: a new method to study the anatomy of the lower urinary tract in urinary stress incontinence. *Br J Urol* 1988;**62**:414–418.

15 Johnson JD, Lamensdorf H, Hollander N, Thurman AE. Use of transvaginal endosonography in the evaluation of women with stress urinary incontinence. *J Urol* 1992;**147**:421–425.

16 Klein HM, Kirschner-Herrmanns R, Lagunilla J, Günther RW. Assessment of incontinence with intraurethral US: preliminary results. *Radiology* 1993;187:141–143.

17 Wise BG, Burton G, Cutner A, Cardozo LD. Effect of vaginal ultrasound probe on lower urinary tract function. *Br J Urol* 1992;70:12–16.

18 Benson JT, Summers JE, Pittman JS. Definition of normal female pelvic floor anatomy using ultrasonographic techniques. *J Clin Ultrasound* 1991;**19**:275–282.

19 Beco J. Echographie dans l'incontinence urinaire de la femme. In: Pelissier J, Costa P, Lopez S, Mares P (eds) *Reeducation Vesico-sphincterienne et Ano-rectale.* Paris: Masson, 1992:42–51.

20 Frea B, Bazzocchi M, Bellis GB, Milocani ML, Perulli A, Clampalini S. L'ecocistouretrografia transvaginale. *Arch Ital Urol Nefrol* 1991;**63**:77–80.

21 Beco J, Jossa V, Lambotte R. 'Prepubien section': a new surgical treatment of frequency, nocturia and urge incontinence? *World J Urol* 1992;10:120–126.

22 Spernol R, Riss P. Paraurethral lidocaine in motor and sensory urgency. Proceedings 12th Annual Meeting of the International Continence Society, Leiden, 2–4 September 1982.

23 The standardization of terminology of lower urinary tract function. *Br J Obstet Gynecol* 1990;Suppl 6:1–16.

24 Beco J, Serilas M. Pouls urétral et échographie endovaginale. In: *Urodynamique et Neuro-urologie*, vol 2. Paris: FIIS, 1990:75–79.

25 Huisman AB. Aspects on the anatomy of the female urethra with special relation to urinary continence. *Contrib Gynecol Obstet* 1983;10:1–31.

26 Serilas M, Gillain D, Lambotte R, Beco J. IUE, pression de cloture et echographie endovaginale. In: *Urodynamique et Neuro-urologie*, vol 2. Paris: FIIS, 1990:63–74.

27 Schick E. Objective assessment of resistance of female urethra to stress: a scale to establish degree of urethral incompetence. *Urology* 1985;**26**:518–526.

28 McGuire EJ, Fitzpatrick CC, Wan J *et al.* Clinical assessment

of urethral sphincter function. *J Urol* 1993;150:1452–1454.

29 Beco J, Serilas M, Schaaps JP. 'Toux maximale' et pression de cloture résiduelle. Leur importance dans le bilan urodynamique. In: *Urodynamique et Neuro-urologie*, vol 2. Paris: FIIS, 1988:73–76.

30 Kil PJM, Hoekstra JW, Van der Meijden APM, Smans AJ, Theeuwes AGM, Schreinemachers LMH. Transvaginal ultrasonography and urodynamic evaluation after suspension operations: comparison among the Gittes, Stamey and Burch suspensions. *J Urol* 1991;146:132–136.

31 Beco J, Emonts P, Lambotte R. Apport de l'échographie endovaginale per-mictionnelle. *Contracept Fertil Sex* 1990;18:461–465.

32 Mouchel J. Traitement chirurgical de l'incontinence d'urine à l'effort chez la femme par soutènement sous-urétral à l'aide d'une bandelette de polytetrafluoroethylene. *Rev Fr Gynecol Obstet* 1990;85:399–406.

33 Vosse M, Lambotte R, Beco J. Ultrasonographic and urodynamic evaluation of a suburethral support using a PTFE strip in stress incontinence. 16th annual meeting of the International Urogynaecological Association, Sydney, 1991.

34 Hodgkinson CP, Hodari AA. Trocar suprapubic cystostomy for postoperative bladder drainage in the female. *Am J Obstet Gynecol* 1966;96:773–781.

35 Donovan WH, Kiviat MD, Clowers DE. Intermittent bladder emptying via urethral catheterization or suprapubic cystocath: a comparison study. *Arch Phys Med Rehabil* 1977;58;291–296.

36 Sutherst JR, Brown MC, Annis D. A hydrogel implant for the treatment of stress urinary incontinence in women. Proceedings of the International Continence Society, 21st annual meeting, Hannover, 1991.

37 Khullar V, Cardozo LD, Abbott D, Hillard T, Norman S, Bourne T. The mechanism of continence achieved with Gax Collagene as determined by ultrasound. Proceedings of the 23rd meeting of the International Continence Society, Rome, 8–11 September 1993.

Section 3
The Breast

Chapter 24 / Breast mass preoperative localization under ultrasound guidance

SYLVIE LÉMERY, VIVIANE FEILLEL and CLAUDINE LAFAYE

Cancer screening and widespread systematic examinations have increased the number of occult breast lesions being found today, many of which were formerly missed because of their small size, the depth of the lump or the volume of the breast. At the same time, breast surgical requirements for minimal and cosmetic glandular excision as well as carcinological safety have increased. When the surgical approach is required for open biopsy confirmation or for complete excision of a suspect breast lesion, a precise localization procedure is needed to guide the surgeon in facilitating removal of the smallest amount of breast tissue.

It is necessary to know the range of possible localization procedures. Ultrasound guidance can be chosen for many lesions because it is easy to perform, comfortable for the patient and highly accurate.

Historical review

Fine-needle biopsies for palpable breast masses were first described by Martin and Ellis in 1930 [1]. Since mammography was shown to demonstrate occult breast lesions, non-invasive and invasive techniques for localization of these small lesions have been widely described. Most of these methods include the use of spot injection and metal localizers. Simon *et al.* [2] have adapted the spot method, first introduced by Rabin in 1941 to localize lung abscesses, using a mixture of Evans blue and Pantopaque. Egan *et al.* [3] preferred the methylene blue injection, while Svane [4] presented carbon marking.

As an alternative to dye solutions, many procedures use insertion of simple needles or hookwires [5–7]. Both techniques have advantages and disadvantages. In addition, with the increased efficacy of ultrasonography for breast mass determination, sonographically guided interventional procedures began to be described: Kopans

et al. [7] performed ultrasound guidance using a hand-held contact system for preoperative wire placement. Meanwhile, we adopted a similar technique, using first hand-held high-frequency probes and then real-time scanners [8].

Technique

Preoperative ultrasound examination

Sonographic breast examination is performed using real-time equipment with only high-frequency transducers (7.5–10 MHz) and usually a linear probe. A water bag is used for the preceding evaluation and is removed for the localization procedure. Even if surgery has been indicated after a complete breast evaluation, which may include clinical, mammographic, sonographic and perhaps cytological or histological studies, a new careful breast ultrasound examination is mandatory. The lesion must be described accurately. A new ultrasound-guided fine-needle aspiration (21 gauge or 19 gauge) has to be attempted every time a cyst is suspected during this preoperative examination so that unnecessary surgery may be avoided. Ultrasound examination will identify other small breast lesions, which can be also removed during the same operation. If the lesion is also visible by mammography (which is a frequent situation), good concordance between the ultrasonographically and mammographically obtained locations must be verified. Every time there is a doubt, mammography with craniocaudal and lateral view must be performed after *in situ* insertion of one ultrasound-guided fine needle. This procedure is particularly necessary for colour marking (Fig. 24.1). The size and the depth of the lesion in the breast in relation to the skin must be noted.

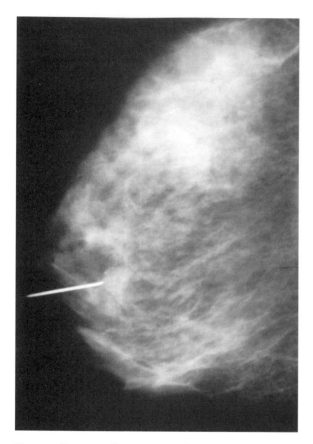

Fig. 24.1 Proper needle position confirmed by mammography.

Patient position and preparation

The patient is placed in a supine position with the arm at 90° from the corporeal axis as it will be during surgery. An oblique position is necessary in the case of peripheral axillary lesions.

Patient consent is obtained after complete information about the procedure is given. The skin is carefully cleaned with alcohol or other disinfectant solution that will be used as acoustic coupling during the localization procedure. Sterile sono-jelly is also available but not mandatory. The transducer is also cleaned with disinfectant solution. Although some physicians cover the transducer with a sterile film, we think this is not necessary if there is no contact between the needle and the transducer. When needling, local anaesthetic is required only if the lesion is directly under the areola as this is a painful area. It is not required in other cases.

Ultrasound guidance

The ultrasound guidance procedure for occult breast mass preoperative localization is the same as the ultrasound guidance technique for percutaneous needle biopsy described by Fornage *et al.* [9,10]. There are two possible ways to reach the target.

1 *Vertical needle insertion* (Fig. 24.2). The suspicious lesion is lying in the midline of the scan. The needle is inserted tangential to the middle of the probe, with a

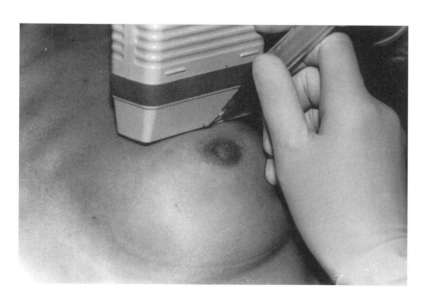

Fig. 24.2 Vertical needle insertion for methylene blue marking.

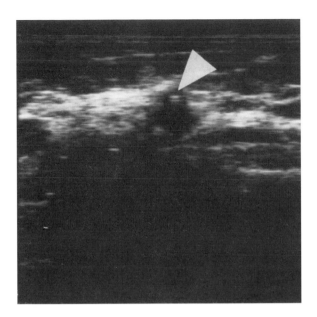

Fig. 24.3 'Tip echo' (arrow).

target on the sonogram. However this is not an obstacle because of real-time control.

2 *Oblique needle insertion* (Fig. 24.4). The suspicious lesion is displayed near the margin of the scan. The needle is inserted close to the middle of the corresponding end of the probe, along the scan plane, with the obliquity depending on the depth of the lesion. Not only the tip is seen but the entire distal portion, from its entry in the scan to the target. Only the first few centimetres of the progression are not visualized. Because of the oblique course of the needle, this technique may be chosen for safety when the lesion lies close to the chest wall.

Needle guides that maintain the needle within the scan plane have been described as convenient for the beginner. This additional equipment is expensive and must be kept sterile. Moreover, the needle must be longer to compensate for the length of the guide and, above all, it can be difficult to relocate the needle if it is advanced out of the scan plane of the target. The free-hand technique is simple and readily performed.

degree of obliquity determined by the depth of the target. With this technique, only the tip of the needle is seen when it is within the lesion, as a bright echo named 'tip-echo' (Fig. 24.3). This technique is preferred by some authors [11] because it offers the shortest route to the target, and also because the site of the needle insertion point is in front of the lesion spot. The difficulty for some beginners is being sure that it is the tip and not a simple section of the needle that is seen inside the

Breast-mass marking: metal localizers or dye injection

Preoperative localization can be achieved with metal devices or dye solutions.

METALLIC LOCALIZERS (see ref. [12])

Today, hookwires are preferred to the simple needles used in the past. They have two parts: a needle used

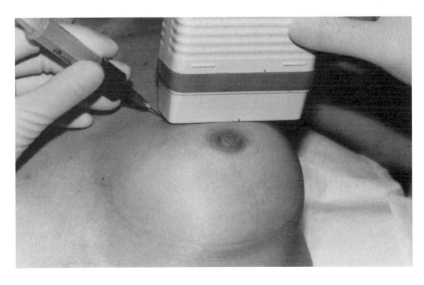

Fig. 24.4 Oblique needle insertion for methylene blue marking.

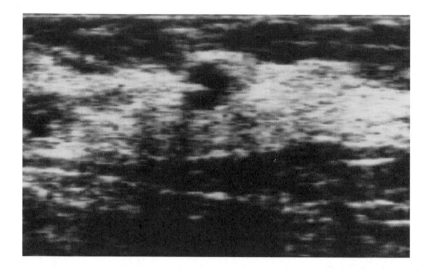

Fig. 24.5 Hookwire advancing into the breast followed on the display (oblique needle insertion).

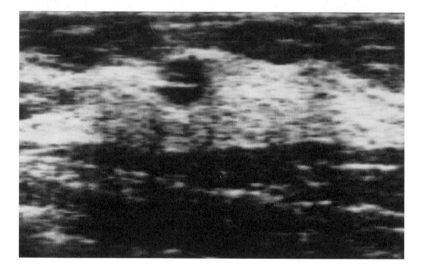

Fig. 24.6 Curved end of the hook released within the target visible on the display.

like a nozzle (20–21 gauge) and a metallic thread with a hook-shaped end that is introduced into the needle.

The ultrasound-guided, bevelled needle is inserted into the breast (Fig. 24.5). During manipulation, the hook is retracted into the needle. When the tip of the needle is correctly placed within the lesion, the wire is advanced and the hookwire is released. The curved extremity of the hook anchors into the target and can be seen on the scan (Fig. 24.6). Several lengths of wire and several shapes of hookwire are available. The most widely used devices used are listed below (Fig. 24.7).

1 Homer Mammalok Plus breast needle/wire localizer (20 gauge) [13] with a curved end (like a J). It is

repositionable if the wire placement is not satisfactory, but its anchorage is not sure and the patient must be operated on rapidly.

2 Kopans spring hook localizer needle: the metallic thread is introduced with a sharp needle (21–22 gauge) and its end is shaped like a V. This hook was found to be accurate for ultrasound-guided procedures [14]. It is not repositionable but risk of displacement is exceptional [7–14].

3 Mammofix device (NycomedIngenior) is a variation on the Kopans hookwire: there are appropriate lengths of needle (20 or 21 gauge) marked with echo pinpoints.

4 Cook 'X' hook is not a recommended device for

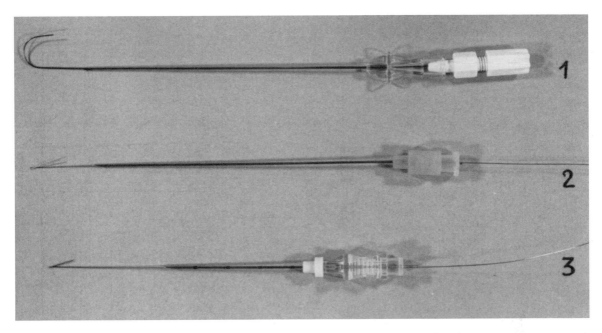

Fig. 24.7 Different breast needle/hookwires used under ultrasound guidance: (1) repositionable J wire (Homer); (2) V wire (Kopans); (3) V wire (Mammofix).

ultrasound guidance because the needle is not sharp enough to penetrate an unsqueezed breast and often a preliminary scalpel nick in the skin is necessary.

When performing an ultrasound-guided hookwire placement, pressure on the breast is less important than in procedures performed under mammographic guidance, where squeezing the breast is a necessity. For this reason, the sharpest and finest devices are chosen for ultrasound procedures because of their ease of penetration. In our breast-imaging clinic, we prefer the Mammofix device 21 gauge/5 or 7 cm.

DYE SOLUTIONS

Localization by dye injection in a non-palpable lesion is easy to perform under ultrasound guidance. A syringe containing dye solution is connected to the 21-gauge bevelled needle. When accurate placement of the needle is confirmed on the real-time ultrasound scanner the dye solution is injected. If there is air in the lumen of the needle, bright echoes are created that shade the target

(Fig. 24.8). However, this phenomenon is not seen when the needle is correctly flushed.

Several coloured solutions can be injected.

1 Methylene blue (1%) is the most commonly employed dye. Pure methylene blue would be painful (burning) and thus it is diluted with an equal volume of local anaesthetic (lignocaine 1%) in order to prevent this pain. About 0.25–0.5 ml of this mixture is injected. The use of methylene blue is sometimes criticized because of its tendency for rapid diffusion; localization should therefore be done within a few hours of surgery, which may not be convenient for departmental scheduling. In our institution, we perform methylene blue injection 1 day before surgery and no surgeon has had trouble in finding the dye [15]. It has also been emphasized that methylene blue disturbs oestrogen receptor evaluation [16]. However this problem seems dependent on the oestrogen receptor evaluation method.

2 Evans blue (Azovan blue) [2–17]. This is a dye that has been used for the determination of blood volume without adverse effects [18].

3 Sulphan blue is a patent blue used to colour lymph vessels. Hypersensitivity reactions have been reported [18]. It does not disturb the histological findings [19].

4 Toluidine blue [20] produces a smaller diffusion radius than methylene blue but preparations ready for injection are not widely available.

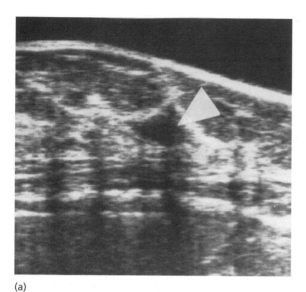

(a)

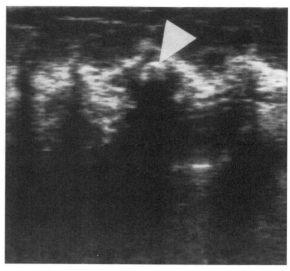

(b)

Fig. 24.8 Localization by dye spot: with air in the lumen of the needle, many bright echoes are created that may shade the target. (a) Fibroadenoma before dye localization (arrow). (b) Same case after dye, showing bright air echoes and shadowing (arrow).

5 Indocyanine green dye [21] seems safe and yields a small diffusion diameter.

6 Carbon marking has the advantage of long-term duration. Tumours treated initially by neoadjuvant chemotherapy can be marked at the beginning of the treatment. Surgery of the residual tumour (or initial site when a very good response carries no residual abnormal tissue) is thus facilitated. Two carbon markers can be used:

(a) India ink (initial studies by Svane [4]: because this preparation is a complex suspension, complications have occurred: inflammatory reactions, too large an extension and distant migration into surrounding parenchyma;

(b) suspension of charcoal seems well tolerated by patients. A suspension of micronized charcoal was developed by Bonhomme *et al.* [22]. In a preliminary study, no inflammation or necrosis were seen. Charcoal is fixed inside histiocytes and can be found by the pathologist. It does not diffuse and thus remains in place for several months.

7 Double mark (dye and metallic wire together) can be performed.

A spot is generally painted on the skin in front of the lesion after completing the invasive localization. In case of vertical needle insertion, this spot corresponds to the needle insertion.

Confirmation of correct localization before surgery

Dye may spill all around the lesion when the mass is very tough to penetrate (e.g. some fibroadenomas). This mass may also not allow the penetration of metallic wires. This is not a failure of the procedure if the hookwire or dye solution is in the vicinity of the tumour and visible to the surgeon. However, it will not be the same in breast localization for cytological aspirations or biopsies, which require exact positioning of the needle in the target for the accuracy of the pathological diagnosis.

Some additional information can be obtained to prove the success of the localization before surgery: (i) when using wire devices, two orthogonal mammographies (face view and profile view) are always performed after placement (Fig. 24.9); (ii) when using any dye solution, if the lesion is detected by ultrasound as well as by mammography two orthogonal mammographies are proposed systematically by some authors as a control for the ultrasound-guided needle placement before dye injection (see Fig. 24.1). We think that this is not always necessary if the lesion on ultrasound is well correlated

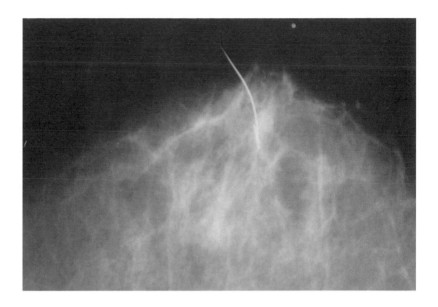

Fig. 24.9 Proper hookwire position confirmed by mammography (Mammofix 21 gauge/5 cm).

with mammograms in the same area and when it is clearly distinguishable from the surrounding parenchyma. This cannot be done if the lesion is only visible by ultrasound. Less frequently, a blue marker mixed with radio-opaque water-soluble contrast may be used for mammographic confirmation [17].

Report of the preoperative localization procedures

Communication between the radiologist and the surgeon is essential. The procedure must always be reported to the surgeon by mentioning the depth of the lesion and describing the relationship of the lesion to the insertion of the device or dye injection, because the insertion is different depending on the ultrasound guidance technique. When using vertical needle insertion, needling is directly in front of the lesion spot; when using oblique needle insertion, it is out of line with the target. Finally, a map of the breast localizing the lesions (one or multiple) to be excised and a set of labelled mammograms if the lesion is visible on X-ray should be assembled. Every document should be taken to surgery.

Perioperative control

If the lesion is visible by mammography, the surgical specimen is radiographed. One view is generally performed (Fig. 24.10). In some questionable cases, confirmation

of the successful biopsy may be improved by an additional orthogonal projection [23]. This perioperative radiography is not an absolute requirement if the nodule is visible and palpable by the surgeon.

An ultrasound scan of the excised specimen placed

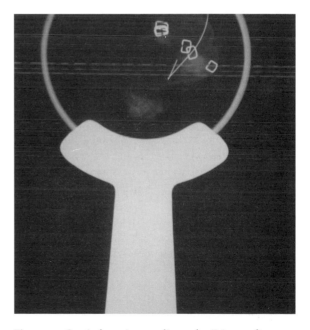

Fig. 24.10 Surgical specimen radiography (Mammofix 21 gauge/5 cm).

in a container with saline may also be performed to confirm the presence of the relevant lesion [24], especially when the lesion in the specimen is not visible by mammography.

Postoperative control

We recommend a postoperative ultrasound examination or mammography after 3 or 6 months to confirm a successful biopsy, especially if histological findings are not compatible with preoperative diagnosis [15].

Indications for ultrasound-guided localization

Sonography cannot replace mammography as a screening method for occult breast lesions. In Gordon *et al*.'s study [25] of 213 malignant lesions only 15 occult cancers (not visible on mammograms) were discovered by ultrasound. In another study, one cancer was present among 796 ultrasound examinations of asymptomatic patients with dense mammography [26]. In these cases, ultrasound is the only guidance possible for directing surgical excision.

If a mass is found on X-ray mammography but is also clearly distinguishable from the surrounding parenchyma by sonography, ultrasound guidance is generally preferred by many workers because of its simplicity, greater convenience to the patient and low cost.

With 'bad palpable' lesions (it is well known that palpation under sonography improves clinical examination), a simple cutaneous spot or an invasive mark under ultrasound guidance will reduce the duration of surgery and is helpful in choosing the appropriate incision.

Advantages and limitations of ultrasound-guided procedures

The advantages include:
1 low cost and widespread use of equipment;
2 rapidity of the procedure (ultrasound localization lasts 5 min on average vs. 15 min for stereotactic procedure);
3 supine position;
4 real-time monitoring of the needle tip during needle insertion;
5 shortest way to the lesion, so vertical needle insertion is preferred;

6 efficacious for lesions lying at the periphery of the breast and that are difficult to project on mammograms;
7 position of the patient is the same as for surgery.

The limitations include: (i) clusters of microcalcifications or some ultrasonographically undetected masses; (ii) the technique is operator dependent and previous experience is recommended for any procedure [27].

Complications

Breast localizations are well-tolerated procedures. No serious complications are generally observed. Mild reactions in the immediate periprocedural period are rare and similar to those observed during fine-needle aspiration under ultrasound guidance [11–28].

Vasovagal reactions have been described: Helvie *et al*., [28] in a prospective study considering all invasive breast-imaging procedures, identified a minority of patients who had vasovagal reactions; these were the youngest and most anxious patients. The use of local anaesthesia did not change the number of vasovagal reactions. They never required specific treatment. Medication before the procedure was not indicated routinely. Under ultrasound guidance these vasovagal reactions are rare and always mild in comparison to those occurring with localization under X-ray guidance [11]. This may be related to both the supine position and lack of compression of the patient's breast. When the procedure is performed in the morning, immediately before the surgery, the patient is fasting and generally more anxious. It seems more advantageous to schedule breast localization the day before surgery with the woman being given reassurance and no specific dietary instructions. Among premenopausal patients, those in the second half of the menstrual cycle have more pain because of their breast tenderness.

Haematomas and ecchymoses are rare, resulting from vessel puncture and without consequences. Infection has not been described but asepsis must be correct.

Localization of very deep lesions close to the chest wall should be delicate due to the risk of needle insertion too far into the chest (wire attached to the pectoralis fascia [11] or pneumothorax). This serious complication is an extremely rare event [28].

Pain has been reported to occur during the period from breast mass localization to the time of surgery. Some patients report pain after use of methylene blue injection (burning sensation). This is variable, and seems more acceptable to patients when they are well informed. Hookwires do not cause any discomfort.

Hookwires may be dislodged from their intended location in the case of excessive fat surrounding the parenchyma. The accidental cutting of the wire is also possible. Hookwire distal fragments may remain in position within the breast indefinitely. However, some authors recommend their removal because of potential distant migration. The disappearance of the wire end into the breast can be avoided by using long wires and by bending and fixing the external wire end to the skin.

Previous investigations have reported failure to excise a non-palpable mammographic abnormality after localization with a frequency of 1.5–10% [6,11,19]. There are not sufficient reports about the failure rate under ultrasound guidance. In our experience, failure rate is about 1.4%. The success rate of biopsies under ultrasound guidance appears to be higher than under X-ray guidance, probably because of the continuous control of the needle during localization. However, because there is a possibility of missing a suspicious lesion, we recommend a postoperative examination.

Choice between dye solution or metallic localizers

Dye is often preferred when there is a possibility of wire dislodgement in cases of excessive fat surrounding the parenchyma. Dye will also be chosen when it is difficult to penetrate a mobile non-palpable fibroadenoma: dye may enclose the lump. In a large number of cases, the surgeon chooses the most cosmetic incision, which is not necessarily lying at the point of hook insertion [29], and he does not dissect along the metallic wire. The wire is sometimes in the way of the dissection tract and the manipulations can increase the risk of hook dislodgement. Overall, the choice depends on the surgeon's habit and selection of the incision. Some surgeons prefer two markers for the same lump and in case of multiple lesions. When two or more localizations are done, dye may be used for the first and a hook for the later.

Our experience

A review of 710 preoperative breast lesion localizations

under ultrasound guidance performed in our breast-imaging department in 587 patients (Centre Jean Perrin, Clermont-Ferrand) [15] identified 196 malignant lesions (size, 11.8 ± 4.8 mm; range 5–35) and 514 benign masses (size, 12.6 ± 4.8 mm; range 5–30). The indication to perform a labelling procedure was a non-palpable lesion (70%) or a very bad palpable lesion (30%); 17 localizations were performed for residual tumour after chemotherapy; 325 localizations (46.5%) were done in patients with other solid palpable or non-palpable lesions in the breast which were excised during the same surgical procedure.

Methylene blue was the most frequently used localization method: methylene blue, 669 (94.22%); hookwires, 32; double mark (methylene blue and hookwires together), 9.

Additional procedures before, during and after localization were used to improve the success of the excision, i.e. control mammography after needling, palpation by the surgeon and specimen radiography. Surgical excision was performed the following day without disappearance of the blue dye. The diffusion of blue dye was not a problem. Minor complications were observed: two haematomas were found and two patients reported pain during the procedure. Ten lesions were missed (failure rate 1.4%): one carcinoma (size 1 cm) and nine benign lesions (mean size 10.1 mm; range 7–13). Of these, no blue dye was detected in three cases. Blue dye was insufficient in seven other cases; in five of them, the lesion was mistakenly found either peroperatively by the surgeon (2 cases) or by the radiologist on the X-ray film of the surgical specimen (3 cases). We successfully performed repeated localization and surgery in four of these patients, and six small fibroadenomas were followed with the same protocol that we used for lesions with a high probability of benignity. We emphasize the importance of meticulous attention to detail at all stages of the procedure by both radiologist and surgeons because of the possibility of failure in localization. We recommend a follow-up 6 months after incisional biopsy.

Conclusions

In spite of the emphasis on guided percutaneous needle biopsies of occult breast lesions (fine-needle and core biopsies) to decrease the number of open biopsies, most abnormalities require surgery for definite and complete diagnosis or for therapy. Sonography can be used to localize and mark a great number of these lesions. The procedure is safe and rapid. Coordinated effort among radiologist, surgeon and pathologist is required at each stage of the procedure in order to obtain total excision of the abnormality with removal of the smallest volume of normal breast tissue for best cosmetic outcome.

Acknowledgements

The authors are grateful to G. Besse, L. Bonhomme, H. Ronayette, Y. Ptak and R. Walher for excellent assistance in this study.

References

1 Martin ME, Ellis E. Biopsy by needle puncture and aspiration. *Ann Surg* 1930;**92**:169–181.

2 Simon N, Lesnick GJ, Lerer WN, Bachman AL. Roentgenographic localization of small lesions of the breast by the spot method. *Surg Gynecol Obstet* 1972;**134**:572–574.

3 Egan J, Sayler C, Goodman J. A technique for localizing occult breast lesions. *CA* 1976;**26**:32–37.

4 Svane G. A stereotaxic technique for preoperative marking of nonpalpable breast lesions. *Acta Radiol Diag* 1983; **24**:145–151.

5 Franck H, Hall F, Steer M. Preoperative localization of non palpable breast lesions demonstrated by mammography. *N Engl J Med* 1976;**295**:259–260.

6 Homer MJ, Pile-Spellman ER. Needle localization of occult breast lesions with a curved-end retractable wire: technique and pitfalls. *Radiology* 1986;**161**:547–548.

7 Kopans D, Meyer J, Lindfors K, Bucchianeri S. Breast sonography to guide cyst aspiration and wire localization of occult solid lesions. *AJR* 1984;**143**:489–492.

8 Travade A, Dauplat J, Ptak Y *et al.* Lésions mammaires infracliniques: repérage préopératoire. Presented at Société française de Sénologie et Pathologie Mammaire, Avignon, 1987.

9 Fornage BD, Coan JD, Cynthia LD. Ultrasound-guided needle biopsy of the breast and other interventional procedures. *Radiol Clin North Am* 1992;**30**:167–185.

10 Fornage B, Peetrons P, Djelassi E *et al.* La ponction échoguidée des masses due sein. *J Belge Radiol* 1987;**70**: 287–298.

11 Rissanen TJ, Mäkäräinen HP, Mattila SI *et al.* Wire localized biopsy of breast lesions: a review of 425 cases found in screening or clinical mammography. *Clin Radiol* 1993;**47**:14–22.

12 Rissanen TJ, Mäkäräinen HP, Kiviniemi HO, Suramo IJ. Ultrasonographically guided wire localization of non palpable breast lesions. *J Ultrasound Med* 1994;**13**:183–188.

13 Homer MJ. Nonpalpable breast microcalcifications: frequency, management, and results of incisional biopsy. *Radiology* 1992;**185**:411–413.

14 Bonifacio A, Kayal R, Bellisari S. Repérage sous guidage échographique des nodules du sein. *J Echographie Méd Ultrasonore* 1994;**15**:33–37.

15 Lemery S, Feillel V, Lafaye C. Breast mass localization under ultrasound guidance. *Ultrasound Obstet Gynecol* 1995; **6** (Suppl. I):22.

16 Hirsch JI, Banks WL, Sullivan BJS, Horsley JS. Effect of methylene blue on oestrogen-receptor activity. *Radiology* 1989;**171**:105–107.

17 Horns JW, Arnt RD. Percutaneous spot localization of nonpalpable breast lesions. *Am J Roentgenol* 1976;**127**: 253–256.

18 *Martindale: The Extra Pharmacopoeia*, 30th edn. London: Pharmaceutical Press. 1993: 684, 938, 943.

19 Delporte P, Laurent JC, Cambier L. Repérage pré-opératoire des lésions mammaires infracliniques par la technique du tatouage stéréotaxique et du 'harpon'. *J Gynecol Obstet Biol Reprod* 1994;**23**:259–263.

20 Czarnecki DJ, Feuder HK, Splittberger GF. Toluidine blue dye as a breast localization marker. *AJR* 1989;**153**:261–263.

21 Berridge DL. Indocyanine green dye as a tissue marker for localization of nonpalpable breast lesions. *AJR* 1995;**164**: 1299.

22 Bonhomme L, Mathieu MC, Seiller M, Bretou M, Fredj G, Alarcon J. Charcoal labeling of mammary tumors in mice prior to chemotherapy and surgery. *Eur J Pharm Sci* 1993;**1**:103–108.

23 Evers K, Troupin RH. Preoperative localization of breast lesions: tailored techniques and potential pitfalls. *Semin Roentgenol* 1993;**28**:242–251.

24 Fornage BD, Ross M, Singletary SE, Paulis DD. Localization of impalpable breast masses: value of sonography in the operating room and scanning of excised specimens. *AJR* 1994;**163**:569–573.

25 Gordon PB, Goldenberg SL, Chan NHL. Solid breast lesions: diagnosis with US-guided fine-needle aspiration biopsy. *Radiology* 1993;**189**:573–580.

26 Rothschild P, Kimme-Smith C, Basset LW, Gold RH. Ultrasound breast examination of asymptomatic patients with normal but radiodense mammograms. *Ultrasound Med Biol* 1988;**14** (Suppl. 1):113–119.

27 Fornage BD, Sneige N, Faroux MJ, Andre E. Sonographic appearance of ultrasound-guided fine needle aspiration biopsy of breast carcinomas smaller than 1 cm³. *J Ultrasound Med* 1990;**9**:559–568.

28 Helvie MA, Ikeda D, Adler DD. Localization and needle aspiration of breast lesions. Complications in 370 cases. *AJR* 1991;**157**:711–714.

29 Dauplat J, Le Bouedec G, Travade A *et al.* Technique chirurgicale pour l'exérèse des anomalies radiologiques infracliniques du sein. *J Chir* 1987;**124**:475–482.

Chapter 25/Interventional ultrasound of the breast

PHILIPPE PEETRONS, ANNE-FRANÇOISE DE POERCK and ANNIE VERHAEREN

There are many situations where the diagnostic tools, including X-ray mammography, diagnostic ultrasound, eventually even colour-coded Doppler, are not accurate enough to determine the nature of breast masses. Moreover, it is often necessary to have a cytological analysis to avoid unnecessary biopsy and to avoid undue delay prior to any conservative or aggressive therapy.

There are many indications for needle puncture under ultrasonic guidance [1,2]:

1 aspiration of cysts;
2 cytological analysis of solid masses;
3 wire localization (harpooning) or dye injection for the localization of subclinical masses prior to open surgery;
4 core biopsy of solid masses.

The puncture procedure will first be explained since it differs little for any of these indications. The few differences between them are detailed later.

Probe characteristics

Linear-array probes are much easier to use than any other system, including mechanical or phased array. The absence of any distortion of the ultrasonic beam, focusing in the near field of investigation, the shape of the probe itself and the possibility of seeing the needle immediately are all reasons to use only linear-array probes. We currently use probes of 7.5 MHz but higher frequencies are now commercially available and give very valuable information about the soft tissues, including the breast.

Ultrasonic pad

An ultrasonic pad is neither required nor is it advised. The nearer the puncture point is to the probe, the better.

Patient position

The supine position, as for diagnostic ultrasound, is required. Sometimes, oblique decubitus is better when the mass is located externally. In all cases, the lesion must be readily accessible for puncture.

Puncture procedure

Antiseptic solution (alcohol, chlorhexidine) is spread over the skin and over the part of that probe in contact with the skin. Chlorhexidine (Hibitane) is preferred over alcohol because of damage to the probe with repetitive applications of alcohol. In addition, chlorhexidine will also act as a conductive agent for the ultrasonic beam. The quantity of liquid applied must be sufficient to last for the entire puncture procedure.

No anaesthesia is required for cytological aspiration, harpooning or dye injection. However, when a core biopsy is required, injection of lignocaine is advisable.

The needle is a common intramuscular 21 gauge, 4–5 cm long, short (or long) bevel. Short bevel, if available, is preferred because of the somewhat larger destruction of tissue due to the inclination of the bevel. It is normally not necessary to use more sophisticated (and more expensive) needles for cytology. However, core biopsies need small Trucut or, in our experience, Bauer needles with automatic gun.

The guidance technique depends on the localization of the lesion and the skill of the operator. The easiest and most frequently used technique is to puncture the skin at the short end of the transducer, pushing the needle obliquely exactly in the axis of the probe, from right to left for a right-handed person and conversely for a left-handed person. When the extremity of the needle reaches the ultrasonic beam, it produces a strong 'metallic' echo, called tip echo. The metallic origin of the echo gives rise to characteristic reverberation echoes, distal to the tip echo. The progression of the needle towards the target is seen on the screen in real time. This technique, called 'hand-free', allows the operator to slightly change the direction of the needle tip before reaching the nodule. If the needle tip is not seen, rotation of the needle is advised to offer the biggest obstacle to the progression of the beam. The orientation of the bevel can sometimes be not reflective enough; by rotating the needle, it can be seen more obviously on the screen. If the needle is still not seen, it means that the needle is not in the correct plane. The needle must be retracted just under the skin and a new attempt carried out, checking that the axis of the puncture is the same as the axis of the transducer. In all cases, it is advisable that the needle is firmly and directly introduced for 1 or 2 cm, depending on the depth of the target, instead of introducing the needle millimetre by millimetre and then trying to see the needle tip. If the target is on the screen, if the introduction point on the skin is in the axis of the transducer and if the needle is introduced in the same axis, there is absolutely no reason to perform a slow and delicate introduction that makes the entire procedure longer than normal. Once again, to reach the target immediately with one pass of the needle is the goal.

Some manufacturers provide a dedicated puncture device, linked to the probe and depicting on the screen the route of the needle. Although this system seems very easy and accurate to beginners, it does not embrace all the possibilities of hand-free punctures, e.g. reaching different parts of the nodule, changing orientation if the nodule slips away, etc.

In some rare cases, puncture at the short end of the transducer may be impossible due to some medially or inferiorly located lesions, or some skin retractions. In some other cases, like wire localization (harpooning), the surgeon sometimes asks, for aesthetic reasons, which is the shortest route from the skin to the lesion. In these cases, it could be advisable to use another kind of technique, called middle axis technique. Here the lesion is depicted exactly in the middle of the transducer and the puncture site is along the long side of the transducer, caudal to it, as near as possible to the middle of the probe itself. The obliquity of the needle depends on the depth of the lesion: the deeper the lesion, the less

obliquity and vice versa. The entire needle cannot be seen on the screen using this route, only the tip echo being depicted. This kind of puncture procedure is somewhat more difficult for beginners, who should be trained beforehand with phantoms. Indeed, when the needle crosses the ultrasonic beam, the tip echo rises (Fig. 25.1); however, if the needle is pushed forward, the tip of the needle can progress distal to the lesion and aspiration can be ineffective, in the normal tissue distally surrounding the lesion.

In the particular case of wire localization, it is advisable that the tip of the needle is placed at the distal end of the lesion, eventually crossing both borders of the lesion. Then, the wire is slightly pushed forward while taking the needle away. This allows the hook end of the wire to go through the target. The surgeon will then be able to find the lesion more easily by following the wire.

In the particular case of core biopsy by means of an automatic gun, the patient *must* be in lateral decubitus, so that the tip of the needle does not penetrate the thoracic wall, which is clearly not recommended. However, the indications for core biopsies under ultrasonic guidance are very few compared with the stereotaxic technique.

Aspiration (Fig. 25.2)

When the tip of the needle is within the target, aspiration is performed with a syringe of 20 ml coupled to the needle. This could be difficult for a single operator, looking at the screen, holding the transducer and aspirating with the syringe. Mechanical guns are often used, allowing aspiration with one hand only. Other authors recommend not to aspirate and to wait until tumoural cells fill the needle by capillarity. However, filling by capillarity is often not accurate enough when dealing with fibrous tissue as found in some fibroadenomas or some squamous carcinomas. We recommend aspiration of all the lesions, with help from a second operator in some cases, where any movements of the needle must be totally avoided, e.g. in very small targets. In the case of larger tumours, the needle can be slightly pushed, pulled and rotated to obtain more material.

Cystic lesions must be totally emptied. The emptying of the cyst is clearly seen in real time on the screen.

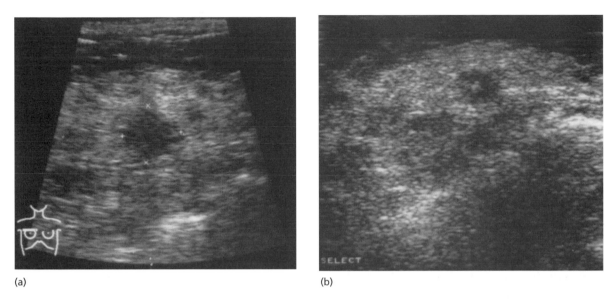

(a)

(b)

Fig. 25.1 Small 11 mm diameter neoplasm: (a) before puncture; (b) tip echo within mass.

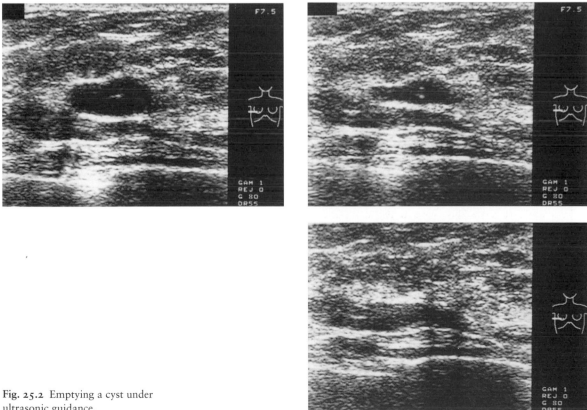

Fig. 25.2 Emptying a cyst under ultrasonic guidance.

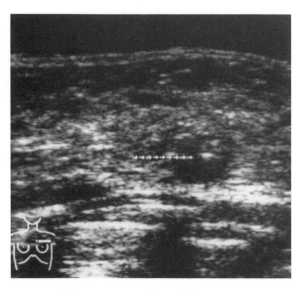

Fig. 25.3 Tip echoes within the mass (arrows).

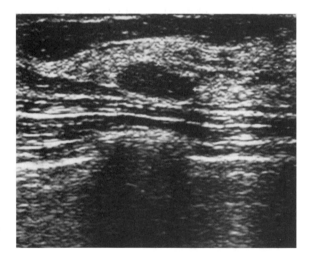

Fig. 25.4 Fibroadenoma in a young patient (see text).

Total emptying is said to avoid local recurrence of the cyst (Fig. 25.2).

Spreading of the material

As in any other cytological aspiration, the material is

Table 25.1 Pathological diagnosis of 220 successive punctures.

Final diagnosis	No.	Palpable	Non-palpable
Cancer	57	34	23 (40%)
Lymph node	3	2	1
Cyst	99	58	41 (41%)
Fibroadenoma	42	19	23 (55%)
Dystrophic lesion	15	4	11
Haematoma	2	1	1
Abscess	2	1	1

spread over glass and fixed with an appropriate fixing solution obtained from the pathology department. The fixation must be immediate, avoiding desiccation of the cells. Commercially available hair sprays can be very effective for fixing the material.

Indications for puncture

Cysts are punctured on rare occasions. We only puncture large, unaesthetic cysts or lesions with internal echoes or non-homogenic structure.

Solid lesions are almost always punctured (Fig. 25.3). The only exceptions are calcified lesions on X-ray mammography, typical of old fibroadenomas, and ovoid, mobile, longer than thicker lesions in patients younger than 30, typically described as fibroadenomas (Fig. 25.4).

Microcalcifications on X-ray mammography are, of course, not an indication for ultrasonic-guided puncture but for stereotaxic core biopsy.

Ultrasonic-guided punctures are clearly superior to palpation-guided procedures. The rate of insufficient material is reduced to 7% in our series [3,4]. Moreover, a negative result means nothing when the puncture is guided by palpation. If the tip of the needle is clearly within the lesion during ultrasonic-guided aspiration biopsy, a negative result (normal galactophoric cells) is much more reliable. In our previous series, 1 of 60 (1.6%) malignancies was classified as benign by the pathologist (Tables 25.1 & 25.2) compared to 7–22% by palpation-guided procedure, as reported in the literature [5].

Final diagnosis	Cytology	Malignant	Dubious	Benign	Inaccurate
Malignancy	60	53 (88%)	6	1 (1.6%)	0
Benign lesion	160	1 (0.6%)	1	143 (89%)	15
Total	220	54	7	144	15

Table 25.2 Final vs. cytological diagnosis in 220 successive punctures.

Conclusions

Interventional procedures in breast pathology using ultrasound are very safe and very accurate techniques. We would recommend that every physician involved in breast pathology and in mammography coupled with ultrasound becomes familiar with these techniques as soon as possible. Aspiration biopsy of a suspicious breast lesion should be offered to every woman as a normal additional diagnostic tool. The numbers of unnecessary and inaccurate open biopsies will be dramatically reduced this way. The delay between the discovery of a lesion and eventual surgical removal will also be reduced, allowing the best possible management of breast malignancies.

References

1 Sickles EA, Filly RA, Callen PW. Benign breast lesions: ultrasound detection, puncture and pneumocystography. *Radiology* 1984;151:467–470.
2 Fornage B, Peetrons P, Djelassi L *et al.* Ultrasound guided aspiration biopsy of breast masses. *J Belge Radiol* 1987;70:287–298.
3 Djelassi L, Peetrons P. Sonography in breast cancer: value of US-guided aspiration biopsy. *J Belge Radiol* 1990;73:357–365.
4 Peetrons P. Echographie mammaire. *Rev Im Med* 1990;2:363–371.
5 Zajdela A, Ghossein NA, Pilleron JP, Ennuyer A. The value of aspiration cytology in the diagnosis of breast cancer: experience at the Fondation Curie. *Cancer* 1975;35:499–506.

Chapter 26/The place of X-rays and ultrasound in interventional mastology

ALAIN ISNARD, ARMELLE TRAVADE and FRANÇOIS SUZANNE

The detection rate of breast lesions has progressively increased with the development of breast screening programmes and improvement of mammographic images. A diagnosis can sometimes be made immediately but in a large number of cases the images are ambiguous and could represent benign, borderline or neoplastic lesions. To avoid performing too many surgical biopsies for benign lesions and overlooking malignant ones, preoperative diagnosis of mammographic lesions must be refined using complementary techniques such as ultrasound, cytology and, more recently, automated needle-core biopsy. If the lesion is visible by ultrasound, cytological or histological samples may be obtained under ultrasound guidance. If the abnormality is purely mammographic, the only alternative is the use of X-ray guidance. Both methods are also used for preoperative localization of masses, guiding the surgeon to impalpable lesions that would be otherwise difficult to excise. In cases where both localization techniques are possible, the choice between them will depend on several factors that are reviewed in this chapter. The shortcomings of one technique can often be made up for by the other if we think of them not as opposed but, on the contrary, as complementary.

X-ray guided fine-needle aspiration cytology and needle-core biopsy

Indications and technique

Needling of breast masses can be done whether they are stellate, nodular, irregular, form clusters of microcalcification or are mixed in nature with dense masses accompanied by microcalcifications. It is important to define the lesions under investigation very clearly because this may explain some of the discrepancies found by different authors. Ultrasonography now elim-

inates typical cystic masses that generally do not need to be punctured. Artefacts must also be ruled out to eliminate pseudomasses produced when the two stereotaxic pictures are not concordant for the lesion. It must be remembered that unlike the standard localization methods using two orthogonal projections, the advantage of stereoataxis is that it can still be used when the lesion is visible from a single projection. Although several X-ray techniques for fine-needle aspiration biopsies have been described [1,2], in this chapter we only describe the stereotaxic method because its reliability and safety have been confirmed by a large number of studies [1,3,4]. The technique allows localization and performance of either fine-needle aspiration cytology (FNAC) or large needle-core biopsy in impalpable mammographic lesions using stereotaxic devices derived from the Nordenstrom apparatus (Sweden). A computer allows the stereotaxic identification of an infraclinical radiological lesion and the positioning of a needle within 1 mm of the lesion. Calculation of the coordinates to puncture a point are based on two mammographic views centred on the lesion: (i) with the X-ray tube inclined to one side and (ii) according to an angle set by each manufacturer. This angle (on average 30°) enables the geometry to be reconstructed in three dimensions. The position for the aspiration guide is then selected by the software.

Currently there are two types of devices available on the market. Some are relatively simple, inexpensive and compact. They are attached to the usual mammography equipment at the time of examination and therefore do not limit its normal use. Others include a complete examination table that integrates an X-ray source and localization computers: they are only used for this type of examination. The former devices, upright add-on stereotactic equipment, require a seated patient with her breast compressed in the same type of position as that usually used during ordinary breast diagnostic procedures [5]. With the latter devices the patient is in prone position with the breast protruding through an opening in the table. Each of these methods has advantages and disadvantages [6,7]. The technique used by these authors for the stereotaxic guidance procedure relies on the upright add-on stereotaxic mammography equipment. The patient is seated and her breast immobilized within the aperture of the compression plate located at the level of the area to be identified. It is important to prepare the patient psychologically because, although the aspiration itself is not very painful, it is unpleasant to have to remain motionless with the breast compressed for the duration of the examination (about 10–20 min). Choice of needle incidence is crucial and is selected according to the position of the lesion

so that there is a minimum amount of tissue to cross and the patient's position is as comfortable as possible. Selection between more than one path for the same lesion will depend on which will later yield the best localization of the centre of the lesion on two small stereotaxic views. In addition, if the procedure is to be completed by needle-core biopsy using an automatic biopsy gun, care must be taken to avoid hitting the Bucky with the needle [8]. The practical sequence of events includes an initial view correctly centred over the lesion to be punctured by inclining the tube-holder arm to one side and then to the other. Based on the two points selected by the radiologist and the two stereotaxic views on a single film, the computer's software will calculate where the aspiration guide should be placed (Fig. 26.1). The point to be targeted by the needle will be calculated by the two small stereotaxic views and must lie in the centre of the radiological anomaly whether it is a cluster of microcalcification or a mass. The needle is then inserted through the guide and two further stereotaxic views made to confirm the correct location (Fig. 26.2). Three possible alternatives then follow: (i) FNAC; (ii) needle-core biopsy using

Fig. 26.1 Stereotaxic guidance localization procedure. (a) Choice of the best incidence. (b) First view: the lesion is localized in the window of the compression plate. (c) The X-ray tube is inclined right then left (30°): two stereotaxic views on the same film, to calculate the point to puncture (the centre of the mass) (GE Medical Systems, stereotaxic device). Well-circumscribed mass in a 62-year-old woman; impalpable; fine-needle aspiration cytology: fibroadenoma.

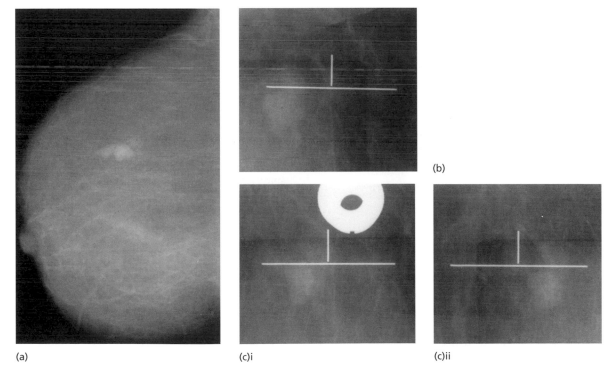

(a) (b) (c)i (c)ii

an automated biopsy gun; and (iii) positioning of a hookwire for preoperative localization of breast masses.

For FNAC the needle is a lumbar puncture-type needle with a stilet. The sample is taken by capillarity or aspiration. It is impossible to move the needle laterally but the depth can be changed by moving the micrometric

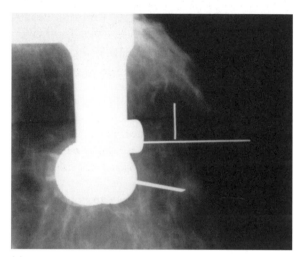

(a)

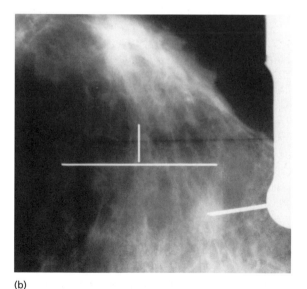

(b)

Fig. 26.2 Stereotaxic views. Two stereo views are obtained to document that the needle is in the lesion. Asymptomatic 45-year-old woman; ill-defined 8-mm mass; fine-needle aspiration cytology (a) and needle-core biopsy (b): invasive ductal carcinoma.

screw 'Z'. Sufficient aspiration is provided using a 20-ml syringe, which must be released before the needle is removed from the breast [9]. Several punctures can be made at the same point or after choosing another point in the lesion. The number of punctures may also explain the discrepancy in results obtained by different authors [10,11].

FNAC may fail to obtain cells and cause false-negative results [12,13]. Therefore, several authors have used the same stereotaxic conditions to complete or even replace FNAC by histological sampling using needle-core biopsy with an automatic biopsy gun (Figs 26.3 & 26.4). This technique has allowed significant improvement in the sensitivity and specificity of needling stereotactic techniques [2,14,15]. The automatic biopsy gun enables very fast movements of the cutting needle, thus protecting the histological sample when it is reintroduced automatically into the device: the speed is impossible to reproduce manually. Furthermore, this high speed makes it possible to punch out a piece of tissue with sharp edges and avoids pushing tumours, such as mobile fibroadenomas, with the needle. There is also less curving of the needle in fibrous tissues. The sample is taken at the exact level of the chosen target and damage to surrounding tissues and patient discomfort is minimal [16,17]. Two or three samples can be taken. Local anaesthesia is necessary to allow a cutaneous incision, which avoids contamination of the sample by shreds of skin. Before and after firing under stereotaxic view, the correct positioning of the biopsy needle, fitted into the automatic biopsy gun, should be determined. The biopsy needle has a notch and comes in various diameters, 20, 18 or even 14 gauge. The choice of needle depends on the type of lesion. However, a large calibre improves the reliability from the histological point of view but is also associated with a greater risk of bleeding [18,19]. The distance to travel will determine the set-up of the biopsy gun. Naturally, this set-up must be taken into account when choosing the initial position so that the needle does not hit the film-holder.

Pitfalls

Small stereotaxic control views may not allow visualization of the tip of the needle within the lesion. If the error is small, the difference in positioning may be

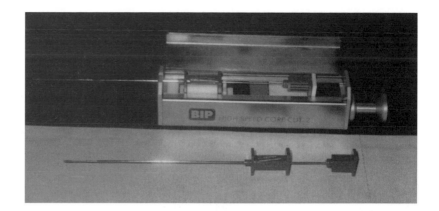

Fig. 26.3 Automatic biopsy gun with biopsy needle (BIP USA Inc., Niagara Falls, New York, USA). Two penetration depths, long throw, short throw, several diameters.

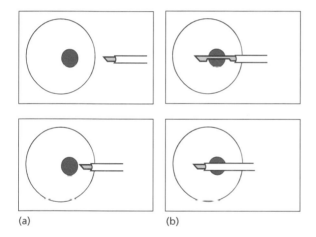

(a)   (b)

Fig. 26.4 Penetration of the biopsy needle, with biopsy gun (pre fire, post fire).

acceptable for preoperative localization because surgery is usually fairly ample. However, in FNAC the procedure must be repeated. Reasons for calculation errors may include the following.

1 Incorrect calibration of the instrument and faulty handling. The technique used must be very strictly followed and this is achieved by training and experience.

2 Patient movements. These can be considerable and are generally due to poor cooperation or faulty compression. There may also be micro-movements, which are both very difficult to prove and sometimes difficult to avoid. The patient is seated in a position that is often uncomfortable and the mammary compression may not be well tolerated. Some cases of vasovagal reaction have been noted [20]. This type of problem can be

kept to a minimum by 'psychological' support with clear explanations given at repeated intervals about the course of the examination and what is to be expected. Once again, this type of problem can be avoided by a dedicated team.

3 Flexibility of the needle. This problem can be partly solved if stiffer needles are used with a double puncture guide. However problems will still remain in very fibrous breast tissues.

4 Poor indication caused by the type of radiological image. Some mammographic images are difficult to use for this type of exploration because a point corresponding exactly to the same anomaly is not found on each stereotaxic view. Polymorphous clusters of microcalcification can easily be identified because one calcification with a recognizable shape is chosen. Similarly, well-defined dense masses, such as stellar lesions, stand out clearly from the surrounding parenchyma and present no problem. However, it can be extremely difficult to locate the same point on both stereotaxic views when dealing with disorganized masses with monomorphous calcification and with subtle architectural distortion. It must be remembered that the quality of stereotaxic views, spatial resolution and kinetic blurring are inferior to those used diagnostically with no grid or 0.1-mm focusing. Diagnostic applications provide enlargement possibilities and less compression, explaining the problems experienced with minimal stereotactic images. We hope that progress in digital imaging technology will lead to the end of this problem.

Prepectoral deep lesions, opposite to the window in the compression plate, may not allow needling [5]. Superficial lesions and those lying near the nipple may also present difficulties in sampling because correct compression cannot be applied if the aperture overlaps with the edge of the breast. In these cases an alternative technique should be used. For example, deep lesions are best explored using an examination table with a dedicated prone equipment.

Complications

If proper aseptic and technical conditions are observed, there is no risk of infection or dissemination of malignant cells. There are several large studies proving the safety of FNAC for neoplastic tumours. Only one case of dissemination along the needle trajectory has been reported after a core-needle biopsy with a 14-gauge needle [21]. When malignancy is diagnosed, treatment should not be delayed.

Bleeding is sometimes seen but is self-limiting or resolves by local compression.

Other possible disadvantages include discomfort due to prolonged breast compression during the procedure as well as due to an awkward position of the neck, especially in patients with cervical arthritis.

Summary of results obtained with FNAC

SMALL UNRECOGNIZED CYSTS

Typical cystic masses are ruled out ultrasonographically. However, small and suspicious masses, due to their irregular shape or long-term follow-up with mammograms, may be missed by ultrasonography. These masses may be hypoechoic and atypical lesions with no proof of fluid content. In a number of cases, aspiration enables the diagnosis of an ordinary cyst or cyst with thick contents to be established, thus avoiding repeated check-ups or unnecessary surgery (Fig. 26.5).

SMALL DENSE TISSULAR LESIONS

If the cytological result is benign, this is as reliable as that obtained in palpable lesions and with the same false-negative rate. Therefore, in specific cases such as round masses with a large number of perfectly identifiable cells, radiological follow-up may be sufficient (e.g. small fibroadenomas or certain benign intramammary lymph nodes with atypical configuration from a radiological point of view).

If the cytological result in stellate or more-or-less regular circumscribed masses proves to be malignant, the reliability of the result is very high. The accuracy of the technique has allowed detection of malignancies of 3–5 mm within these mammographic lesions.

The cytological result may be inconclusive in up to one-third of cases due to technical problems at sampling, type of radiological image or histological nature of the lesion in question. Because cells may not be obtained or the result may represent a false-negative, FNAC has almost been replaced by needle biopsies using an automatic biopsy gun.

Results obtained with an automatic core biopsy gun

The rate of positive results depends on the number of samples taken, the size of the lesion and its histological type. Comparison of results from various studies [14] demonstrates that failure occurs more frequently with small lesions (e.g. < 1 cm, clusters of microcalcification or *in situ* carcinoma).

In cases of neoplastic lesions, the quality of the sample taken usually enables an exact histological analysis with the possibility of ascertaining the SBR stage. Investigation of hormonal receptors and cell proliferation markers can also be carried out.

If the histological result proves benignity, simple follow-up management is allowed, provided the following conditions are met.

1 The radiological image itself must also be clear. The histological result must be compared with the radiological appearance of the lesion. Images that are statistically unlikely to be neoplastic can be followed radiographically (e.g. the risk of carcinoma in rounded, well-circumscribed masses is 2–4%). Images that are far more likely to correspond to malignant lesions, such as stellate lesions and very suspicious clusters of microcalcifications, should be managed more aggressively.

2 There must be proof that the sample was indeed taken from the lesion in question. This is why it is an advantage to have stereotaxic views with the needle in place.

3 The various elements of histological analysis and the appearance of the radiological image must be coherent: calcification, fibrous tissue, etc.

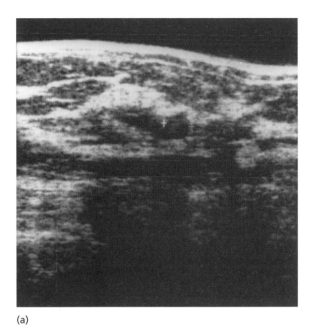

(a)

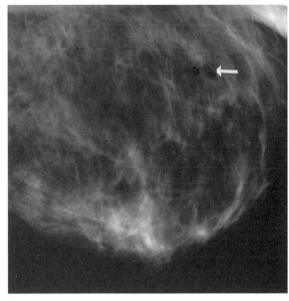

(b)

Fig. 26.5 Screening in a 50-year-old woman with familial history. Mammogram: a round 6-mm mass, not seen on previous mammogram. (a) Sonography: a small (6-mm) hypoechoic lesion with internal echoes. It is not a typical cyst. Stereotaxic guided fine-needle aspiration: fluid cyst. This is confirmed by pneumocystography (b).

4 The patient must accept regular follow-up because a low risk of false-negative results still remains, especially in deep lesions located against the pectoral muscle where there is a risk of the breast slipping and thus affect the reliability of the biopsy sample.

Association of FNAC and needle-core biopsy

Given that needle-core biopsy gives a histological result and is thus more reliable than simple cytology, it is questioned whether it is necessary to continue to associate the two types of sample or if the fine-needle phase should be eliminated. Some authors report a curious paradox between cytology and histology, where false-negatives by needle biopsy have been demonstrated by positive cytology. In the case of clusters of micro-calcification the two techniques must continue to be

associated systematically because biopsy can overlook carcinoma *in situ*, whereas cytology, due to its aspirative nature, enables loose cells to be detached with improvements of the results [14]. As previously mentioned, a biopsy is unnecessary in previously unrecognized small cysts, especially if not seen by ultrasonography or are misleading in appearance. In this situation, aspiration cytology may be both diagnostic and therapeutic [22]. Finally, the cutting needle used for biopsy does not permit aspiration or pneumocystography.

Preoperative localization of breast masses

Accurate preoperative localization of breast masses provides a guide to the surgeon. This will allow the excision of the smallest amount of tissue, avoiding a large and non-aesthetic quadrantectomy. In addition, the pathologist's task is easier because he or she can multiply the number of sections over a smaller area. Localization of the mass is essential for the excision of small, deep lesions in a large breast.

Classic localization procedures

The usual mammographic views show the mammary

gland in just one plane. Therefore, two orthogonal images can locate the anomaly at the intersection of their two planes the third dimension being the missing depth. To localize the lesion the breast must be imagined as a graph with the nipple at point 0. The horizontal coordinates (*x*) are measured from the front, with the lesion located by specifying internal or external relative to the nipple. The vertical coordinates (*y*) are measured on a strict profile incidence, specifying upper or lower sector relative to the nipple. With the *x* and *y* coordinates transferred to the breast the lesion is localized. The mammographic measurements are more important than the real measurements because of the compression and alterations secondary to the X-ray technique. The coordinates must therefore be interpreted before making the appropriate skin marking. How great a reduction must be applied depends on a number of factors, including the mammographic apparatus, the type of breast, its volume, density and the degree of compression and compressibility. Simple marks can be made on the skin, which constitutes a 'planimetry'.

Several authors use modified compression plates consisting of multi-perforated plexiglass plates or plates with a rectangular aperture with radio-opaque centimetre graduations around the edges (coordinate-grid compression plate) [1,23,24].

A fine needle can be guided to the intersection of the two selected planes, confirming the position by two additional orthogonal mammographic views. If the needle is more than 10–20 mm away from the lesion, and depending on the volume of the breast, the procedure may need to be repeated. After confirmation of the correct location of the needle there are three alternatives: (i) the needle is left in place and the surgical excision performed immediately; (ii) injection of a colouring material such as methylene blue and surgical excision as the colouring material diffuses in the tissue; and (iii) introduction of a needle wire system that is hook-shaped. This localization can be carried out the day before surgery.

Stereotaxic localization procedures

As previously mentioned, stereotaxic localization enables three-dimensional identification of the lesion to be biopsied. After the needle is confirmed to be inside the lesion, the procedure can be ended either by injecting a colouring material or, more frequently, by implanting a hookwire. The latter case requires two additional orthogonal views to determine the correct position of the hook. The surgeon now has an overall view of the breast with the hook in place, improving evaluation of the relationships between radiographic images, opaque markers and mammary gland. There is, however, a risk for the hookwire to move and it must be carefully anchored to the skin. Compared with the classic local-

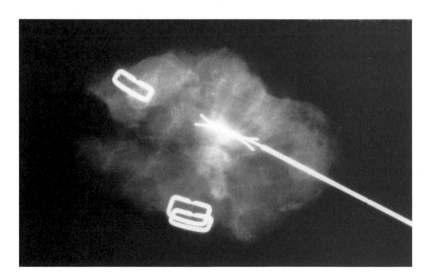

Fig. 26.6 Specimen radiograph. X-shaped hookwire left in the lesion; 5-mm invasive ductal carcinoma. Mammogram: impalpable ill-defined 5-mm mass visible only on profile views, 90° and oblique mediolateral 60°, too high to be seen on the craniocaudal view. Not seen with sonography. The only method for guidance is stereotaxic guidance.

ization procedure, preoperative stereotaxic localization has brought about a decrease in the volume of excised tissue (an obvious advantage), a drop in the number of repeat incisions and a reduction of the failure rate. Repeat incisions are required when intraoperative radiographic studies on surgical specimens demonstrate that all or part of the lesion has been left behind. Even the most experienced groups know how difficult this type of surgery can be and have witnessed a certain number of failures due to lesions remaining visible at the post-excisional evaluation (Fig. 26.6).

Complementarity of ultrasound and X-ray for management of breast masses

Ultrasound-guided techniques are reviewed elsewhere in this book. However, we would like to stress that ultrasonographic and X-ray techniques are not exclusive. Some abnormalities can only be visualized by one of the two methods of investigation. For example, clusters of microcalcification are rarely seen by ultrasonography and localization can only be made radiologically. Other lesions can be seen by ultrasound and have no equivalent visibility on mammography due to breast density or because of the type of breast. In the latter cases, localization may only be possible under ultrasound guidance. In general, and when there is a choice, FNAC under ultrasonography is the first option because it is a simple procedure in trained hands [25]. In small ultrasonographically detected lesions that are deep or have poor contrast, stereotaxy is the first option depending on breast volume, location of the lesion and the operator's experience or skill.

Stereotaxic needle-core biopsy can be used initially or may be required after an aspiration if the cytological sample has insufficient or no cells. Ultrasound-guided methods of core biopsy are difficult to perform on a routine basis and do not permit visualization of the needle in real time. Stereotaxic techniques are more reliable and easy to implement by trained personnel. Furthermore, only relatively voluminous lesions (> 10–12 mm) can be punctured under ultrasound guidance, whereas stereotaxy enables images of only 5 mm to be punctured [26].

For preoperative localization ultrasound guidance may be the best alternative. However, in those cases where the lesions are small or difficult to visualize it may be desirable to confirm the concurrence of the ultrasound and X-ray images: a needle can be positioned under ultrasound and checked by two orthogonal mammograms before its removal.

References

1 Helvie MA, Ikeda DM, Adler DD. Localization and needle aspiration of breast lesions: complications in 370 cases. *Radiology* 1990;**174**:657–661.
2 Isnard A, Travade A. Biopsie stereotaxique: alternative a la chirurgie diagnostique. Octobre 1992, 14emes Journees Nationales de la S.F.S.P.M. Marseille.
3 Haehnel P, Kleitz C, Chantreuil J, Renaud R. Stereotaxic breast puncture: an indispensable complement to the detection of breast cancers within the framework of a screening program. *Recent Results Cancer Res* 1990;**119**: 105–108.
4 Lofgren M, Andersson I, Lindholm K. Stereotactic fine-needle aspiration for cytologic diagnosis of nonpalpable breast lesions. *AJR* 1990;**154**:1191–1195.
5 Diadone MG, Orefice S, Mastore M, Santoro G, Salvadori B, Silvestrini R. Comparing core needle to surgical biopsies in breast cancer for cell kinetic and ploidy studies. *Breast Cancer Res Treat* 1991;**19**:33–37.
6 Evans WP. Fine-needle aspiration cytology and core biopsy of nonpalpable breast lesions. *Curr Opin Radiol* 1992;**4**: 130–138.
7 Jackson VP. The status of mammographically guided fine needle aspiration biopsy of nonpalpable breast lesions. *Radiol Clin North Am* 1992;**30**:155–166.
8 Dronkers DJ. Stereotaxic core biopsy of breast lesions. *Radiology* 1992;**183**:631–634.
9 Logan-Young WW, Hoffman NY, Janus JA. Fine-needle aspiration cytology in the detection of breast cancer in nonsuspicious lesions. *Radiology* 1992;**184**:49–53.
10 Fajardo LL, Jackson VP, Hunter TB. Interventional procedures in diseases of the breast: needle biopsy, pneumocystography, and galactography. *Am J Radiol* 1992;**158**:1231–1238.
11 Mitnick JS, Vazquez MF, Roses DF, Harris MN, Schechter S. Recurrent breast cancer: stereotaxic localization for fine-needle aspiration biopsy. *Radiology* 1992;**182**:103–106.
12 Ciatto S, Dell Turco MR, Braveti P. Non palpable breast lesions: stereotaxic fine needle aspiration cytology. *Radiology* 1989;**173**:57–59.
13 Travade A, Isnard A, Gimbergues H. Anomalies mammaires impalpables. Apport de la ponction cytologique par reerage stereotaxique. *J Radiol* 1989;**70**:443–446.
14 Dowlatshahi K. Nonpalpable breast lesions: findings of stereotaxic needle-core biopsy and fine-needle aspiration cytology. *Radiology* 1991:**181**:745–750.

15 Lifrange-Colin C. Diagnostic des lesions mammaires non palpables: contribution des biopsies a l'aiguille stereoguidee (a propos de 148 cas). *J Le Sein* 1992;2:6–75.

16 Parker SH, Lovin JD *et al*. Stereotactic breast biopsy with a biopsy gun. *Radiology* 1990;**176**:741–747.

17 Travade A, Isnard A, Gimbergues H. Techniques de localisation stereotaxique it echographique. Cytology. Microbiopsie. Octobre 1993. XV emes journees Nationales de la Societe Francaise de Senologie et de Pathologie Mammaire. Clermont-Ferrand. Sauramps Ed. 1993.

18 Hopper KD, Baird DE *et al*. Efficacy of automated biopsy guns versus conventional biopsy needles in the pygmy pig. *Radiology* 1990;**176**:671–676.

19 Parker SH, Lovin JD *et al*. Nonpalpable breast lesions: stereotactic automated large-core biopsies. *Radiology* 1991;**180**:403–407.

20 Helvie MA, Ikeda DM, Adler DD. Localization and needle aspiration of breast lesions: complications in 370 cases. *AJR* 1991;**157**:711–714.

21 Harter LP, Swengros Curtis J, Ponto G, Craig PH. Malignant seeding of the needle track during stereotaxic core needle breast biopsy. *Radiology* 1992;**185**:713–714.

22 Franquet T, Cozcolluleal R, DeMiguel C. Stereotaxic fine-needle aspiration of low-suspicion, nonpalpable breast nodules: valid alternative to follow-up mammography. *Radiology* 1992;**183**:635–637.

23 Hann L, Ducatman BS, Wang HH, Fein V, McIntire JM. Non palpable breast lesions: evaluation by means of fine-needle aspiration cytology. *Radiology* 1989;**171**:373–376.

24 Teixidor HS, Wojtasek DA, Reiches EM, Santos-Buch CA, Minick CR. Fine-needle aspiration of breast biopsy specimens: correlation of histologic and cytologic findings. *Radiology* 1992;**184**:55–58.

25 Ciatto S, Catarzi S, Morrone D, Del Turco MR. Fine-needle aspiration cytology of non palpable breast lesions: US versus stereotaxic guidance. *Radiology* 1993;**188**:195–198.

26 Elvecrog EL, Lechner MC, Nelson MT. Non palpable breast lesions: correlation of stereotaxic large-core needle biopsy and surgical biopsy results. *Radiology* 1993;**188**:453–455.

Index